Queen Elizabeth Hospital

UH00004530

D1756854

Perioperative Nursing

An introductory text

UHB TRUST LIBRARY
WITHDRAWN FROM STOCK

DATE DUE

			PRINTED IN U.S.A.

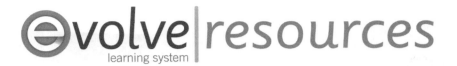

⊖volve|resources
learning system

Evolve – the Latest Evolution in Learning

Evolve provides online access to **free learning resources** and activities designed specifically to enhance the textbook you are using in your class.

Visit this website and start your learning Evolution today!
Login: http://evolve.elsevier.com/AU/Hamlin/perioperative/

Evolve online courseware for *Perioperative Nursing* **offers the following features:**

- **case studies** — Designed to enhance critical thinking in clinical settings and also provides analytical questions

- **self assessment questions** — multiple choice questions with answers and rationales provided in an interactive format

- **further readings** — optional readings corresponding to chapters in the textbook

- **weblinks** — offer useful links to websites carefully chosen to supplement the content of the textbook.

- **image collection** — collection of photographs and figures from the text to bring concepts and techniques clearly to life

- **glossary** — fully searchable and comprehensive list of key words

Think outside the book...evolve.

Perioperative Nursing

An introductory text

Editor-in-Chief
Lois Hamlin

Editors
Marilyn Richardson-Tench
Menna Davies

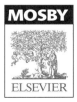

Sydney Edinburgh London New York Philadelphia St Louis Toronto

Mosby
is an imprint of Elsevier

Elsevier Australia, ACN 001 002 357
(a division of Reed International Books Australia Pty Ltd)
ELSEVIER Tower 1, 475 Victoria Avenue, Chatswood, NSW 2067

© 2009 Elsevier Australia. Reprinted 2010.

This publication is copyright. Except as expressly provided in the Copyright Act 1968 and the Copyright Amendment (Digital Agenda) Act 2000, no part of this publication may be reproduced, stored in any retrieval system or transmitted by any means (including electronic, mechanical, microcopying, photocopying, recording or otherwise) without prior written permission from the publisher.

Every attempt has been made to trace and acknowledge copyright, but in some cases this may not have been possible. The publisher apologises for any accidental infringement and would welcome any information to redress the situation.

This publication has been carefully reviewed and checked to ensure that the content is as accurate and current as possible at time of publication. We would recommend, however, that the reader verify any procedures, treatments, drug dosages or legal content described in this book. Neither the author, the contributors, nor the publisher assume any liability for injury and/or damage to persons or property arising from any error in or omission from this publication.

National Library of Australia Cataloguing-in-Publication Data

Perioperative nursing : an introductory text / editors,
Lois Hamlin ; Menna Davies ; Marilyn Richardson-Tench.

ISBN: 978 0 7295 3887 9 (pbk.)

Includes index.
Bibliography

Operating room nursing
Post anesthesia nursing.

Hamlin, Lois
Davies, Menna
Richardson-Tench, Marilyn

610.73677

Publisher: Libby Houston
Developmental Editor: Sabrina Chew
Publishing Services Manager: Helena Klijn
Editorial Coordinator: Lauren Allsop
Edited by Carolyn Pike
Proofread by Kerry Brown
Index by Mei Yen Chua
Cover design by Trina Mcdonald
Internal design and typesetting by Midland Typesetters
Printed in China by 1010 Printing International Limited

CONTENTS

FOREWORD

For decades, perioperative nurses in Australia have had to rely on international textbooks to provide reference and theoretical support for our dynamic, principle-based specialty. While the principles behind perioperative practice may be the same across the world, many nuances exist locally. *Perioperative nursing: an introductory text* has been written for and by Australian and New Zealand perioperative nurses and, by addressing those nuances, meets our local needs.

With over 70 years of experience between them—both locally and internationally—I believe the editors of this textbook are not only academically qualified but professionally and clinically well placed to meld the input from a range of expert perioperative nurse contributors into a wonderful resource.

It was not the intention of the editors to reproduce or replicate works that currently exist and, as such, this textbook does not seek to detail all surgical procedures but, rather, to provide a contemporary resource that outlines the essential information, particularly for undergraduate nursing students, postgraduate students of perioperative nursing and anyone with an interest in our specialty. This textbook covers a broad cross-section of our practice, from roles and responsibilities, including medicolegal aspects, to more clinical and technical aspects, such as wound care, patient positioning, scrubbing, gowning and gloving. It will provide a comprehensive resource for everyday use.

I commend those involved for bringing us a geographically relevant, contemporary work that is based on well-researched evidence, which I have no doubt will assist us in providing safe and effective care for our patients.

James A. Harrison
President
International Federation of Perioperative Nurses

PREFACE

Perioperative nursing is one of the oldest nursing specialties. It has featured in the nursing curriculum within Australia and New Zealand for more than 100 years, and longer elsewhere. It has evolved into a highly specialised, indeed, unique area of nursing, both within Australasia and globally. Although many aspects of perioperative nursing are universal and readily understood by all who work in this environment, the application of fundamental (as well as advanced) principles is highly contextual. Even in our respective states, territories and regions it varies; in fact, such is the nature of the practice that perioperative nursing can be understood and practised differently in two operating suites within the same locale. Notwithstanding these idiosyncrasies, the need for an Australasian perioperative text that addresses the sociopolitical and legal milieux, as well as the clinical practice issues within this region, was clear. It is to these ends that this text has been developed.

Perioperative nursing: An introductory text addresses the core aspects of contemporary perioperative nursing care in Australia and New Zealand, and reflects the expertise of the 23 contributors—all practising perioperative clinicians, managers, educators or academics from both countries. It has been developed for use by practising perioperative registered nurses and enrolled nurses, especially those new to the perioperative environment. Senior undergraduate nursing students with an interest in all phases of surgical patient care, or those who have an opportunity to experience a clinical practicum in the perioperative setting, will also find this book a valuable resource.

The text focuses on the principles of perioperative nursing wherever it is delivered— traditional operating suite, day surgery or endoscopy centre—but it is equally applicable to newer, evolving practice arenas, such as radiology and imaging suites. Although it does not address the particulars of any given surgical specialty, it does outline the fundamental principles associated with caring for patients in the preoperative, intraoperative and postoperative phases of their surgery or procedure. The perioperative care and practices described here are derived from the professional practice of the contributors and are underpinned by contemporary professional standards, local and national health policies and pertinent legal principles. Wherever possible, the text incorporates recent research findings. Notwithstanding this, in a world of continually developing knowledge and technology, the book represents a 'moment in time' of our understanding and practice of perioperative nursing. Consequently, the reader is directed to utilise the resources and websites listed at the end of each chapter, and to identify and use other contemporary sources, so as to remain abreast of changing and evolving practices.

Perioperative nursing in Australia and New Zealand is a vibrant specialty. It is represented by a national professional association in each country and each entity has a long and proud history. The Australian College (formerly confederation) of Operating Room Nurses (ACORN) and the Perioperative Nurses College of the New Zealand Nurses Organisation (PNCNZNO), both members of the International Federation of Perioperative Nursing (IFPN), play a major role in developing perioperative nursing practice via their many activities. These include developing standards and competencies that underpin patient care and perioperative nursing practice, and supporting the education of perioperative practitioners via their respective journals and conferences. These organisations, along with the IFPN, are important beacons in the many challenging environments where surgery is conducted. The delivery of perioperative care in the third millennium is no easy task and we trust this text assists perioperative nurses to care for patients during the most vulnerable time of their surgical experience.

Lois Hamlin
Marilyn Richardson–Tench
Menna Davies
July 2008

EDITORS

Dr Lois Hamlin

Dr Lois Hamlin is a senior lecturer at the University of Technology, Sydney (UTS), where she is the Director of Postgraduate Programs and Coordinator of Perioperative Education. She worked in the operating room for many years, as well as practising in coronary care, intensive care and high-dependency medical/surgical ward settings. Her research interests include the role of professional perioperative associations, competency development, advanced practice, and factors impacting on recruitment and retention in the operating room.

Dr Hamlin was a member of the executive committee of the NSW OTA Inc. for more than 10 years and President in 1998/1999. She also served on the executive of the Board of ACORN. She is past editor of *ACORN Journal* and is a member of the editorial review panel, as well as a member of the Editorial Board of *AORN Journal* and the *Journal of Perioperative Practice*.

Dr Hamlin has presented numerous papers locally, nationally and internationally as well as published articles and book chapters.

She was the inaugural winner of the NSW OTA *Excellence in Perioperative Nursing Award* in 2004.

Dr Marilyn Richardson-Tench

Dr Richardson-Tench is a Senior Lecturer in the School of Nursing and Midwifery, Victoria University, Melbourne. She obtained an operating room qualification from the Royal Melbourne Hospital and has practised operating room nursing in Melbourne and in the United Kingdom, specifically at the Hospital for Nervous Diseases, London; Hospital for Sick Children, London, and University College Hospital, London. Dr Richardson-Tench obtained her Clinical Teaching Certificate in the United Kingdom and her BAppSc (Adv Nsg), MEdStud and PhD in Melbourne. Her PhD study explored operating room nursing practice. Her current research projects cover areas such as day surgery and nursing ethics. Dr Richardson-Tench has presented papers at national and international conferences.

Menna Davies

Menna Davies is Clinical Nurse Consultant in the Operating Suite at Prince of Wales/Sydney Children's Hospitals. Menna has also worked as a Nurse Educator at Westmead Hospital and The College of Nursing, during which time she assisted in the development of the first postgraduate distance education perioperative nursing course in Australia, and coordinated the program for 10 years.

Menna is an active member of the NSW Operating Theatre Association and served two terms as President. She was NSW representative on the ACORN Board and Conference Convener for the ACORN National Conference in 1995 in Sydney. Menna was a member of the ACORN Competency Working Party and has scripted and produced a number of educational videos on behalf of ACORN, including Scrubbing, Gowning and Gloving.

Menna has presented papers at state, national and international perioperative nursing conferences, published articles and contributed to perioperative nursing texts, received the inaugural ACORN Excellence in Perioperative Nursing Award in 2004 and is an Honorary Fellow of ACORN.

CONTRIBUTORS

Leigh Anderson, RN, MN (Hons), NZNO
Perioperative Nurse Educator Adult & Emergency Operating Rooms, Auckland City Hospital, Auckland, New Zealand

Lyell Brougham, RN, MNSc, BNurs(Clinical), Dipl App Sc, ICCert, MACORN
Clinical Service Coordinator, Postanaesthesia Recovery Unit, Royal Adelaide Hospital, Adelaide, South Australia; Clinical Lecturer, Faculty of Health Sciences, School of Population Health and Clinical Practice, Discipline of Nursing, University of Adelaide, South Australia

Serena Cole, RN, Military Perioperative Certificate, Anaesthetic & Recovery Room Certificate, MACORN, ACORN
Registered Nurse, Nambour Hospital, Sunshine Coast, Queensland

Lisa Conlon, RN, BSc (Nursing), MClinNurs, DNurs (Candidate), Cert OR Management, MACORN
Lecturer and Deputy Director of International Activities, Faculty of Nursing, Midwifery and Health, University of Technology, Sydney, New South Wales

Menna Davies, RN, CM, BHlth Sc (Nsg), MHlth Sc (Nsg), COTN, Cert Sterilising Technology, FACORN, FCN
Clinical Nurse Consultant, Operating Suite, The Prince of Wales/The Sydney Children's Hospitals Randwick, New South Wales

Brigid Gillespie, RN Cert Periop, BHth Sc (Hons) PhD
Lecturer & Research Ethics Adviser, School of Nursing and Midwifery, Griffith University, Gold Coast, Queensland

Toni Gwynn-Jones, RN, MN (Acute Care), Grad Cert Clinical Teaching,
Educator, Staff Development Unit, ACT Health, Canberra, Australian Capital Territory

Prue Hames, RN, BN, MN (Hons), Cert of Tertiary Teaching, NZNO
Perioperative Nurse Educator Adult & Emergency Operating Rooms, Auckland City Hospital, Auckland, New Zealand

Lois Hamlin, RN, DNurs, BN, MN (Nurse Ed), ICCert, OTCert, FRCNA, Foundation Fellow, ACORN, FCN
Senior Lecturer and Director, Postgraduate Nursing Programs;
Coordinator, Graduate Certificate in Perioperative Nursing and Anaesthetics & Recovery Room Nursing Courses
Faculty of Nursing, Midwifery and Health, University of Technology, Sydney, New South Wales

Beth Hooper, RN, Critical Care Cert, BNsc, Grad Cert Anaes/Recovery, Grad Dip Anaes/Recovery, MACORN, SAPNA committee since 2001
Clinical Manager Anaesthetics/Recovery and Day Services, Ashford Hospital, South Australia

Marika Jenkins, RN, BN, MN
Lecturer, Faculty of Nursing, Midwifery and Health University of Technology, Sydney, New South Wales

Celia Leary, RN, MRCNA, President, Day Surgery Nurses Association NSW,
Past President, Australian Day Surgery Nurses Association,
Surgery Centre Development Director, Cortez Enterprises Pty Ltd, New South Wales

Michelle Loth, RN, BN, Grad Cert Nursing (Periop)
Nurse Educator, Perioperative and Procedural Areas, The Prince Charles Hospital, Brisbane, Queensland

Ann Parkman, RN, BN, Grad Cert (Perioperative), MPET, VPNG
Lecturer & Post Graduate Clinical Course Co-ordinator—Nurse Educator (Perioperative), Austin Health/La Trobe University, Clinical School of Nursing & Midwifery, Melbourne, Victoria

Jennifer Rabach, RN, OpThCert, BAppSci (AdvNsg), MEd, FRCNA
Past President Australian College of Operating Room Nurses;
Lecturer and Coordinator Acute Care, School of Nursing and Midwifery, Faculty of Health Sciences and Engineering, Victoria University, Melbourne, Victoria

Lynn Rapley, RN, ACGEN, MRCNA, Grad Certificate Perioperative, Grad Certificate Gastroenterology, MN Clinical Practice (Periop)
National Director of Education, Gastroenterological Nurses College of Australia;
Conjoint Lecturer, School of Nursing & Midwifery, Faculty of Health, Newcastle University, New South Wales;
Clinical Associate, The College of Nursing, New South Wales

Marilyn Richardson-Tench, RN, RCNT(UK), PhD, MEdStud, BappSc (Adv Nsg), Cert Clin Teach (UK), Cert.Anaes. (UK),Cert.OR Tech. & Man.
Senior Lecturer—Acute Care, School of Nursing & Midwifery, Faculty Health, Science & Engineering, Victoria University, Melbourne, Victoria

Emma Robbins, RN, BN, GradCert Acute Care, MACORN
Part-time Clinical Nurse Educator Adult Recovery Unit, Part-time After Hours Clinical Support Nurse
Prince of Wales Hospital, Randwick, New South Wales

Leonie Robertson, RN, Midwife, OTCert, Grad Cert (Perioperative Nursing)
Nursing Unit Manager, Prince of Wales/Sydney Children's Hospital Operating Suite, New South Wales

Narelle Sommerfeld, RN, RM, BHSc(Nsg), COTM, Cert IV Workplace Training & Assessment, MRCNA, MACORN
Nurse Educator—Transition to Practice Nurse Education Programs Statewide Support, Queensland Health, Brisbane, Queensland

Sally Sutherland-Fraser, RN, MEd, BEd (Adult Ed), PeriopCert, MACORN, MRCNA, MCN
Clinical Nurse Consultant for Perioperative Practice Development in the South Eastern Sydney Illawarra Area Health Service, St Vincent's Hospital, Sydney, New South Wales

Julie Walters, RN, RM, Graduate Certificate in Anaesthetic and Recovery Room Nursing, Certificate IV in Training and Assessment, MACORN
Clinical Nurse Educator, Anaesthetics, Prince of Wales and Sydney Children's Hospitals

Elizabeth Welstead, RN, BNg (postreg), OTCert, GradCert LGTC, MACORN
Education Coordinator, Perioperative Services, Calvary Health Care Tasmania, Hobart, Tasmania

REVIEWERS

Judith Berry, RN, BN, MNsg, Dr of Nursing, ACORN, AFPP, AORN
The Australian and New Zealand Institute of Health, Law and Ethics, Sterilizing, Research and Advisory Council of Australia
Nursing Director, Operating Room Services, Royal Adelaide Hospital, Adelaide, SA

Sandra de Rome, BN, CNOR, MRCNA, MACORN, VPNG; ASPAAN, DSSIG, GENCA, RCNA, AORN
Perioperative Nursing, Course Convenor, Deakin University, Melbourne, Vic.

Lynda Mitchell, RN, RMN, Grad Cert Perioperative Nursing, Diploma of Nursing Education, Cert IV Workplace Training and Assessment, MACORN, ANTS, CON
Nurse Educator, Perioperative Services, Westmead Hospital, Sydney, NSW

Sonya Osborne, RN, MN, BSN (USA), BS Psychology (USA), Grad Cert (Perioperative Nursing), Grad Cert (Higher Education), CNOR, MRCNA, MACORN
Lecturer, School of Nursing, Faculty of Health, Queensland University of Technology, Brisbane, Qld

Kathryn Taaffe, RN, COTN, BN, Grad Cert Adult Ed
Clinical Nurse Consultant, Operating Theatres, Royal Prince Alfred Hospital, Sydney, NSW

ACKNOWLEDGMENTS

We acknowledge our chapter contributors—thank you for your commitment in meeting deadlines while developing the depth and quality of content that is both relevant and up to date. We also acknowledge the work of our external reviewers, who provided insightful suggestions to improve the text. We feel sure that the students and clinicians who use this book will benefit from the thorough approach that has been adopted to the preparation and completion of this book.

We are especially grateful to many people at Elsevier Australia for their support throughout this project. In particular, we would like to thank Debbie Lee (previous Publishing Editor) for her enthusiastic response to the proposal for an introductory perioperative textbook. Further, we would like to thank Sabrina Chew, Debra Gooley, Andreea Heriseanu, Helena Klijn and Lauren Allsop for their support and guidance. We would like to especially thank Carolyn Pike, our editor, who ensured that the quality of this book is of such a high standard.

Finally to our respective loved ones—Chris, Ryan and Alex Lewis, Edward and Matthew Tench, Lorelle Kinsey—thank you for your patience and support throughout the writing of this book.

Lois Hamlin
Marilyn Richardson-Tench
Menna Davies

1

Perioperative nursing

Brigid Gillespie and Marilyn Richardson-Tench

The authors wish to acknowledge Prue Hames RN MN (Hons), Unit Manager, Short Stay Surgical Unit, Greenlane Clinical Centre, Auckland, and Leigh Anderson RN MN (Hons), Nurse Educator, Adult and Emergency Operating Rooms, Auckland City Hospital, for their contribution on cultural safety to this chapter.

LEARNING OBJECTIVES

After reading this chapter, you should be able to:

- discuss the philosophy that underpins perioperative nursing practice
- describe the patient care roles of the perioperative nurse
- identify in what circumstances these roles may overlap in the management of the patient undergoing surgery
- explain the importance of cultural safety in the perioperative environment
- identify prominent features of perioperative culture and examine the ways in which they influence perioperative nurses' socialisation and clinical practice.

KEY TERMS

communication	nursing roles	perioperative nursing
cultural safety	patient care	teamwork
culture	perioperative culture	
multidisciplinary	perioperative nurse	

INTRODUCTION

The purpose of this chapter is to introduce the beginning perioperative nurse to the key concepts used in perioperative nursing. It examines issues that are fundamental to understanding the context and culture that frames the perioperative nurses' professional roles. Specifically, this chapter addresses issues related to the history and philosophy of perioperative nursing, the concept of cultural safety, and the multifaceted aspects of workplace culture. Chronic skills shortages in perioperative nursing mean that retention and recruitment of nurses to this specialty remains a crucial imperative for the profession if it is to advance in the current healthcare climate. Additionally, the nursing workforce is ageing. Addressing crucial issues associated with these concerns are key aspects of perioperative nursing knowledge.

HISTORY OF THE PERIOPERATIVE SPECIALTY

Perioperative nursing in Australia is one of the oldest nursing specialties and has existed as a distinct entity for almost a hundred years, dating back to 1910 (Richardson-Tench, 2002). Operating room nursing underwent considerable change throughout the 20th century. The advent of sophisticated anaesthesia with its associated complexity of surgical procedures and the increased use of technology required the operating room nurse to develop commensurate knowledge and skills. In the 1970s, the term 'perioperative nursing' gained acceptance with a shift in emphasis away from the traditional geographic boundaries inside the operating suite to the temporal boundaries of preoperative patient assessment, intraoperative care and postoperative evaluation. The advancing technology and changes in the healthcare system has impacted upon perioperative nursing practice, providing the professional nurse with a variety of roles to practice. Perioperative nursing practice is flexible, with the scope of practice inclusive of all aspects of care of the surgical patient (Richardson, 2000).

Historically, surgical interventions have taken place in the traditional environment of the hospital operating suite. Advances in surgical technology and procedures, improvements in anaesthetic techniques and changes in the healthcare environment have altered where and how surgery is performed.

PERIOPERATIVE NURSING AS A CONCEPT

The **perioperative nurse** is a professional who provides complex care for patients in a high-dependency situation. The care encompasses safe and effective management in collaboration with other health team members; the nurse also safeguards the patient's integrity by acting as an advocate for patients during their perioperative experience. Furthermore, the perioperative nurse explores strategies for the enhancement of practice through continuing education, research and habits of lifelong learning.

Professional nursing in the operating room has been defined in the United States as:

> the identification of the physiological, psychological and sociological needs of the patient, and the implementation of an individualised program of nursing care that co-ordinates the nursing interventions, based on a knowledge of the natural and behavioural sciences, in order to restore, or maintain, the health and welfare of the patient before, during, and after surgery (Atkinson & Fortunato, 2000, p 22).

Even though the literature is replete with descriptions of the role of Australian perioperative nursing, there does not appear to be an explicit definition. Richardson-Tench (2002) describes the role of the perioperative nurse as follows:

The perioperative nurse is in a unique and privileged position as s/he assists with the surgical procedure. S/he is the consciousness of the unconscious patient. The perioperative nurse maintains the personhood of the patient by the provision of psychological care and by making ordinary the extraordinary event of surgery. S/he designs, co-ordinates and delivers care comprised of nursing knowledge and psychomotor skills which are a blend of thinking and doing, to meet the needs of the surgical patient. While scientific nursing techniques underpin perioperative nursing practice, competent fulfilment of the role is based on the knowledge and critical application of the biological, physiological, behavioural and social sciences (p 37).

Perioperative nursing is a highly skilled specialty with subspecialties, and a clearly defined role in terms of the surgical team and the patient. It requires nurses to be educated in nursing theory and the health sciences and to have attained appropriate interpersonal **communication** skills. The delivery of perioperative **patient care** requires complex knowledge and skills to effect safe outcomes for the surgical patient (Richardson-Tench, 2002).

PHILOSOPHY OF PERIOPERATIVE NURSING

Ideally, perioperative nursing practice is based on a written stated philosophy, which blends with the hospital's mission statement and describes values and beliefs that pertain to professional nursing practice. Perioperative nurses' primary professional responsibility is to the patients for whom they care. In the perioperative setting, healthcare personnel from different professional disciplines work together for a common objective: to provide competent, skilled and appropriate patient care. The philosophy of perioperative nursing encompasses a holistic, **multidisciplinary** approach that is concerned with:

- the need to provide a safe physical environment
- the protection of patients from adverse events
- the achievement of optimal patient outcomes
- promoting the knowledge and skills of all multidisciplinary team members to enable cost-effective, research-based health care delivery
- the acknowledgement of the dignity of persons with diverse physical, emotional and cultural backgrounds.

Thus, perioperative nurses possess unique knowledge and skills. They provide holistic care and are particularly aware of the fears and anxieties of the patient, as well as their physical needs (e.g. warmth and comfort), spiritual needs (e.g. support from staff) and sociological needs (e.g. acquaintance with staff and environment). Perioperative nurses constantly analyse, reflect and evaluate their performance. In other words, how they deliver patient care reflects their professionalism.

CARING ROLE VERSUS TECHNICAL ROLE

The technical dominance that defines **perioperative culture** inevitably links the evolution of nurses' roles to the development of technology. Technology can be best understood in terms of knowledge, skills, techniques, artefacts and resources (Barnard, 2007). Of necessity, perioperative nurses need to have technical aplomb for the wide array of machinery and equipment used in the provision of patient care. Moreover, some research suggests that there is still theoretical distancing of perioperative nursing from mainstream nursing based on conventional notions of the nurse–patient relationship that develops between people (Yamaguchi, 2004). Defining nursing care in the perioperative setting within this narrowly conceived traditional model has contributed to stereotypical perceptions that cast nurses as 'handmaidens' to the surgeons (Gruendemann, 1970), and positions the specialty as task-orientated and technical (Sandelowski, 1999). These descriptions imply that nurses' interpersonal relationship with patients in the perioperative setting is restricted; and that the nature of 'caring' is considerably diminished because of the differences in role orientation. There is continuing debate about whether perioperative nursing can even be considered nursing (Sandelowski, 1999), or even if nurses need to be present in the operating suite (Bull & FitzGerald, 2006).

For example, one field study found that perioperative nurses experienced role confusion as they were socialised to perform exclusively as technicians and assistants to the surgeons, not as nurses (Yamaguchi, 2004). This study demonstrated that nurses' roles in the perioperative environment were more technically focused and task-orientated, and substantiates the struggle that many perioperative nurses have working within a non-traditional area of nursing. The apparent conflict between caring and technical roles as the level of technology increases in the perioperative context has the potential to distance nurses from their patients, and erode the quality of care that patients receive (Bull & FitzGerald, 2006). Likewise, technical competence is often recognised and rewarded in the perioperative setting, and nurses with these attributes are held in high esteem—they are trusted and consulted (Bull & FitzGerald, 2006; Gillespie et al., 2008b). Consequently, perioperative nurses may find themselves faced with something of a predicament because of the dual nature of their perioperative role. The caring aspect of their role is what makes them 'real nurses' and yet the technological component is what earns perioperative nurses professional respect (Bull & FitzGerald, 2006). An example of the conflict that nurses experience between the technical and caring roles is emphasised in research conducted by Richardson-Tench (2007), presented in Box 1-1.

Box 1-1 Dialectic between caring and technical roles

Findings from Richardson-Tench's (2007) field study illustrate the tensions that perioperative nurses experience in their dual roles as carers and technicians. It appeared that for some of the lesser experienced nurses, the caring role was subsumed in the technical imperative that was associated with learning the surgical procedure. Consequently, for the novice, 'humanistic caring' could not take place until there was mastery of the psychomotor skills that defined the technical aspect of the perioperative role.

Patient care presents many challenges as perioperative nurses often have minimal time to establish rapport or provide reassurance, as well as obtain important clinical and/or psychosocial information. Perioperative nurses must have the ability to assess the patient quickly and become attuned to the patient's verbal and non-verbal cues. In many instances, the nurse is the last person that patients see before they are anaesthetised (Sigurdsson, 2001). For perioperative nurses, the central purpose of the patient–nurse relationship is to ensure the safe passage of patients during the perioperative period (Bull & FitzGerald, 2006). Perioperative nurses are in a unique position, as they must ensure a safe therapeutic environment for patients by maintaining practice standards (Richardson-Tench, 2007). Patients are at their most vulnerable when they enter the operating suite and are profoundly reliant on the skills and expertise of the nurses who care for them. In combining the technical and caring aspects of their perioperative role, nurses are the human conduits that provide the physical link between the patient and the machine (Glaze, 1999; Sandelowski, 1999).

Perioperative care roles

Nursing roles in the perioperative setting are based on both behavioural and technical components of clinical competence. The perioperative nurse plans and directs nursing care for patients undergoing operative and other invasive procedures. The scope of practice may include (but is not limited to) preadmission nurse, anaesthetic nurse, circulating nurse, instrument nurse, postanaesthetic recovery unit (PARU) nurse, perioperative nurse surgeon's assistant (PNSA), manager, educator and researcher. The roles of anaesthetic nurse and PARU nurse are usually exclusively designated—that is, nurses working in these roles do not routinely undertake other perioperative roles—but this may be dependent on staffing levels and skills. However, the traditional intraoperative roles of circulating nurse and instrument nurse are undertaken interchangeably throughout the day's operating list. Importantly, perioperative and surgical outcomes are influenced by the standard of care delivered by the nurse working within each of these roles (ACORN, 2006; PNCNZNO, 2005).

Preadmission nurse

The preadmission nurse plays an important role in the preparation of the patient for surgery by functioning in a screening role, detecting medical or physical conditions that may generate a referral to the surgeon or anaesthetist.

Anaesthetic nurse

The presence of an appropriately educated anaesthetic nurse/assistant is integral for the safe and efficient administration of anaesthesia (ACORN 2006; ANZCA 2003; PNCNZNO 2005). Specifically, the role of the anaesthetic nurse is to collaborate with the anaesthetist to provide patient care and procedural support (ANZCA, 2003). If an anaesthetic technician is required to fulfil this role briefly, then they require the appropriate professional education.

A registered nurse (RN) or enrolled nurse (EN) (Division 2 Registered Nurse, Victoria/Western Australia) may perform the anaesthetic nurse role. Perioperative nurses who work in this role have an option to obtain specialty education through an accredited postgraduate program. The Australian and New Zealand College of Anaesthetists recommends 150 contact hours (ANZCA, 2003). Enrolled nurses must work within their defined scope of practice as determined by the relevant state registration board authority (ACORN 2006; PNCNZNO 2005). Some of the role responsibilities of the anaesthetic nurse are outlined in Box 1-2.

Box 1-2 Role responsibilities of the anaesthetic nurse

- Collaborate with and assist anaesthetist during preparation, induction, maintenance and emergence phases of anaesthesia.
- Anticipate and provide equipment/supplies for routine and emergency anaesthetic procedures.
- Assist patient to maintain a clear airway.
- Patient assessment and monitoring.
- Assessment/documentation of fluid balance.
- Assist with patient transfer and positioning before and after surgery.
- Patient advocate, especially when anaesthetised.
- Evaluate effectiveness of planned care.
- Collaborate with PARU staff to provide patient care.

ACORN (2006); PNCNZNO (2005)

Circulating nurse

Perioperative nurses' primary role in the operating room is that of the circulating nurse. This is a complex role encompassing management of nursing care of the patient within the operating room and coordination of the needs of the surgical team and other care providers necessary for the completion of surgery (Matson, 2001). The circulating nurse's duties are performed outside the sterile area. Using critical thinking skills, the circulating nurse observes the surgery and the surgical team from a broad perspective and assists the team to create and maintain a safe and comfortable environment for the patient. The circulating nurse assesses the patient's condition before, during and after the operation to ensure an optimal outcome for the patient. Most patients undergoing surgery are anaesthetised or sedated and are powerless to make decisions on their own behalf during the intraoperative phase.

The critical importance of the circulating nurse cannot be understated (Matson, 2001). The circulating nurse serves as patient advocate while patients are least able to care for themselves. However, they have limited time to establish a bond with the patient before the procedure in order to be an effective advocate. Some of the role responsibilities of the circulating nurse are summarised in Box 1-3.

Box 1-3 Role responsibilities of the circulating nurse

- Anticipate the needs of the surgical team before/during surgery.
- Monitor any breach in aseptic technique and initiate corrective action.
- Perform the surgical count with the instrument nurse.
- Correct handling and labelling of surgically removed human tissue and explanted items.
- Advocate for the anaesthetised patient.
- Documentation of intraoperative nursing care.

ACORN (2006); PNCNZNO (2005)

Instrument nurse

The instrument nurse works directly with the surgeon within the sterile field, passing instruments, packs and other items needed during the procedure. Both the circulating and instrument nurses have a dual role in checking to ensure that all appropriate sterile instrumentation and surgical supplies are available and functional before the start of the list (ACORN, 2006; PNCNZNO, 2005). During surgery, the instrument nurse's role should be distinct from, and not overlap with, the role of the first surgical assistant, that is, the person assisting the surgeon. While there may be situations where there is a transient overlap of these roles (e.g. patient haemorrhage, difficult access), this situation should not occur routinely. Knowledge in relation to standards of perioperative practice (e.g. standards for cleaning and practice, aseptic technique, infection control, medicolegal requirements, anatomy/physiology, surgical procedures) is essential to perform these roles safely and effectively. To assist nurses to develop a broad knowledge base, specialty perioperative education through an accredited program is recommended (ACORN, 2006; PNCNZNO, 2005). Depending on the policy of the particular hospital, the instrument nurse may be an RN or an EN. ENs must work within their defined scope of practice as determined by the relevant state regulation authorities and must be under the supervision of an RN (ACORN, 2006). The role responsibilities of circulating/instrument nurse(s) may overlap a little with that of the anaesthetic nurse, depending on the policy of the relevant operating room department, scope of practice of individual nurses within the team and the structure of the surgical team. For instance, in some operating suites, it is the role of the anaesthetic nurse to check the patient's details (i.e. correct identity/surgical site, consent, allergies, etc.) when they arrive, whereas this duty may be incorporated in the role of the circulating nurse in other departments. Box 1-4 highlights some of the responsibilities associated with the instrument nurse role.

Box 1-4 Role responsibilities of the instrument nurse

- Prepare the instruments and equipment needed in the operation.
- Anticipate the needs of the surgical team before/during surgery.
- Adhere to and maintain aseptic technique throughout the procedure.
- Monitor any breach in aseptic technique and initiate corrective action.
- Perform the surgical count with the circulating nurse.
- Correct handling of surgically removed human tissue and explanted items.
- Documentation of intraoperative nursing care.

ACORN (2006); PNCNZNO (2005)

Perioperative nurse surgeon's assistant

It has been recognised for many years that nurses have acted as assistants to surgeons in the capacity of first assistant, where the nurse provides skilled assistance but not surgery (McGarvey et al., 2000). However, more recently, changes in health care delivery have precipitated the emergence and recognition of an extended practice role for RNs in the perioperative setting (ACORN, 2006). The PNSA role in Australia incorporates the preoperative, intraoperative and postoperative phases of care. Within its most limited scope of practice, the PNSA role may be restricted to the intraoperative phase (Riley & Peters, 2000). The Australian College of Operating Room Nurses endorses the ongoing development and expansion of the PNSA as a Nurse Practitioner role (ACORN, 2006), which would require educational preparation to a Masters degree. Essentially, the scope of practice within the PNSA role is determined by state and federal legislation. Box 1-5 details some of the role responsibilities undertaken by the PNSA.

Box 1-5 Role responsibilities of the PNSA

- Undertake physical patient assessment, including medical history, and, in collaboration with the surgeon, organise required clinical investigations.
- Collaborate with patient, surgeon and other health care team members to develop a clinical pathway.
- Develop education programs for patients/staff.
- Assist with skin preparation, draping, haemostasis, cutting sutures/ligatures, retracting organs and skin closure.
- Provide postoperative care in wound management, education, dressing application, etc.

ACORN (2006)

Postanaesthesia recovery unit nurse

The PARU nurse is an important member of the perioperative team and provides patient care immediately following an anaesthetic, surgical or other procedure (ACORN, 2006; PNCNZNO, 2005). The role of the PARU nurse is to ensure patient safety through a trajectory of unconsciousness and instability to consciousness and stability, following the transfer of the patient from the operating room to the PARU. Vigilance is crucial in achieving the intended outcome as the patient is at increased risk during this trajectory.

In some health care facilities, the PARU and anaesthetic nurse roles are interchangeable, with nurses working across both subspecialties. Where direct patient care is given by an EN, an RN must supervise it. ENs must work within their scope of practice as determined by the relevant state registration authority and departmental policy. Specialty education through an accredited postgraduate program is recommended. Box 1-6 features some of the role responsibilities performed by the PARU nurse.

Box 1-6 Role responsibilities of the PARU nurse

- Patient assessment and airway management.
- Patient observation/monitoring.
- Perform resuscitation.
- Management of acute pain, nausea and vomiting.
- Management of patient's fluid balance.
- Documentation of nursing care during the immediate postoperative period.
- Prompt acting on and reporting aberrant changes in the patient's condition to anaesthetist/surgeon.
- Provision of a comprehensive patient handover to the nurse caring for the patient in the receiving unit.

ACORN (2006); PNCNZNO (2005)

CULTURAL SAFETY

Cultural safety is a concept that arose in the context of post-colonial countries, such as Australia, Canada and New Zealand. It emerged in health care as a means of engendering a critical understanding of colonial structures and their impact on contemporary Indigenous populations (Dyck & Kearns, 1995). The concept of cultural safety emphasises that health care is not merely provided for individuals but for members of minority ethnic groups whose care is inevitably defined and influenced by social disadvantage. The Nursing Council of New Zealand (NCNZ) (2002, p 7) defines cultural safety as:

> The effective nursing practice of a person or family from another culture, and is determined by that person or family. Culture includes, but is not restricted to age or generation, gender, sexual orientation, occupation and socioeconomic status, ethnic origin or migrant experience, religious or spiritual belief, and disability.

Therefore, cultural safety encompasses a person's socioeconomic status, age, gender, sexual orientation, ethnic origin, migrant/refugee status, religious belief or disability to enable the delivery of safe, appropriate and acceptable nursing care. Cultural safety relates to the experience of patients as recipients of nursing care, and extends beyond cultural awareness and cultural sensitivity. While the terms 'cultural awareness' and 'cultural sensitivity' are used synonymously with 'cultural safety', they are not interchangeable with cultural safety (Ramsden, 2002). These are separate concepts that are positioned on a continuum that ultimately leads to cultural safety.

It is important that health care professionals involved in patient care consider the cultural implications of their practice on others. Within the literature, cultural safety may also be referred to as cultural competence. Cultural competence is a way of being sensitive to the differences in culture and acting in a way that is respectful of the values and traditions of the patient while performing those activities or procedures necessary for the patients well-being (de Chesnay, 2005).

As a result of the fundamental differences in the personal characteristics and backgrounds of the patient and the nurse, cultural safety provides care within a framework that affirms and respects these individual differences (Milnes et al., 2007). It is the nurses' responsibility to engender trust; and the patient determines whether sufficient trust has been established for cultural safety. Accordingly, a culturally safe nurse does not need to be culturally similar to patients; however, it is considered culturally safe because patients believe that their own values are accepted rather than discounted. For instance, in Māori culture, all body parts are highly revered and are either disposed of according to *tikanga* practices and/or returned to patients and their *whanau* (extended family) (Waikato District Health Board, 2006). *Tikanga* refers to the customs and traditions that have been passed down through generations and guides general behaviour. Box 1-7 describes a practice example where observance of this cultural belief has implications for the disposal of resected organs or tissues postoperatively.

Box 1-7 Respect for traditional values and religious beliefs

Huatare, a 53-year-old Māori man, has been scheduled to have a left lower leg amputation. Prior to the surgery, at the request of his *whanau*, two members from the perioperative team met to discuss the possibility of returning the amputated limb back to Huatare. Explicit consent and informed acceptance was obtained from Huatare and his *whanau* regarding their intentions for removal, retention and return of Huatare's amputated limb. The family wanted the amputated limb so they could 'return to the earth what has come from the earth'. A notation of the discussion and its outcome was documented in Huatare's chart.

During surgery, handling of the amputated limb reflected *tikanga* practices. The perioperative team made the necessary arrangements regarding the appropriate handling and prompt return of the amputated limb to family members.

Cultural safety is also concerned with recognising the inherent power imbalances that exist between the health care provider and the people who use the service. Within the hospital setting, the use, control and language of clinical information have contributed to a disproportionate power base in favour of health care professionals (Ramsden, 2002). Nurses' clinical, biological and technical knowledge and their access to resources have clearly created and maintained inequities within the nurse–patient relationship (Milnes et al., 2007). The potential for disparity in power relations between nurses and their patients is acutely evident in the perioperative context as patients enter the alien environs of the operating suite. Not only are patients stripped of the vestiges of their personal and social identities through the donning of operating room attire, they have been relocated to an environment where medical technology is an omnipresent feature, and the esoteric language of surgery is fluently spoken. In this context, cultural safety recognises that perioperative nurses have greater access to power because of their professional and technical knowledge. Box 1-8 presents a practice example to illustrate this.

Ramsden (2002) suggests that cultural safety is about the nurse rather than the patient, meaning the enactment of cultural safety is about the nurse, while for the patient it is a mechanism that allows the recipient of care to say whether the service is safe for them to approach and use. The Nursing Council of New Zealand (2005)

Box 1-8 Recognising powerlessness and power

A 19-year-old Indigenous woman from the Tjapukai mob, north of Cairns, arrived at the operating suite reception area and was scheduled to have surgery for an excision and drainage of a Bartholin's cyst. The anaesthetic nurse greeted the young woman and briefly explained the 'checking-in' process, and then proceeded to ask the woman questions based on the preoperative checklist. The nurse noticed that the young woman was not accompanied by a relative and was very reluctant to speak. Upon completion of the check-in process, the nurse asked the young woman to verify the procedure to which she had given written consent. The young woman's reticent and incomplete responses indicated that her understanding of the surgery and the perioperative process was very limited. At that moment, the anaesthetist and operating orderly arrived and introduced themselves as they began to wheel the young woman into the operating room.

Unfortunately, there was no family member or interpreter to intervene and assist the young Indigenous woman to negotiate through the maze of these dilemmas during this crucial time.

---

asserts that cultural safety may provide consumers of nursing services with the power to comment on practices and contribute to the achievement of positive health outcomes and experiences. Mistakenly, when questioned about cultural safety, health professionals may answer that they treat all their patients equally. In terms of cultural safety, the response of equal treatment is not appropriate as this does not allow for the unique needs of each patient. Unsafe cultural practice may lead to the disempowerment of the cultural identity or well-being of an individual (NCNZ, 2005).

Within the preoperative phase of a patient's journey, cultural safety may be demonstrated in numerous ways. Examples may include ensuring that the patient has the appropriate support person or family with them during the consultation period, or that the patient has the services of a medical interpreter if required. Aspects of the physical examination may also require gaining permission from the patient to touch their head, as in some cultures the head area is deemed sacred. When unsure of a patient's beliefs, the best approach is to ask the patient if the care they are receiving is appropriate to their beliefs. While obtaining surgical consent, consideration may be required by the patient as to whether they would like their body parts/tissue returned to them postoperatively, regardless of whether laboratory investigations are required. The wishes of the patient are to be clearly documented on the surgical consent/agreement to treatment form. Individual hospital guidelines and policy are required to guide practice with any such request.

The concept of cultural safety has had a powerful ideological influence on health education and practice. The 'cultural safety' model was developed by Māori nurse leader, Irihapeti Ramsden (NCNZ, 2002). The tenets of this model are outlined in Box 1-9.

CONTEXT AND CULTURE OF THE PERIOPERATIVE ENVIRONMENT

The relevance of **culture** to workplaces is becoming increasingly important because of its psychosocial impact on group dynamics. Culture has been symbolically described as the universal 'glue' that binds the members of a workplace together through mutual patterns of meaning, conveyed through language (Chao et al., 1994). Professional socialisation involves developing the necessary skills, attitudes and behaviours that are expected and reinforced by the collective. Research conducted in Australia and overseas indicates that the extent to which new staff members are accepted into complex work environments, such as the perioperative setting, generally depends on: (a) their ability to

---

Box 1-9 Tenets of the cultural safety model

- Cultural safety provides care that is mindful of individual differences. Patients are viewed as individuals who may share information based on the establishment of trust.
- 'Emic' (insider's view) Indigenous context.
- Concerned with the transfer of power and establishment of trust.
- Acknowledges the experience of colonisation; therefore, nurses need to examine their own attitudes and the realities they bring to each patient they encounter in their everyday practice.
- Nurses who are culturally safe are deemed as such by the people they care for.
- Cultural knowledge belongs to the culture.
- Interactions are bicultural.
- Negotiated and equal partnership model.

Ramsden (2002)

---

acclimatise to the contextual subtleties of the workplace; and (b) the level of professional (e.g. education/preceptorship) and social support (e.g. included in the team) given as new staff members acquire the required specialty knowledge and develop their clinical skills (Bull & FitzGerald, 2006; Gillespie et al., 2008b; Richardson-Tench, 2007; Silén-Lipponen et al., 2004).

Based on research conducted in Australia, North America and the United Kingdom, pertinent aspects of perioperative culture have been identified: specialty knowledge; social organisation; teamwork and communication; and the caring versus the technical role. The following sections present a discussion on each of these aspects.

Specialty knowledge

Recent Australian research has indicated that specialty knowledge is a critical attribute of perioperative culture (Gillespie et al., 2008b). Operating suites are characteristically fast-paced clinical environments where specialty knowledge and clinical judgement are highly valued. Nursing practice in this unique setting includes specialty knowledge related to standards of perioperative practice, principles related to infection control and aseptic technique, and the management of instruments and equipment. For example, the way that instruments should be laid out on the sterile trolley for efficient use, how instruments should be passed in a dextrous manner so that the surgeon does not have to reposition the instrument before it is used, and the timely and intuitive response given to the surgeon's request is underpinned by specialty knowledge. Therefore, for nurses to develop the knowledge and skills to assume the role of instrument nurse, they are 'double-scrubbed' with a more experienced member of the nursing staff to provide physical and psychological support, and to enable close observation and appraisal of the novice's skills (Riley & Peters, 2000). Additionally, perioperative nurses need specialty knowledge in relation to the wide array of machinery and equipment used to provide patient care.

However, more implicit forms of specialty knowledge are also developed as a function of experience, familiarity and time. Perioperative nurses necessarily develop an intimate knowledge of the requirements of the surgeons and anaesthetists with whom they work closely (Riley & Manias, 2007). Perioperative nurses possess detailed knowledge relating to the minute aspects of clinical practice; for instance, surgeons' habits and preferences, such as which way to load a needle on the needle holder or how abdominal packs are to be folded. The importance of technical instrumentation knowledge and knowing the surgeon's preferences is an important aspect of specialist knowledge for the perioperative nurse (Richardson-Tench, 2002). As well as a knowledge of surgeons' technical preferences, perioperative nurses also develop knowledge of whether surgeons are fast or slow during surgery, the time they usually take to perform a specific procedure, whether they are punctual or habitually late, and their degree of flexibility during surgery (Riley & Manias, 2007). Having such knowledge informs the organisation of the nurses' work activities in the operating rooms, such as when to commence the instrument set-up, who would be best placed in the role of the circulating and instrument nurse, and when to send for the next patient (Riley & Manias, 2007).

Language is another salient feature of workplace culture and influences the ways in which individuals are socialised. As a form of knowledge, language frames the clinician's technical dialogue, which consists of acronyms, nomenclature and vernacular that are unique to the health care setting (Chao et al., 1994). When perioperative nurses are conversant in the specialty language, they are more likely to communicate effectively with other members of the team (Gillespie et al., 2006). When nurses were unable to understand and use this language effectively to converse, other members frequently became frustrated and this increases tensions within the team. Recent research conducted by Gillespie et al. (2008b) illustrated the difficulties perioperative nurses had when they were not familiar with the specialty language. The potential consequences this presented are highlighted in Box 1-10. Other researchers suggest that specialty language also determines professional and social boundaries (Lingard et al., 2002b; Tanner & Timmons, 2000). Therefore, the perioperative nurse's sense of professional identity, which is constructed through language, is forged during the early socialisation period.

Box 1-10 Specialty language

In a recent Australian field study that examined perioperative culture, Gillespie et al. (2008b) identified that nurses' ability to understand and use the specialty language associated with perioperative practice was influenced by their level of knowledge and clinical experience. Effective communication depended on nurses' ability to interpret and act on subtle verbal and non-verbal messages given by other team members who assumed, to some degree, that all team members would have this form of knowledge. When participants were unable to use this specialty language proficiently, they felt that they were not able to contribute to the team, and some even reported feelings of social isolation.

Social organisation

The impact of socialisation is particularly evident in operating room culture, where the traditional hierarchical model has historically defined social organisation (Richardson-Tench, 2007). Seminal research described the traditional, medically dominated social structure that has dictated the direction of authority in the perioperative environment (Goffman, 1972). Subsequent research has identified that power and culture were reflected in the conversations between medical and nursing staff in the operating suite (Tanner & Timmons, 2000). Conversation among doctors was often serious and intellectual, whereas conversation with the nursing staff was jocular and superficial. However, this research also indicated that the professional identities, and therefore the social status of members, were concealed through the uniformity of dress, enabling hierarchy to be suspended.

More recent research conducted in Australia and North America has challenged the prevailing myth of a 'pecking order', historically captained by the surgeon (Gillespie et al., 2008b; Lingard et al., 2002a). For instance, Gillespie et al.'s (2008b) Australian field study noted that while traditional authority gradients do exist in the perioperative context, they are momentarily manipulated to fit the needs of the situation. There are instances when the situation dictates that the person who is ultimately responsible for a specific patient treatment—the anaesthetist or surgeon—carries out coordination of a particular activity. Alternatively, the most qualified person who is not easily distinguishable by professional status may be more appropriate than the attending doctors on specific aspects of patient care in a particular situation. An example of this in the operating room is during the positioning of the patient prior to surgery. It is usually the operating room technician who is designated as being responsible for retrieving and using equipment required to position the patient (e.g. hip joint replacement surgery). In this instance, the operating room technician is recognised by other members of the surgical team as being the most informed and should therefore coordinate this activity. Clinical practice in the perioperative setting tends to encourage a certain amount of flexibility of authority, which is determined by the situation and the people involved.

Workplace bullying and harassment

Workplace bullying and harassment have been described in the literature as prevalent features that have influenced social organisation in the perioperative context (Dunn, 2003; Gillespie et al., 2008c; Gilmour & Hamlin, 2003). It is also contended that regressive behaviours, such as sabotage, social exclusion and withholding of vital information, limits the extent to which individuals can participate as team members. These types of behaviours have historically constrained the development of perioperative nursing and, in doing so, have reinforced nursing's subordination to medicine (Dunn, 2003). It has also been suggested that workplace bullying and harassment in the perioperative setting reinforces the 'pecking order' of the culture (Gillespie et al., 2008c).

Bullying appears to flourish in environments where there is a strict hierarchical order and where there is a high value placed on the skills required to perform work roles competently (Hughes, 2003). Some authors have attributed the prevalence of bullying in the perioperative setting to its geographic isolation, the high stress associated with the nature of the work, the familiarity and the bonding that develops between staff, and the dated belief that nurses are 'handmaidens' to surgeons and anaesthetists (Dunn, 2003; Gilmour & Hamlin, 2003). Bullying has been described in relation to decreased job satisfaction, diminished work performance, low staff morale, burn-out and attrition (Dunn, 2003; Hughes, 2003).

Emphasis is placed on preventing workplace bullying and, in many health care institutions, primary prevention is underpinned by education and training of staff. The Australian College of Operating Room Nurses (ACORN) has published a position statement that details the obligations of individuals and organisations in relation to the prevention and management of workplace bullying, and the imperative to promote 'a culture of zero tolerance' in perioperative environments (ACORN, 2006, PS3).

Teamwork and communication

Embedded in perioperative culture is the notion of teamwork. **Teamwork** is defined as a group of individuals who share common goals, work together interdependently to perform tasks, and who manage their relationships and clinical roles across professional boundaries (DiPalma, 2004). Teamwork is underpinned by factors related to effective communication, team formation, leadership, resource management, workload prioritisation and distribution, and coping with stress (Aggarwal et al., 2004).

In the perioperative setting, a number of professionals with differing clinical backgrounds and expertise perform a variety of activities directed towards a common goal—the well-being of the patient (Schaefer et al., 1995). Every team member has a specialised role: the anaesthetist's focus is to maintain life-support measures during surgery; the surgeon's role is to perform surgery to improve the patient's physical status in some way; the technician's role is to support the anaesthestist; and the nurse's role centres on providing safe patient care by ensuring that all team members adhere to professional standards and practices that are circumscribed by the context. Within this team culture, optimal patient outcomes are dependent on the performance of individuals.

The perspective for measuring a team's performance in the perioperative setting has traditionally focused on assessing the skill of the surgeon alone (Aggarwal et al., 2004), with little acknowledgement given to the role of the perioperative nurse. However, the increasing reliance on complex surgical technologies in perioperative nursing has led to nurses being recognised as valued members of the multidisciplinary team since they must possess a comprehensive knowledge of how the equipment is prepared, used and maintained (ACORN, 2006).

Contribution of effective team communication to patient care

There is growing evidence that supports the need for better communication among surgical teams. The role of effective communication in maintaining patient safety is increasingly being recognised as essential in high-risk environments, such as the perioperative setting (Undre et al., 2006). Surgical teamwork involves complex interpersonal dynamics among highly specialised professionals—specifically, nurses, anaesthetists, surgeons and technicians.

There is much evidence to suggest that communication failures can have devastating results, leading to the potential for human error (Reason, 2005; Schaefer et al., 1995). Recent data from the Australian Institute of Health and Welfare suggests that up to 50% of adverse events in Australian hospitals occur as a result of communication failures between health care professionals, in particular, nurses and doctors (AIHW, 2007). In the operating room specifically, communication failures have been identified as the primary cause in 80% of perioperative sentinel events (JACHO, 2004). Retained sponges, wrong-site surgery, and mismatched blood transfusions and organ transplants can be the result of interpersonal dynamics, where communication failures occur among members of the perioperative team (Giles et al., 2006). Therefore, the performance of the collective is the key to good surgical care and a predictor of optimal surgical outcome (Flin et al., 2003; Giles et al., 2006). Box 1-11 illustrates the dynamics needed for effective communication during surgery.

Box 1-11 Dynamics of communication in surgery

During surgery, effective communication between the surgeon and the perioperative nurse depends on:

- a two-way exchange of information and objects
- appropriate timing of exchanges (i.e. information/objects)
- verbal exchanges that are clear, comprehensible and of an appropriate tone and volume
- the instrument nurse anticipating the surgeon's procedural needs
- the surgeon appreciating that the nurse depends on other team members (i.e. circulating nurse).

A communication breakdown between the nurse and the surgeon has the potential to adversely affect the care of the patient during these critical intraoperative moments.

Communication is not standardised in the perioperative setting and will vary depending on the rapport among team members (Gillespie et al., 2008a; Healey et al., 2006). Communications among the multidisciplinary team may be based on previous professional and social relationships, and may have the potential to hinder team effectiveness (Lingard et al., 2002b). This is particularly true when team members are transitory and there is a significant reliance on casual or agency staff. Additionally, nurses and doctors have been socialised into different communities of practice and, therefore, have different foci and communication styles. For example, doctors tend to approach a clinical situation using a diagnosis-and-treatment model, whereas nurses operate from a different contextual frame, using a provision-of-care model (Dayton & Henriksen, 2007). Accordingly, there is the potential for communications to derail, resulting in communication breakdowns (Gillespie et al., 2008a; Leonard et al., 2004; Lingard et al., 2006). The potential for the loss of vital information as a result of poor communication among team members is highlighted in research conducted by Lingard and colleagues, presented in Box 1-12.

Box 1-12 Communication failures

In a series of Canadian observational studies, Lingard et al. (2004; 2005; 2006) identified problematic issues in relation to team communication in the perioperative setting. Communication was often too late to be effective, the content was inconsistent or incomplete, issues were left unresolved until the point of urgency and key personnel were excluded from discussions. Consequently, up to 30% of procedurally relevant information exchanges were obscured or lost as a result of communication failures among members of the surgical team.

Negotiating the flow of the operating list

The operating list is an artefact that represents a structured means of communication. The list indicates the sequencing and priority of surgical procedures used by members of the surgical team (Riley & Manias, 2007). It communicates the surgical procedures undertaken in each operating room and the subsequent nursing actions that maintain it. The list may be typewritten, and the information is arranged to correspond to the numbered operating rooms, beginning with the morning sessions, followed by the afternoon sessions. All work in the operating room revolves around the written operating list. Further, members of the team frequently refer to it as 'the list', acknowledging its iconic role in the communication of essential information. Nevertheless, situations frequently arise that necessitate a change in the order of the list based on the availability of particular instruments or unplanned surgical emergencies. Consequently, negotiating the flow and priority of the operating list is based on a complex set of interactions among various key team members.

Unplanned (urgent or semi-urgent) surgery presents the surgical team with competing individual and organisational challenges, especially when there is an increasing queue of patients requiring surgery (Lum & Fitzgerald, 2007). Prioritisation involves clinical assessment and a process for deciding the order of patients and competing teams. Negotiations surrounding these clinical issues may be inherently problematic as surgical emergencies present contemporaneously. Often, determining surgical priority ultimately rests with the surgeon, who liaises with the anaesthetist. However, there may be occasions when disagreement arises between these two professional groups based on competing priorities. Barriers to communication occur when there is an absence of, or ineffective, communication, differing perceptions about the same event, or when there is a lack of leadership. Collectively, this situation is problematic not only for those team members from different disciplines, but also for those from the same discipline.

CONCLUSION

This chapter introduced the beginning perioperative nurse to the key concepts used in perioperative nursing. The chapter addressed issues related to the history and philosophy of perioperative nursing, and the concept of cultural safety, which guides appropriate and sensitive patient care. A discussion of nursing roles within the perioperative specialty was presented. Additionally, issues that are fundamental to understanding the context and culture that frames the perioperative nurses' socialisation into professional roles were identified and explored. Specifically, specialty knowledge, social organisation, teamwork and the caring versus technical role have defined operating room culture. Moreover, safe patient care depends on the ways in which team members communicate with each other.

CRITICAL THINKING EXERCISES

1. Perioperative practice

The perioperative role allows operating room nurses to extend their influence beyond the technical duties of the operating room.
• Critique this statement in relation to your view of perioperative nursing.

2. Teamwork in the operating room

The operating room represents the epitome of teamwork. When members become part of the perioperative team, many dimensions of group dynamics come into play and members' behaviours are often influenced by the situation and the ways in which information is exchanged.
• What are the qualities of a cohesive team?
• Reflect on some of the factors that may sabotage effective teamwork.
• Consider strategies that you could use to enhance teamwork and communication among team members.

3. Communication in the operating room

You are a new graduate working in the orthopaedic trauma operating room. You have been asked to scrub for a right knee washout and debridement. During the procedure, the surgeon asks you to take a 'sprinkler system' onto your set-up. You are feeling a little out of your depth because you are unfamiliar with this term of speech.
• What course of action should you take in this situation?

4. Negotiating the flow of the operating room list

It is 10.30 pm and Dr Smith, an orthopaedic surgeon, has been waiting in the operating room department to perform an open reduction and internal fixation of a fractured hip. Unfortunately, there are three other patients requiring emergency surgery who are considered by the anaesthetist as 'more urgent' by the anaesthetist. Dr Smith approaches you—he is angry at being kept waiting and insists that another operating room be opened to allow him to perform the procedure.
• What course of action should you take in this situation?

RESOURCES

Australian Nursing & Midwifery Council
www.anmc.org.au
Association of Perioperative Registered Nurses
www.aorn.org
New Zealand Health Workforce Statistics
www.nzhis.govt.nz
Royal College of Nursing, Australia
www.rcna.org.au
The Joint Commission
www.jointcommission.org

REFERENCES

ACORN. (2006). *ACORN standards for perioperative nursing: including nursing roles, guidelines, position statements and competency standards.* Adelaide: Australian College of Operating Room Nurses.

Aggarwal, B., Undre, S., Moorthy, C., Darzi, A. (2004). The simulated operating theatre: comprehensive training for surgical teams. *Quality and Safety in Health Care, 13,* 27–32.

AIHW. (2006). *Nursing and midwifery labour force 2004: national health labour force series, number 31.* Canberra: Australian Institute of Health & Welfare.

AIHW. (2007). *Sentinel events in Australian public hospitals 2004–05.* Australian Institute of Health and Welfare and the Australian Commission on Safety and Quality in Health Care. Canberra. Retrieved April 17, 2008, from http://www.aihw.gov.au/publications/index.cfm/criteria/Sentinel%20events.

Atkinson, L., & Fortunato, N. (Eds). (2000). *Berry and Kohn's introduction to operating technique* (9th ed.). New York: Mosby.

ANZCA. (2003). *Professional documents of the Australian and New Zealand College of Anaesthetists. Guidelines for the assistant for the anaesthetist.* Canberra: Australian and New Zealand College of Anaesthetists.

Barnard, A. (2007). Advancing the meaning of nursing and technology. In A. Barnard, & R. Locsin (Eds.), *Technology and nursing practice concepts and issues.* Basingstoke, UK: Palgrave Macmillan.

Bull, R., & FitzGerald, M. (2006). Nursing in a technological environment: nursing care in the operating room. *International Journal of Nursing Practice, 12,* 3–7.

Chao, G., O'Leary, A., Wolf, S., Klein, H., Gardiner, P. (1994). Organisational socialisation. *Journal of Applied Psychology, 79(5),* 730–743.

Dayton, E., & Henriksen, K. (2007). Communication failure: basic components, contributing factors, and the call for structure. *Joint Commission Journal on Quality and Patient Safety, 33(1),* 34–47.

de Chesnay, M. (2005). *Caring for the vulnerable.* Sudbury, MA: Jones & Bartlett.

DiPalma, C. (2004). Power at work: navigating hierarchies, teamwork and roles. *Journal of Medical Humanities, 25(4),* 291–308.

Dunn, H. (2003). Horizontal violence among nurses in the operating room. *Association of Operating Room Nurses Journal, 78(6),* 977–985.

Dyck, I., & Kearns, R. A. (1995). Transforming the relations of research towards culturally safe geographies of health and healing. *Health and Place, 1(1),* 137–147.

Flin, R., Fletcher, P., McGeorge, P., et al. (2003). Anaesthetists attitudes to teamwork and safety. *Anaesthesia, 58,* 233–242.

Giles, S., Rhodes, P., Cook, G., Hayton, R., Maxwell, M., Sheldon, T., et al. (2006). Experience of wrong site surgery and surgical marking practices among clinicians in the UK. *Quality and Safety in Health Care, 15,* 363–368.

Gillespie, B. M., Wallis, M., Chaboyer, W. (2006). Clinical competence in the perioperative environment: implications for education. *ACORN, 19(3),* 19–26.

Gillespie, B. M., Chaboyer, W., Lizzio, A. (2008a). Teamwork in the OR: enhancing communication through team-building interventions. *ACORN Journal, 21(1),* 14–19.

Gillespie, B. M., Wallis, M., Chaboyer, W. (2008b). Operating room culture—implications for nurse retention. *Western Journal of Nursing Research, 30(2),* 259–277.

Gillespie, B. M., Wallis, M., Chaboyer, W. (2008c). Response by Gillespie, Wallis & Chaboyer. *Western Journal of Nursing Research, 30(2),* 281–283.

Gilmour, D., & Hamlin, L. (2003). Bullying and harassment in perioperative settings. *British Journal of Perioperative Nursing, 13(2),* 79–85.

Glaze, J. (1999). Part 5: Reflecting on interpersonal knowledge and professional knowledge. *British Journal of Theatre Nursing, 9(2)*, 64–69.

Goffman, E. (1972). *Encounters: two studies in the sociology of interaction*. Harmondsworth: Penguin University Books.

Gruendemann, B. (1970). Analysis of the role of the professional staff nurses in the operating room. *Nursing Research, 19*, 349–353.

Healey, A., Undre, S., Vincent, C. (2006). Defining the technical skills of teamwork in surgery. *Quality and Safety in Health Care, 15*, 231–234.

Hughes, A. (2003). Being bullied. *British Journal of Theatre Nursing, 13(4)*, 166–172.

Joint Accreditation Commission of Healthcare Organisations. (2004). *Sentinel event statistics: December 17, 2003*. Oakbrook Terrace: JACHO.

Leonard, M., Graham, S., Bonacum, D. (2004). The human factor: the critical importance of effective teamwork and communication in providing safe care. *Quality and Safety in Health Care, 13*, 85–90.

Lingard, L., Reznick, R., De Vito, I., Epsin, S. (2002a). Forming professional identities on the health care team: discursive constructions of the 'other' in the operating room. *Medical Education, 36*, 728–734.

Lingard, L., Reznick, R., Epsin, S., Regehr, G., De Vito, I. (2002b). Team communications in the operating room: talk patterns, sites of tension, and implications for novices. *Academic Medicine, 77(3)*, 323–237.

Lingard, L., Garwood, S., Poenaru, D. (2004). Tensions influencing operating room team function: does institutional context make a difference? *Medical Education, 38*, 691–699.

Lingard, L., Epsin, S., Rubin, B., et al. (2005). Getting teams to talk: development and pilot implementation of a checklist to promote interprofessional communication in the OR. *Quality and Safety in Health Care, 14*, 340–346.

Lingard, L., Regehr, G., Epsin, S., Whyte, S. (2006). A theory-based instrument to evaluate team communication in the operating room: balancing measurement authenticity and reliability. *Quality and Safety in Health Care, 15*, 422–426.

Lum, M., & Fitzgerald, A. (2007). Dialogues of mediating priorities in unplanned emergency surgical queues. In R. Iedema (Ed.), *The discourse of hospital communication: tracing the complexities in contemporary health care organisations* (pp. 90–108). Hampshire: Palgrave.

Matson, K. (2001). The critical "nurse" in the circulating nurse role—registered versus unlicensed supervision. *AORN Journal, 73(5)*, 971–975.

McGarvey, H., Chambers, M., Boore, J. (2000). Development and definition of the role of the operating department nurse: a review. *Journal of Advanced Nursing, 32(5)*, 1092–1100.

Milnes, P., Fenwick, C., Truscott, K., St John, W. (2007). Working in a cross-cultural setting. In W. St John, & H. Keleher (Eds.), *Community nursing practice: theory, skills and issues* (pp. 289–308). Sydney: Allen & Unwin.

NCNZ. (2002). *Guidelines for cultural safety, the Treaty of Waitangi, and Māori health in nursing and midwifery education and practice* (p. 24). Auckland: Nursing Council of New Zealand.

PNCNZNO. (2005). *Recommended standards, guidelines, and position statements for safe practice in the perioperative setting*. Wellington: Perioperative Nurses College of New Zealand Nurses Organisation.

Ramsden, I. (2002). *Cultural safety and nursing education in Aotearoa and Te Waipounamu*. Wellington: Victoria University.

Reason, J. (2005). Safety in the operating theatre—Part 2: Human error and organisational failure. *Quality and Safety in Health Care, 14*, 56–61.

Richardson, M. (2000). Advanced practice: what does this mean for perioperative nursing? Paper presented at ACORN National Conference, Adelaide.

Richardson-Tench, M. (2002). Unmasked! The discursive practice of the operating room nurse: a Foucauldian feminist analysis. Unpublished PhD thesis, Monash University.

Richardson-Tench, M. (2007). Technician or nurturer: discourses within the operating room. *ACORN Journal, 20(3)*, 12–15.

Riley, R., & Manias, E. (2007). Governing the operating room list. In R. Iedema (Ed.). *The discourse of hospital communication: tracing the complexities in contemporary health care organisations* (pp. 67–88). Hampshire: Palgrave.

Riley, R., & Peters, G. (2000). The current scope and future direction of perioperative nursing practice in Victoria, Australia. *Journal of Advanced Nursing, 32(3)*, 544–553.

Sandelowski, M. (1999). Troubling distinctions: a semiotics of the nursing/technology relationship. *Nursing Inquiry, 6*, 198–207.

Schaefer, R., Helmreich, R., Scheidegger, D. (1995). Safety in the operating theatre—Part 1: Interpersonal relationships and team performance. *Current Anaesthesia and Critical Care, 6*, 48–53.

Sigurdsson, H. (2001). The meaning of being a perioperative nurse. *AORN Journal, 74(2)*, 202–217.

Silēn-Lipponen, M., Tossavainen, K., Turunen, H., Smith, A. (2004). Learning about teamwork in operating room clinical placement. *British Journal of Nursing, 13(5)*, 244–253.

Tanner, J., & Timmons, S. (2000). Backstage in the theatre. *Journal of Advanced Nursing, 32(4),* 975–980.

Undre, S., Sevdalis, N., Healey, A., Darzi, A., Vincent, C. (2006). Teamwork in operating theatres: cohesion or confusion. *Journal of Evaluation in Clinical Practice, 12(2),* 182–189.

Waikato District Health Board. (2006). *Guidelines: Tikanga recommended best practice.* Waikato: Waikato District Health Board. Retrieved April 9, 2008, from www.waikatodhb.govt.nz.

Yamaguchi, S. (2004). Nursing culture of an operating room. *Nursing and Health Sciences, 6,* 261–269.

FURTHER READING

Andre, S., Sevdalis, N., Healey, A., Darzi, S. A., Vincent, C. (2005). Teamwork in the operating theatre: cohesion or confusion? *Journal of Evaluation in Clinical Practice, 12(2),* 182–189.

Lingard, L., Reznick, R., DeVito, I., Esprin, S. (2002). Forming professional identities on the health care team: discursive constructions of the 'other' in the operating room. *Medical Education, 36,* 728–734.

McGrath, P., Howela, H., McGrath, Z. (2006). Nursing advocacy in an Australian multidisciplinary context: finding a medico-centrism. *Scandinavian Journal of Caring Sciences, 20,* 394–403.

Riley, R., & Manias, E. (2002). Foucault could have been an operating room nurse. *Journal of Advanced Nursing, 39(4),* 316–324.

Sevdalis, N., Healey, A., Vincent, C. (2007). Distracting communications in the operating theatre. *Journal of Evaluation in Clinical Practice, 13,* 390–395.

Sutherland-Fraser, S. (2006). It's time to examine alternatives to the traditional staffing mix and role allocation in the perioperative environment. *ACORN Journal, 19(4),* 22–23.

CHAPTER 2

Preadmission and preoperative patient care

Leigh K Anderson and Prudence V M Hames

LEARNING OBJECTIVES

After reading this chapter, you should be able to:

- explore the purpose of preoperative assessment
- describe the components of preoperative assessment
- examine the physical, psychological and educational preparation of the surgical patient
- review the activities completed during preoperative admission.

KEY TERMS

patient teaching

preadmission

preoperative assessment

preoperative care

preoperative preparation

preoperative screening

INTRODUCTION

Preoperative care encompasses the unique holistic physical, psychological, emotional and spiritual preparation of patients prior to their surgery. Adequate **preoperative preparation** can lead to optimal outcomes for the surgical patient. Preoperative care is a complex and dynamic field; however, much of the literature and clinical guidelines lacks evidence. This leaves room for debate on what constitutes optimal patient care (Solca, 2006). The perioperative nurse plays a critical role with patient assessment, preparation, management and evaluation of care.

This chapter explores the preadmission and preoperative care of the perioperative patient. Specifically, elements of preoperative assessment are identified and discussed. Preoperative care of the patient, once in a health care organisation, starts in the preoperative ward and continues into the preoperative holding area. The increasing role of the preadmission clinic is presented, along with the development of nurse-led clinics. The importance of patient education is highlighted. Preoperative tests and examinations and the effects of preoperative smoking are discussed. Discussion includes the importance of the preoperative check for the surgical patient.

PREADMISSION

The **preadmission** stage of a patient's surgical journey is critical in the preparation of the patient for surgery. The requirement to increase the number of patients receiving surgery (maximising theatre utilisation) and reduce waiting lists and waiting times has determined the need for patients to be fully prepared, thus minimising the risk of cancellations or delays (Beck, 2007). The need for increased efficiency has been driven largely by government and policy, such as the New Zealand Health Strategy (Hodgson, 2006) and those developed by the Australian Department of Health and Ageing (2007). The effectiveness of preadmission clinics is demonstrated in an associated reduction in cancellation of cases, shortened length of hospital stay related to increased patient well-being and improved patient satisfaction (Correll et al., 2006; Ferschl et al., 2005; Halaszynski et al., 2004). The preassessment clinic plays an important role in minimising cancellations by having the patient appropriately assessed, investigated and prepared for the surgery (Rai & Pandit, 2003).

Preoperative assessment

Preoperative assessment is the clinical investigation that precedes anaesthesia for surgical or non-surgical procedures and which provides data for the selection of an appropriate anaesthetic strategy (van Klei et al., 2004). Preoperative assessment may be required for surgery that takes place in a variety of practice settings, including, hospitals, clinics, doctors' rooms and dentists' rooms, both in the public and private settings.

Traditionally, patients were visited on the wards by the anaesthetist the day before surgery. However, if significant comorbidities were present, this could result in cancellation of surgery. A late cancellation is distressing for the patient and results in under-utilisation of the operating room as it may not be possible to schedule another patient (Van Klei et al., 2002). The provision of preoperative/preadmission clinics has enabled an opportunity to manage comorbidities, provide quality safe perioperative care and reduce cancellations. Box 2-1 outlines the objectives of preoperative assessment.

The principles of assessment vary and include ensuring that the consultation occurs at an appropriate time and place. The environment should provide adequate privacy for the patient, such as a single-bed consulting room, and the consultation should occur without interruption. Ideally, the consultation should occur several weeks before surgery. This

UHB TRUST LIBRARY QEHB

Box 2-1 Preoperative assessment objectives

- Reduction of fears and anxieties by giving a full explanation of the procedure and making sure that patients understand what is going to happen to them.
- Assessment of the patient's fitness for the impending anaesthesia and surgery, with appropriate interventions.
- Obtaining the patient's informed consent for the anaesthetic and surgical procedures.
- Assessment of whether the patient is suitable for day surgery or requires inpatient admission.
- Identification of specialist requirements (e.g. critical care beds).
- Providing preoperative and postoperative instructions.
- Establishing a point of contact.
- Providing an opportunity for health promotion and patient teaching.
- Assessment of patient needs post-discharge.

Oakley (2005)

---

is particularly important if there are significant comorbidities requiring management, special laboratory tests or procedures to be ordered, or planning/management of any anaesthetic concerns, and to allow time for patient education (Barnett, 2005; Garcia-Miguel et al., 2003). Each patient is unique and requires the opportunity to express concerns, ask questions and be supported in their decision-making, even if that means changing their minds as to the intended surgical procedure.

The Australian and New Zealand College of Anaesthetists acknowledges that it is not always possible to plan early consultation and assessment of patients, particularly in cases of emergency; however, it stresses that the consultation must not be modified except when the overall welfare of the patient is at risk (ANZCA, 2003). It also recommends that the assessment of patients prior to anaesthesia is the primary responsibility of the anaesthetist and, where practical, is to be conducted by the anaesthetist who is to perform the anaesthesia (ANZCA, 2003). This differs from Europe and the United States, where nurse anaesthetists or anaesthetic non-physician practitioners may also take part in the preoperative assessment and provide anaesthetic services to patients under the direct supervision of a consultant anaesthesiologist. Wilkinson (2007, p 168) describes the non-physician practitioner role requirement to:

> … assess the patients preoperatively, identify any co-morbidity that would render the patient unsuitable for care by an anaesthetic practitioner; form a plan for the anaesthetic in discussion with their supervisor; induce anaesthesia under supervision; maintain the anaesthetic and hand the patient over to recovery staff with a plan for their immediate postoperative care.

However, nurse-led clinics are developing and provide competent preoperative assessments of patients. A study by Kinley et al. (2003) concluded that preoperative assessments by qualified nurses were equal in quality to assessment by pre-registration medical residents. Further discussion on nurse-led clinics is given below.

A number of different health care professionals may be involved in the care and preparation of the patient prior to surgery; for example, preadmission nurse, anaesthetist, dietician, physiotherapist, pharmacist, social worker or occupational therapist. Assessment involves a two-way preadmission interview between the patient and health practitioner so that the patient is assessed physically, psychologically and socially for surgery (Walsgrove, 2006). The preadmission interview is scheduled once the patient returns a completed medical/health questionnaire, and provides the opportunity for information sharing and for education to occur.

The preadmission nurse plays a vital role in the assessment and preparation of the patient for surgery. Assessment by the preadmission nurse includes clarification of the medical/health questionnaire; taking a nursing history; recording of baseline observations; recording of height and weight and the patient's body mass index (BMI); ordering of preoperative diagnostic and other tests, such as spirometry and electrocardiography (ECG); review of the patient's current medication, including the use of herbal and complementary medicines; and referral to the anaesthetist or other consultant if required. Venepuncture accreditation for registered nurses allows the preadmission nurse to collect blood samples ordered for required testing.

Nurse-led clinics

Preadmission clinics may be staffed by nurses whose role includes patient **preoperative screening**. This may detect medical or physical conditions that may generate a referral to the surgeon or anaesthetist, as discussed above (Finegan et al., 2005). Within nurse-led clinics, policies and protocols provide guidance as to when referral may be made to others within the multidisciplinary health care team. Nurse-led clinics may prevent inappropriate admission of unfit patients and reduce late cancellations (Hilditch et al., 2003; Kinley et al., 2003).

The responsibilities and activities of the preadmission nurse may vary between different health care agencies. A major responsibility is to ensure that patients are available and prepared for their allocated surgery. This includes communicating with patients by telephone regarding preoperative diagnostic tests, organisation of the preoperative assessment consultation and detailed patient education so that the patient is prepared for the planned surgery. A study by van Klei et al. (2002) demonstrated that the preadmission nurse can undertake the patient's health assessment independently, provided the anaesthetist is available to perform additional assessment for patients who are categorised as requiring further assessment.

To be effective, this advanced role requires clinical nurse specialists to be educated to a Master's level, with skills and knowledge in anatomy, clinical assessment and decision-making (Ormrod & Casey, 2004). Some authors argue that the role is not one of a nurse specialist but rather that of an advanced Nurse Practitioner. The Nurse Practitioner has similar educational qualifications; however, the scope of practice in a speciality field is generally broader (Barnett, 2005). Nurse Practitioners must be able to collect, identify and interpret important information. They provide preoperative information and education, order and review diagnostic test results, perform physical examinations and take medical histories independently, and work collaboratively with other health care providers, such as anaesthetists (Barnett, 2005).

Even though most preoperative assessments are carried out in clinics, some aspects are completed over the telephone. Trials in Britain have demonstrated success in telephone assessment of patients, with the result that more patients can be assessed in a timely manner (Digner, 2007). Strict selection criteria are required to identify patients who are suitable to be assessed via telephone. Suggested criteria include:

- diastolic blood pressure <95 mmHg
- body mass index <35
- aged over 16 and under 60 years
- no obvious medical condition.

The format, policy and protocol of the telephone assessment should be the same as for face-to-face assessment. Consent must also be obtained for telephone assessment, and identification of the correct patient confirmed using unique patient identifiers, such as mother's maiden name or date of birth.

The types of questions asked during consultation may vary and Table 2-1 provides some examples of preoperative questions. Following consultation, a written summary is included in the patient's health record.

The American Society of Anesthesiologists' (ASA) physical status classification system is commonly used to assist in preoperative assessment of patients (Table 2-2). Devised in the 1960s, the system was meant to assess the degree of sickness or the physical state of a patient prior to selecting the anaesthetic or prior to performing surgery. It is not a tool to be used to determine or measure operative risk (ASA, 2002).

Table 2-1 Preoperative assessment questions

Preoperative assessment questions	Rationale
History	
1. Have you ever had an anaesthetic? 2. Were there any problems related to the anaesthetic?	Knowledge of problems with a previous anaesthetic enables the anaesthetist to prepare for such problems.
3. Have you or any member of your family had any problems with an anaesthetic?	This may be indicative that the patient may have the same problem.
4. Have you had any previous surgery?	Provides a baseline for education.
5. Do you ever get any chest pain or shortness of breath?	May require the patient to undergo diagnostic tests prior to surgery.
6. Have you have taken illicit drugs? If yes, how recently? 7. What is your alcohol intake?	Taking of illicit drugs and/or excessive alcohol intake may necessitate increased amounts of anaesthetic agents.
8. Do you smoke? If so how much, how often?	Smoking effects on pulmonary function.
9. Do you have any allergies to any medications? 10. Are you on any regular medicines?	Will affect choice of medications given.
11. Do you take any non-prescription medications? If so, what are they? 12. Are you taking any complementary therapies?	Certain medications, including herbal and complementary therapies, may have consequences for the anaesthetic or surgical procedure.
13. Do you have any medical problems?	Certain comorbidities require specific preparation before surgery. Prior history may indicate potential medical problems or undiagnosed diseases.
Physical	
1. Do you have any dentures or loose teeth, caps or crowns?	Necessary knowledge for induction of anaesthesia and intubation.
2. What is your approximate weight? 3. What is your approximate height?	Provides data for body mass index (BMI) calculation for anaesthetic.

(contd)

Psychosocial	
1. Do you have any cultural beliefs that we should be particularly aware of, such as Jehovah's witness?	Ensures cultural safety is observed.
2. Do you have any questions or would you like me to discuss any aspect of the anaesthetic?	Alleviates/minimises anxieties and fears.
3. Is there anything else your surgeon or anaesthetist should know?	Provides opportunity to identify outstanding issues or concerns.

Adapted from Solca (2006)

Table 2-2 ASA physical status classification system		
ASA category	**Preoperative health status**	**Comments/examples**
ASA 1	A normal healthy patient	Patient able to walk up one flight of stairs without distress. Little or no anxiety. Little or no risk.
ASA 2	A patient with mild disease	Patient able to walk up one flight of stairs but will need to stop after completion of exercise due to distress. History of well-controlled disease states, including non-insulin-dependent diabetes, pre-hypertension, epilepsy, asthma or thyroid conditions
ASA 3	A patient with severe systemic disease	Patients able to walk up one flight of stairs but will have to stop en route because of distress. History of angina pectoris, myocardial infarction (MI), cerebrovascular accident (CVA), heart failure (HF) over 6 months ago.
ASA 4	A patient with severe systemic disease that is a constant threat to life	Patient unable to walk up one flight of stairs. History of unstable angina pectoris, MI, CVA, HF within last 6 months.
ASA 5	A moribund patient who is not expected to survive without the operation	Generally, hospitalised, terminally ill patients.
ASA 6	A declared brain dead patient whose organs are being removed for donor purposes	–

American Society of Anesthesiologists (2007)

While preoperative assessment cannot claim to be the answer to all of the potential problems faced by elective surgical patients, it is vital that health care professionals involved in patient care prepare and coordinate their efforts to ensure the best possible outcome for the patient. Box 2-2 highlights the importance of assessment before admission for surgery.

Box 2-2 Preadmission care of the patient

A systematic review identified two major findings that are useful in suggesting practices to improve the preadmission process for both patients and the day surgery unit. These were the use of preoperative telephone screening or questionnaires, and a preadmission appointment a few days prior to admission. Both of these measures were used to prepare patients for their upcoming operation, whether adults or children, and to create an opportunity for nurses to screen those in whom surgery should be postponed.

Pearson et al. (2004)

Preoperative investigations

In the past, all patients received standard testing regardless of their physical condition. Tests that were directly, indirectly or even remotely related to the planned surgery were ordered. While the tests proved useful as baseline values for those caring postoperatively for the patient, in the current era of cost containment, such testing is not financially practical (Halaszynski et al., 2004). Furthermore, current evidence supports the view that change in patient management rarely occurs as a result of routine testing (Bryson et al., 2006; Johnson & Mortimer, 2002).

Evidence-based guidelines have been developed which rationalise the use of preoperative tests, leading to a reduction of tests ordered with no compromise to patient safety occurring, and the added benefit of reducing costs to both the patient and the health care system (Ferrando et al., 2005; Finegan et al., 2005; Johnson & Mortimer, 2002). Even in patients who are older than 70 years, routine preoperative testing has been shown to be of little benefit (Bryson et al., 2006). Although some authors suggest that routine testing can be completely eliminated, others propose that testing should be based on the patient's medical condition (Yaun et al., 2005). Each health care institution should develop policies and procedures regarding preoperative assessment and screening.

Medical history

A complete medical history of the individual is required. This includes details of past surgical history, family medical history and current intake of medication. Social history must also be examined, noting alcohol intake, smoking habits, use of illicit drugs and use of non-prescription medications and/or complementary medications. Also noted are the support systems available to the patient following surgery, such as family, church or other community groups (van Klei et al., 2004).

Chest X-rays

The benefit of chest X-ray examinations as part of the preoperative examination is unproven; even when abnormalities are detected the information is not necessarily useful. Furthermore, routine chest X-rays are ineffective in detecting asymptomatic tuberculosis or cancer. Therefore, a preoperative chest X-ray is not recommended in asymptomatic patients, regardless of age (Finegan et al., 2005; Joo et al., 2005).

Electrocardiography

The ordering of a routine 12-lead ECG has been common practice for all adult patients before an operation involving regional or general anaesthesia but there is growing consensus that it is of little benefit and only needed for a subset of patients with cardiac signs and older patients (Ho, 2007). Commonly, an ECG is not routinely needed for asymptomatic males younger than 45 years and females younger than 50 years, and should be based on the clinical needs of the patient. Abnormalities on preoperative ECGs in older patients are common but are of limited value in predicting postoperative cardiac complications (Lui et al., 2002).

Obtaining preoperative ECGs based on an age cut-off alone may not be indicated because ECG abnormalities in older people are prevalent but non-specific and less useful than the presence and severity of comorbidities in predicting postoperative cardiac complications. However, in the elderly, silent myocardial infarction is not uncommon and the availability of a baseline ECG is helpful in the subsequent diagnosis and management of any suspected cardiac event (Finegan et al., 2005; Yuan et al., 2005).

Blood investigations

Traditionally, routine blood tests prior to surgery have been carried out for all patients. This has included a full blood count (FBC), urea, electrolytes and glucose. This practice was expensive for individuals and health care institutions, and offered little advantage to the patient. A study by Johnson and Mortimer (2002) found that, commonly, results were not in the patient's notes on arrival at the operating room and, when abnormalities were detected, there was little change in patient management.

To ensure appropriate ordering of tests, it is recommended that a detailed history and physical examination is performed. For major surgery, a blood group test and screen will also be required to ensure the availability of blood should a transfusion be required. Informed consent is required from patients for authorisation of a blood transfusion prior to a surgical procedure. Documentation of such is recorded in the patient's health record and/or on the surgical Consent/Agreement to Treatment form. Table 2-3 lists the tests recommended by the National Institute for Clinical Excellence.

Table 2-3 Recommended preoperative screening for ASA grade 1 adults for grade 2 surgeries				
Test	Age (years)			
	16–<40	40–<60	60–<80	>80
Chest X-ray	Not recommended	Not recommended	Not recommended	Not recommended
ECG	Not recommended	Consider	Consider	Recommended
Full blood count	Not recommended	Consider	Recommended	Recommended
Haemostasis	Not recommended	Not recommended	Not recommended	Not recommended
Renal function	Not recommended	Not recommended	Consider	Consider
Random glucose	Not recommended	Consider	Consider	Consider
Urine analysis	Consider	Consider	Consider	Consider

National Institute for Clinical Excellence (2003)

Smoking

An assessment of patient smoking habits is ascertained well before surgery and is undertaken by the primary person making the surgical referral. Smoking is a risk factor for postoperative wound dehiscence, wound infections and delayed healing (Warner, 2005b). Smoking also results in a higher incidence of perioperative respiratory and cardiovascular complications compared to non-smoking (Kuri et al., 2005; Warner, 2005a). The optimum length of time a smoker should cease smoking prior to surgery remains unclear; times range from 12 hours to several weeks, with all such cessation showing improvement in, for example, rates of postoperative wound healing (Kuri et al., 2005; Warner 2005a, 2005b). However, there is no absolute evidence that cessation of smoking before surgery reduces complications (Box 2-3).

Box 2-3 Interventions for preoperative smoking cessation

The results of a systematic review showed that preoperative smoking interventions are effective for changing smoking behaviour perioperatively. Direct evidence that reducing or stopping smoking reduces the risk of complications is based on two small trials with differing results. The impact on complications may depend on how long before surgery the smoking behaviour is changed, whether smoking is reduced or stopped completely, and the type of surgery.

Moller & Villebro (2005)

Opportunity may be taken by the preoperative health professional to encourage total smoking cessation. For the patient about to undergo surgery, health care professionals need to stress the importance of smoking cessation and provide an explanation of the possible consequences of not stopping smoking. Box 2-4 provides examples of the type of educational information that may be provided to patients preoperatively by health care professionals.

The governments of both New Zealand and Australia have produced strategies and reviews to reduce overall smoking in the general population (Australian Ministerial Council on Drug Strategy, 2004; NZ Ministry of Health, 2004; Wilson, 2007). Options for patients coming into the hospital environment may include nicotine gum, lozenges or patches, which have been found to be effective in helping smokers quit the habit (Shiffman, 2007; Shiffman et al., 2002). All health care organisations are now smoke-free. To assist the patient, health professionals may check their local organisation's policy regarding the availability of nicotine patches, free of charge to patients who normally smoke, during hospitalisation. Advice available to the patient may take the form of written information or speaking with nurses who specialise in smoking cessation.

Other perioperative considerations

It is necessary to check if the patient has any special needs during the perioperative period (e.g. an interpreter or presence of a carer or significant other). Supporting the patient's unique needs protects their dignity and allows consumers of health care to maintain control over what is happening to them.

PATIENT EDUCATION AND INFORMATION

Preoperative education supports patients by giving a clear and consistent message of the impending surgery from all members of the multidisciplinary health team. Patient education allows informed decisions to be made, with time to reflect on information already given, and provides opportunities to ask questions. Providing preoperative information also helps decrease postoperative pain, reduce length of stay, decease anxiety and increase patient satisfaction (Garretson, 2004).

Fear of the unknown and anxiety are common feelings for many patients and these fears may be eliminated, or at least minimised, with patient education and teaching. Familiarisation with the hospital environment, equipment, procedures, anaesthesia, surgical routine and postoperative expectations provide a locus of control for the patient. This reduces vulnerability, increases confidence and provides an improved overall experience and better outcomes. Patient involvement may also mean ensuring that

---

Box 2-4 Preoperative information that may be provided to patients who smoke

Smoking cessation for surgery

Why quit for surgery?

- Deceases your chances of problems during surgery
- Helps you heal faster after surgery
- Helps prevent complications after surgery, such as pneumonia, heart trouble and wound infection

What should you do?

- Set a quit date right now
- Stop smoking at least 12 hours prior to surgery
- Use nicotine patches instead of smoking on the morning of surgery
- Stay smoke-free for at least a week following surgery

Want to stay smoke-free for life?

It is tough to quit but surgery is a great time to try because:

- you cannot smoke in the surgical facility
- most people are free of cravings right after surgery
- you may be more motivated to change your lifestyle

What are the benefits of a smoke-free life?

- Reduced risk of dying early
- Reduced risk of developing lung cancer
- Reduced risk of coronary heart disease and stroke
- Reduce risk of dying from chronic bronchitis and emphysema
- Improvement in respiratory symptoms, such as cough and shortness of breath
- Reduced risk of other cancers related to smoking
- Reduced risk of complications in pregnancy and childbirth
- Improvement in some mental health symptoms
- Fewer sick days off work
- Save money!

How can you get help?

- Ask us—we can help!
- Call Quit line toll free New Zealand 0800 778 778 or www.quit.org.nz
- Call Quit line Australia 131 848 or www.quitnow.info.au

Warner (2005a)

---

caregivers and family are briefed on what to expect. A systematic review of knowledge retention from preoperative patient information identified that preadmission teaching is more effective compared to post-admission teaching and knowledge retention (Joanna Briggs Institute, 2000). Group teaching is just as effective as individual teaching and has the added advantage that it is more efficient for health care workers. However, Johansson et al. (2005) argue that a lack of systematic evidence exists about the quality and effectiveness of patient education.

Patient teaching can take several forms, for example, from informal sitting down and conversing with a patient at admission to the ward/perioperative unit, to more formalised, structured teaching/information sessions. Nursing staff play a vital role in the provision of education to the patient. Follow-up communication may be by telephone to ensure that the patient understands all of the preparation requirements, such as fasting or specific surgical preparations.

It is important that the education/information is provided at an appropriate health literacy level for the patient. In other words, it is important to speak clearly without the use of medical jargon, while using active listening skills. A variety of media and tools may be used to provide patient information, including written pamphlets (provided in a variety of languages), videos and practical sessions with equipment, talks, visits and website instruction. A systematic review published by The Joanna Briggs Institute (2000) suggested that the use of pamphlets was particularly beneficial in terms of knowledge of the condition and surgical procedure, exercise or skills performance and the time taken to learn the exercises or skills. Coupled with verbal information provided prior to admission, pamphlets are vital tools in the resources available to empower patients. Notwithstanding the importance of written material, there are disadvantages—they are costly to print, cumbersome to file and store, and hard to keep up to date. Some organisations have moved to developing electronic patient education materials, allowing staff to download and print this or e-mail it to patients (Agre, 2007). Table 2-4 summarises a patient and family teaching guide for preoperative preparation.

Preoperative visiting

Commonly, patients come into hospitals on the day of surgery, which reduces opportunities for perioperative staff to spend time with patients to ensure that their concerns or issues are addressed. Patient notes and files are generally unavailable until the patient arrives at the operating suite. One of the main advantages of preoperative visiting is the opportunity it provides to plan individual patient care. A preoperative visit allows information to be gained regarding the patient's physical or mental status, for example, obese patients may require extra or different types of equipment, such as used for positioning, or instruments for their surgery. With preoperative visiting, a collaborative strategy and management of care can be achieved with members of the health care team.

In emergency situations, preoperative visiting becomes a low priority; however, a visit to the emergency department may provide essential information, such as the extent of the injuries, thus allowing planning time for case requirements and estimated time of arrival to the operating room (Wicker & O'Neill, 2006). Management of the care of a trauma patient is vital in order to provide the most efficient and effective treatment to allow maximum chances of outcome and survival.

The concept of preoperative visiting has been considered an important aspect of the perioperative nurse's role and a way of articulating the patient-centred focus. Although the importance of preoperative visiting is recognised, it is rarely, if ever, undertaken. Advancing technology, changes in the health care system, changing models of care and the predominance of 'day of surgery' admission have negated the opportunity for the perioperative nurse to undertake a preoperative visit (Richardson-Tench, 2002).

PREOPERATIVE SURGICAL SITE PREPARATION

Surgical site infection (SSI) is a serious complication of surgery and can be the cause of long illness and, less frequently, death among surgical patients. Preventing a postoperative SSI through preoperative skin preparation has a long history. Bathing with an antiseptic solution and hair removal are two procedures currently undertaken preoperatively to reduce or prevent an SSI.

Table 2-4 Patient and family teaching guide for preoperative preparation

Sensory information

- Holding area is often noisy.
- Drugs and cleaning solutions may be smelled.
- Operating room can be cold; warm blankets are available.
- Talking may be heard in the operating room but will be distorted because of masks. Questions should be asked if something is not understood.
- Operating room bed will be narrow.
- Lights in the operating room can be very bright.
- Machines (ticking and pinging noises) may be heard when awake. Their purpose is to monitor and ensure safety.

Procedural information

- What to bring and what type of clothing to wear to the day surgery centre.
- Any changes in time of surgery.
- Fluid and food restrictions.
- Physical preparation required (e.g. bowel or skin preparation).
- Purpose of frequent vital signs assessment.
- Pain control and other comfort measures.
- Why turning, coughing and deep breathing postoperatively are important; practice sessions need to be done preoperatively.
- Insertion of intravenous lines.
- Procedures for anaesthesia administration.

Process information

Information about general flow of surgery
- Admission area.
- Preoperative holding area, operating room and recovery area.
- Families can usually stay in holding area until surgery.
- Families may be able to enter recovery area as soon as patient is awake.
- Identification of any technology that may be present on awakening, such as monitors and central lines.

Where families wait during surgery
- Patient and family members need to be encouraged to verbalise concerns.
- Operating room staff will notify family when surgery is completed.
- Surgeon will usually talk with family following surgery.

Brown & Edwards (2008, p 386)

Preoperative bathing

Preoperative bathing has been practised since the 19th century for the purpose of removing debris and residues and reducing the flora around the surgical site (Seal & Paul-Cheadle, 2004; Webster & Osborne, 2007). The provision of an antiseptic solution to patients for preoperative bathing is widely practised in the belief that it reduces the incidence of SSI. The Centers for Disease Control and Prevention (CDC) recommends that patients shower or bathe with an antiseptic agent the night before the operative day, as a nine-fold reduction in skin microbial colony counts has been shown as a result (Seal & Paul-Cheadle, 2004). However, a systematic review conducted by Webster and Osborne (2007) found that six trials, including over 10,000 patients, did not show clear evidence of benefit for the use of chlorhexidine solution over other wash products in the prevention of SSI.

Preoperative hair removal

The removal of hair from the intended surgical wound site has been accepted practice, with different hair-removal methods recommended throughout the world. The CDC guidelines strongly recommend that hair should not be removed preoperatively unless it obscures the incision site. If this is the case, clipping is recommended as shaving causes micro-abrasions, which provides a portal of entry for microorganisms. Furthermore, the CDC recommends that preoperative hair removal takes place as close as reasonable to the time of surgery, preferably less than 2 hours prior to surgery to lessen the opportunity for SSI (CDC, 1999). These guidelines have not been updated.

A systematic review conducted by Kjønniksen et al. (2002) found that there was no strong evidence to advocate against hair removal. However, there was strong evidence to recommend that when hair removal is considered necessary, shaving should not be performed. Instead, a depilatory cream or electric clipping, preferably immediately before surgery, should be used. The findings of Kjønniksen et al. (2002) are supported by the findings of the systematic review by Tanner et al. (2006), who suggest that there is insufficient evidence to state whether removing hair affects SSI rates or when is the best time to remove hair. However, if it is necessary to remove hair, then either clipping or depilatory creams result in fewer SSIs than shaving using a razor. Debate continues regarding hair removal from the intended surgical site.

PREOPERATIVE CARE IN THE OPERATING SUITE

Hospital policy designates the exact procedure that should be followed when admitting the patient to the holding area and the operating suite. A general routine includes initial greeting, extension of human contact and warmth, and proper identification. Accompanying documentation, such as the patient's health record and diagnostic results (e.g. blood and urine testing, chest X-ray and ECG results) are reviewed. Box 2-5 presents the requirements for admission to the operating suite. Detailed admission procedures are discussed below.

Box 2-5 Requirements for preoperative admission

- Patient is to be dressed in hospital-supplied theatre gown with all other clothing, including undergarments, removed.
- The correct patient identification bracelet to be worn.
- All jewellery to be removed or taped to prevent loss.
- Denture container and reading glasses case if required.
- Patient health record, including signed Agreement to Treatment form, observations chart, drug chart and completed preoperative checklist.

Duncan (2008)

Admission to the preoperative holding room

The preoperative holding area is an area specifically allocated for receiving patients. Characteristically, the environment is quiet, provides privacy and is staffed by an appropriately qualified registered nurse (RN) with skills in patient assessment, decision-making and an understanding of perioperative process and procedure. Some preoperative areas may provide calm, quiet music to minimise patient anxiety. A reassessment of the patient should take place, with time allowed for last-minute questions. A warm blanket, pillow or position adjustment is provided if the patient is uncomfortable (Duncan, 2008).

It is the responsibility of the RN, enrolled nurse (EN) or Registered Anaesthetic Technician (AT) (in New Zealand) to 'check in' patients prior to surgical procedures. The perioperative nurse or AT will introduce themselves to the patient and receive the handover from the ward nurse, systematically working through the preoperative checklist to ensure that the patient is ready for surgery. Figure 2-1 shows a patient being checked into an operating suite.

Figures 2-2 and 2-3 show examples of a preoperative checklist. While these differ between hospitals, their aim is the same: to ensure patient safety and timely care.

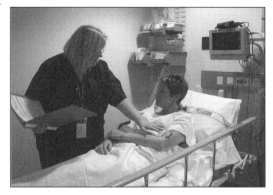

Figure 2-1 A perioperative nurse checking a patient into an operating suite.

Patient identification

The preoperative nurse is required to ensure the correct identity of the patient. The identification process includes asking patients to state their name, their surgeon's name, and the operative procedure and location. This information is checked against the patient health record plus their patient identification bracelet/s. Preoperative nurses need to ensure that they are admitting the:

- correct patient
- for the correct surgery
- correctly prepared
- at the correct time (ACORN, 2006; Duncan, 2008).

Consent

Informed consent is the process whereby a patient is fully informed regarding their surgery. Patients require balanced information about the procedure, risks involved and alternatives to having surgery. The need for informed consent springs from the legal and ethical right of patients to have total control over what happens to their body (Staunton & Chiarella, 2008) and from the ethical duty of doctors to involve patients in their own health care (Association for Perioperative Practice, 2007; Health and Disability Commissioner, 2007; PNCNZNO, 2005). Ideally, surgical and anaesthetic consent is signed prior to the patient entering the operating suite. It is undesirable for consent to treatment to be gained in the preoperative area. Patient consent is not required in an emergency. Any discrepancies regarding the Consent/Agreement to Treatment form must be queried with the surgeon or anaesthetist prior to transfer to the operating room.

The Consent/Agreement to Treatment form is written in plain English. Interpreter services must be available for patients whose first language is other than English. Only recognisable and agreed upon abbreviations, identified by local policy, may be used to describe procedures. The side of the operation must be written in full, for example, 'right' must not be abbreviated to 'R' (Queensland Health, 2005). This form is signed by the surgeon, anaesthetist and patient or legal representative. The concept of informed consent is discussed further in Chapter 11.

OPERATIVE CHECKLIST

The ALFRED

Pre Procedure Ward

Post Procedure Ward

U.R.

Surname

Given Names

Please circle Yes or No

WARD NURSING STAFF			HOLDING ROOM NURSE			PACU STAFF		
1. PATIENT IDENTIFICATION			**Time into H.R.**			Correct patient identification label in place		
Patient identification label checked against patient record	Yes	No		Yes	No		Yes	No
2. CONSENT FOR SURGERY	Yes	No		Yes	No			
3. ALLERGIES/SENSITIVITIES	Yes	No		Yes	No		Yes	No
IF YES – State Details								
4. PATIENT PREPARATION				Checked	N/A			
Fasted from _____ hours								
Morning Medication Administered	Yes No N/A			Yes	No			
State Details								
Premedication ordered and given	Yes	No		Yes	No			
Teeth – natural, caps, crown	(circle)							
LOOSE TEETH – State Details								
Dentures – sent to OR	Yes	No	Denture in situ Yes		No	Denture in situ Yes		No
IF YES – State Details eg full, upper, lower, partial			If no state location			State details		
Hearing Aid/Spectacles (circle)	Yes	No						
IF YES – sent to OR	Yes	No		Yes	No		Yes	No
Prosthesis	Yes	No						
IF YES – State Details								
Valuables/Jewellery – sent to OR	Yes	No	Valuables/Jewellery Present Yes		No	Valuables/Jewellery Present Yes		No
IF YES – State Details			If yes state details			If yes state details		
Patient belongings – sent to OR	Yes	No	Stored in PACU Yes		No	Patient belongings present		
IF YES – State Details							Yes	No
On ward	Yes	No						
IF YES – State Details								
Sent to other ward	Yes	No						
IF YES – State Location								
5. CHARTS								
Patient Labels	Yes	No		Yes	No		Yes	No
Perianaesthesia Record MR P32	Yes	No		Yes	No		Yes	No
Patient History	Yes	No		Yes	No		Yes	No
Medication Record MR M50	Yes	No		Yes	No		Yes	No
Intravenous Orders MR M60	Yes	No		Yes	No		Yes	No
Fluid Balance Chart MR R40	Yes	No		Yes	No		Yes	No
Diabetic Chart MR M45	Yes	No		Yes	No		Yes	No
Observation Charts	Yes	No		Yes	No		Yes	No
Day Surgery Procedure S40-L	Yes	No		Yes	No		Yes	No
Clinical Pathway Document	Yes	No		Yes	No		Yes	No
Periop Nursing Care Record MR P33							Yes	No
6. RADIOLOGICAL FILMS								
X-Rays	Yes	No		Yes	No		Yes	No
CT/MRI Scan	Yes	No		Yes	No		Yes	No
Ultrasound	Yes	No		Yes	No		Yes	No
Nuclear Medicine	Yes	No		Yes	No		Yes	No
Private X-Rays	Yes	No		Yes	No		Yes	No
RN/EN Signature			RN/EN Signature			RN/EN Signature		
Date/Time			Date/Time			Date/Time		

OPERATIVE CHECKLIST

MR P-31

Figure 2-2 Australian preoperative checklist (The Alfred Hospital, Melbourne).

AUCKLAND DISTRICT HEALTH BOARD
Te Toku Tumai

Preoperative Checklist

SURNAME: _____ NHI: _____

FIRST NAMES: _____

DATE OF BIRTH: ___ / ___ / ___ SEX: _____

Please attach patient label here

PREOPERATIVE ASSESSMENT	
First Language	English / Maori / Other:
Interpreter	Provided / Not required / Not available
Psychological	Orientated / Disorientated to Place and Time:
Impairment	Vision / Hearing / Speech / Mobility (details)
Isolation	Nursed in Isolation (details)
Diabetes	Blood Sugar Level – @

WD   OR
✓ - Yes   X - No   n/a - not applicable

PLEASE FILL IN RELEVANT SECTIONS

		PATIENT PREPARATION	
		Name Verbally Identified	
		Identification Band correct according to Front Sheet	
		Operation Consent Form signed	
		Anaesthetic Consent Form signed	
		Operation site marked	☐ Hair Clipping checked
		Patient/Family Requests Return of Body Parts/Tissue	☐ **Release Form signed**
		Last ate (time)	
		Last drank (time)	
		Metalware / Implants:	
		Urine voided (time)	
		Urinary catheter in situ	
		Bowel preparation completed	
		Anti-embolism Stockings	

		MEDICATION
		Premedication given (details)
		Allergies (details)
		Medic Alert Bracelet worn (details)
		Medication due in the next 4 hours
		Medication with patient (state)

		LABORATORY
		ECG Present
		Haematology Results
		Biochemistry Results
		Blood – Group and Screen or Cross Match:

		DOCUMENTATION
		X-Rays with patient
		Old Notes: with patient / on CRIS
		Additional Items: Labels, Fluid Balance Chart, Medication Record

		PATIENT CARE	
	Teeth	Own or Dentures T / B : Partial Plate / Caps / Loose:	
	Skin Integrity	Intact / Broken / Bruised (details)	
	Jewellery	Rings / Earrings / Body Piercing – removed / taped	
	Extra	Hair pins / Nail polish / Make up – removed / Toy	
	Vision	Glasses with patient / Contact lenses removed	

ADDITIONAL INFORMATION

☐ Escort Home   ☐ Overnight support   ☐ Parent/Guardian/Caregiver   ☐ LMP/Pregnancy

	WARD NURSE SIGNATURE	PREOPERATIVE STAFF SIGNATURE	INTRAOPERATIVE STAFF SIGNATURE
Name			
Signature			
Designation			
Date / Time			

PREOPERATIVE CHECKLIST

CR4048

PAGE 1
03/06

Figure 2-3 New Zealand preoperative checklist (Auckland District Health Board).

Allergies and sensitivities

Any allergies or sensitivities that a patient reveals require listing, with the type of reaction noted on the preoperative check-in sheet. This should include non-drug as well as drug reactions/sensitivities. All care is taken during the perioperative continuum to avoid contact with or administration of these allergens. It is common practice for patients to wear an identifying bracelet to highlight any such conditions. The patient with a history of any allergic responsiveness has a greater potential for demonstrating hypersensitivity to drugs administered during anaesthesia (Naismith, 2008). Previous unfavourable reactions to anaesthesia, blood transfusions, latex, iodine and tapes are noted.

Latex allergy

The incidence of latex allergy has increased significantly as the use of rubber gloves in health care settings has increased. Airborne latex particles that adhere to the cornstarch used to powder gloves are a major cause of respiratory symptoms and a source of sensitisation. Those at high risk of latex allergy include health care workers and those undergoing repeated surgeries, especially early in life. Symptoms of latex allergy may progress rapidly and unpredictably to anaphylaxis. All patients coming to the operating rooms are assessed with purposeful questions to identify the risk of latex allergy. If the patient is identified as being at risk, the following steps are required:

1. History plus potential or actual risk must be clearly documented in case notes.
2. Latex-sensitive patients are to be placed first on the operating list so that there is less risk of exposure to aerosolised latex particles.
3. Inform multidisciplinary team of sensitivity.
4. Before the patient enters the operating room, identify all known latex-containing items and isolate them to prevent accidental use. Use latex-free products only.
5. Make sure that there are clear signs on the doors of the operating room which state that the patient is latex-sensitive.
6. Maintain a latex-free environment throughout the perioperative journey and ensure a thorough handover of sensitivity to the PARU and ward (AORN, 2004; Davis, 2002).

Preoperative fasting

Preoperative fasting is an essential component of patient preparation. The rationale of fasting preoperatively is to empty the stomach and, therefore, reduce the risk of the stomach contents being regurgitated and then aspirated into the lungs (Baril & Portman, 2007), which is a rare but dangerous and potentially fatal complication of anaesthesia.

The Australian and New Zealand College of Anaesthetists (2006) recommendations for fasting times in adults who are having day surgery are that limited solid food may be taken up to 6 hours prior to anaesthesia and unsweetened clear fluids of not more than 200 mL in adults may be taken up to 2 hours prior to anaesthesia.

Body fluid depletion due to excessive fasting should be avoided. However, it is not unusual for the patient to be fasted from midnight before the surgery, regardless of whether they are first on the list or booked in for the afternoon. In a 'healthy' adult having elective (planned) surgery, this is unnecessary and can cause dehydration, headaches, irritability, electrolyte imbalance and malaise (Napoli, 2002). Unrestricted free fluids given 3 hours prior to surgery do not significantly increase gastric volume or affect the stomach pH. There is no indication that the volume of fluid permitted during the preoperative period results in a different outcomes from those participants that follow standard fasting regimens. Flexible and suitable fasting times in relation to scheduled operating times have been identified as improving patients' postoperative recovery (Brady et al., 2003).

On assessment, some people may be considered to be more likely to regurgitate while under anaesthetic, such as those who are pregnant, on opioids, are obese, or have a neurological deficit, a hiatus hernia or abdominal disorder (Brady et al., 2003). Also, patients who are acutely ill or have been involved in some unexpected event, such as a car accident, requiring them to have surgery, will be treated as though they have a full stomach. The assessment of risk to the patient is made by the anaesthetist, who needs to be fully informed by the preoperative nurse of exactly what the patient has recently had to eat and drink.

Box 2-6 Preoperative fasting

Findings from a recent systematic review indicated that, for local and general anaesthesia, a majority of anaesthetists would allow a patient undergoing general anaesthesia to consume clear liquids up to 2 hours before surgery, a light breakfast 6 hours before surgery and solid food up to 8 hours before surgery.

Richardson-Tench et al. (2005)

Surgical site marking

If the patient is to undergo surgery on a limb, or any other body part where the potential for operating on an incorrect site exists, such as a kidney, breast or digit, the patient may not proceed to the operating room unless the surgical site is clearly marked (Carney, 2006). The surgeon marks the site with a single-use indelible pen. Alternatively, a variety of commercially produced marking tools are available. The marking consists of an arrow close to, but not directly on, the site of the incision, which must remain visible to the operating room staff when the patient has been draped. If the details of the intended operative procedure differ between the operating list and Consent/Agreement to Treatment form, surgical site marking on the patient or patient opinion, the surgeon is informed prior to transfer to the operating room. When the Consent/Agreement to Treatment form has been completed prior to admission to hospital, the surgeon or delegated registrar is to mark the surgical site of the operation before the patient is moved to the operating room (ACORN, 2006; The Joint Commission, 2003).

Premedication and medications

Special consideration needs to be given to the patient who has been administered a premedication as they may need close observation and surveillance. Once the premedication has been administered on the ward, the Consent/Agreement to Treatment form cannot be amended. Also, if the patient is due other medications while in the operating suite, this needs to be communicated to the operating room staff to ensure timely administration. Regular medications taken orally may be continued unless documented by the anaesthetist (Association for Perioperative Practice, 2007).

An assessment of all current medications and their schedules is undertaken in the preoperative area. Special attention is given to antihypertensive, antianginal, antiarrhythmic, anticoagulant, anticonvulsant and insulin medications (Keglovitz & Kraft, 2002). An assessment of when these medications were last given and next due is prudent and included in the handover to operating room staff.

Diabetic patients who have been fasting preoperatively are monitored closely to ensure they maintain stable perioperative glucose control. The aims of management of diabetic patients are:

- stable perioperative glucose control
- prevention of ketosis and hypokalaemia
- promotion of wound healing and the reduction of infection
- ability to cope with postoperative nausea and vomiting (Auckland District Health Board, 2003).

Implants

All implants within the patient must be documented on the preoperative form and highlighted during handover. This ensures that the perioperative nurse is alerted to their presence when considering electrosurgical unit (ESU) pad placement. Some implants are large and will have scar tissue encircling them. Scar tissue is high in resistance and placing a return electrode (diathermy plate) over this area may result in a temperature increase underneath the pad (Valleylab, 2003). If the patient has an internal or external pacemaker, bipolar diathermy may need to be used, as monopolar diathermy interferes with the pacemaker signals, potentially causing it to enter an asynchronous mode or block the pacemaker entirely. If the patient has an internal cardiac defibrillator, the cardiologist may need to be consulted (Valleylab, 2004). Consideration is also required with patients with cochlear implants. Diathermy must never be used over the implant as this can cause tissue damage or permanent damage to the implant.

Return of body parts or hair

The patient must give informed consent prior to the surgical procedure for the removal of any body part/tissue. Although not commonplace in Australia, it is routine in New Zealand that in every case where hair, specimens or tissue are removed, patients are offered the opportunity to have their body part returned to them on completion of histology or other required testing. The wish to have their body part returned must be clearly documented on the preoperative check form and tissue return form (Fig 2-4). When patients choose to have their body part/tissue returned to them, staff will ensure that the body part/tissue is returned with written instructions if preserved in formalin. In the case of emergency surgery where no wishes have been noted, any body part/tissue removed is retained for subsequent return to the patient.

Jewellery and piercings

The presence of body piercing and jewellery requires attention from the perioperative nurse during the preoperative assessment period and ideally should be removed. This is to minimise the risk of infection, traumatic removal or loss of jewellery. If the jewellery remains in place, such as a wedding band, it needs to be taped to prevent its loss. All mouth, tongue, nasal and facial jewellery must be removed as they create a risk to patients undergoing anaesthetic and operative procedures. Other body jewellery is removed if it is within the operative field or is at risk of being traumatically removed, causing pressure damage, or if it provides an alternate pathway for ESU current. Genital piercing does not have to be removed if the surgery is elsewhere on the body (Association for Perioperative Practice, 2007). If there are any doubts, these should be discussed with the anaesthetist and surgeon. Removed jewellery is given to a family member or labelled and locked away in the ward or hospital safe.

Prevention of deep vein thrombosis

Deep vein thrombosis (DVT) is a clot within a vein, usually occurring in the leg. DVT can occur in surgical patients as a result of their inability to move and change position during anaesthesia compounded with reduced mobility during the postoperative period.

Body Part or Tissue Release

AUCKLAND
DISTRICT HEALTH BOARD
Te Toka Tumai

SURNAME: _____ NHI: _____

FIRST NAMES: _____

DATE OF BIRTH: _____ / _____ / _____ SEX: _____
Please attach patient label here

RETURN OF BODY PART OR TISSUE TO PATIENT or FAMILY

To be used in all cases where the patients/child's family has requested return of the body part/tissue.
Section on Agreement to Treatment form also to be ticked.

Return of Body Part or Tissue to Patient or Family

Describe body part / tissue to be returned _____
(staff to complete)

☐ **Yes** I wish to take my / my child's body part or tissue immediately following surgery

Comments _____

☐ **Yes** I wish to retain my / my child's body part or tissue following laboratory examination. I wish to have it stored until I collect it from Lab Plus laboratory on the Grafton site. I understand that the laboratory will dispose of the body part or tissue if I have not collected it within one month of the tissue being available. I understand that I will be contacted prior to disposal.

Patient / Guardian / Parent's Name: _____
(Please print)

Patient / Guardian / Parent's Signature: _____ Date: _____

Staff Member's Name: _____ Designation: _____
(Please print)

Staff Member's Signature: _____ Date: _____

Contact Number: _____ Ward / Unit: _____

Confirmation of Body Part / Tissue Return

Please complete this section when the body part / tissue is returned to the patient or family.

☐ I have received instructions on the proper transport and disposal of body parts.

Patient / Guardian / Parent's Name: _____
(Please print)

Patient / Guardian / Parent's Signature: _____ Date: _____

Staff Member's Name: _____ Designation: _____
(Please print)

Staff Member's Signature: _____ Date: _____

This form is to remain with the body part when it is transported to the laboratory. On completion of the form by the staff member and person receiving the body part / tissue, the form is then to be sent to be filed in the patient's Clinical Record. A copy may be given to the person receiving the body part / tissue.

PAGE 1
01/03

BODY PART OR TISSUE RELEASE

CR2547

Figure 2-4 Body parts or tissue release form (Auckland District Health Board).

A consequence of reduced mobility is the impaired physiological mechanisms for returning blood to the heart from the peripheral circulation. This can lead to stasis of blood in the deep leg veins and the potential development of a DVT. Fragment clots can dislodge and lead to pulmonary or cerebral emboli. These complications are associated with a high rate of morbidity and mortality (Byrne, 2002; Heizenroth, 2003).

To encourage venous return during the perioperative period, anti-embolism stockings are put on the patient preoperatively. This is discussed in detail in Chapter 4.

Preoperative patient warming

All patients have their temperature measured and recorded prior to admission to the operating suite to act as a baseline. Preoperative management of normothermia involves assessing the patient for risk factors of unplanned (inadvertent) perioperative hypothermia. Risk factors include a temperature lower than 36°C on admission, the very young and very old (Association for Perioperative Practice, 2007; Wagner et al., 2006). Inadvertent hypothermia may have detrimental effects on the patient undergoing surgery and has been associated with:

- poor clotting times
- increased risk of wound infection
- delayed healing
- decreased drug metabolism and clearance
- increased blood loss
- postoperative myocardial ischaemia
- impaired immune function
- delayed postanaesthesia recovery
- lengthened hospital stay.

It also interferes with the perception of comfort during patients' perioperative experience. A further discussion is detailed in Chapter 4.

CONCLUSION

This chapter has explored the preadmission and preoperative care of the patient through the perioperative continuum. Specifically, elements of preoperative assessment have been identified and discussed. Discussion has included activities undertaken in the preoperative period and the potential consequences for the patient.

The importance of the preoperative phase becomes crucial in the provision of effective and efficient patient care within the environment of shorter hospital stays, an increasing complexity of surgery and comorbidities, longer waiting lists and fiscal constraints.

CRITICAL THINKING EXERCISES

1. Preadmission anxiety

At the preadmission clinic Mrs Heath states that she is feeling anxious about the upcoming planned surgery and has a number of questions to ask.

- How can you assist Mrs Heath to ensure that she is fully informed of the anaesthetic and surgical procedures?
- How can you relieve her anxieties?

2. Improving patient understanding

Mr Chang has come into the preoperative area with the ward nurse. English is Mr Chang's second language and he is unable to answer your questions in a way that demonstrates he understands them.

- What steps do you take to assist Mr Chang to ensure that he is able to understand proceedings?

3. Patient consent

Mrs Andrews is a 73-year-old Māori woman who has been admitted to the preoperative area in readiness for a total hip joint replacement. You note that her Consent/Agreement to Treatment form does not indicate whether she wishes to have her tissue returned to her postoperatively.

- What steps do you take to ensure that Mrs Andrew's wishes are communicated to the surgical team?

4. Medication use

Mrs Diakomonalis, who is scheduled for a hysterectomy, reports using ginkgo biloba to improve her memory.

- Of what relevance is this information to Mrs Diakomonalis's surgery?
- What do you do with this information?

RESOURCES

Australian Department of Health and Ageing
  www.health.gov.au
National Institute for Health and Clinical Excellence
  www.nice.org.uk
New Zealand Health and Disability Commissioner
  www.hdc.org.nz
New Zealand Ministry of Health
  http://www.moh.govt.nz/moh.nsf/wpg_Index/Publications-Index

REFERENCES

ACORN. (2006). *ACORN standards for perioperative nursing including nursing roles, guidelines, position statements and competency standards. PS6. Ensuring correct patient, correct site, correct procedure* (pp. 1–3). Adelaide: Australian College of Operating Room Nurses.

Agre, P. (2007). Downloading patient-education materials. *American Journal of Nursing, 107(7)*, 66–69.

American Society of Anesthesiologists. (2002). Using the ASA physical status classification may be risky business. Retrieved November 5, 2007, from http://www.asahq.org/Newsletters/2002/9_02/vent_0902.htm.

American Society of Anesthesiologists. (2007). ASA physical status classification system. Retrieved November 5, 2007, from http://www.asahq.org/clinical/physicalstatus.htm.

ANZCA. (2003). *Professional documents of the Australian and New Zealand College of Anaesthetists. PS7. Recommendations on the pre-anaesthetic consultation.* Retrieved November 5, 2007, from http://www.anzca.edu.au/resources/professional-documents/professional-standards/ps7.

ANZCA. (2006). *Professional documents of the Australian and New Zealand College of Anaesthetists. PS15. Recommendations for the perioperative care of patients selected for day care surgery—2006.* Retrieved November 20, 2007, from http://www.anzca.edu.au/resources/professional-documents/professional-standards/ps15.html/?searchterm=fastingadults.

AORN. (2004). Latex guidelines. *AORN Journal, 79(3)*, 653–672.

Association for Perioperative Practice. (2007). Standards and recommendations for safe perioperative practice. Retrieved November 5, 2007, from www.afpp.org.uk.

Auckland District Health Board. (2003). Clinical guidelines: Diabetic patients—management of. Retrieved November 5, 2007, from http://www.adhb.govt.nz/_vti_bin/shtml.dll/search/search.htm.

Australian Department of Health and Ageing. (2007). National demonstration hospitals program (NDHP).

Retrieved November 6, 2007, from http://www.health.gov.au/internet.wcms/publishing.nsf/Content/health-hospitals-dem.

Australian Ministerial Council on Drug Strategy. (2004). National tobacco strategy, 2004–2009: the strategy. Canberra: AMCDS.

Baril, P., & Portman, H. (2007). Preoperative fasting: knowledge and perceptions. *AORN Journal, 86(4),* 609–617.

Barnett, J. S. (2005). An emerging role for nurse practitioners—preoperative assessment. *AORN Journal, 82(5),* 825–834.

Beck, A. (2007). Nurse-led preoperative assessment for elective surgical patients. *Nursing Standard, 21(51),* 35–38.

Brady, M., Kinn, S., Stuart, P. (2003). Preoperative fasting for adults to prevent perioperative complications. *Cochrane Database of Systematic Reviews, 4,* CD004423.

Brown, D., & Edwards, H. (Eds.). (2008). *Lewis's medical–surgical nursing: assessment and management of clinical problems* (2nd ed.) Sydney: Elsevier.

Bryson, G. L., Wyand, A., Bragg, P. R. (2006). Preoperative testing is inconsistent with published guidelines and rarely changes management. *Canadian Journal of Anesthesia, 53(3),* 236–241.

Byrne, B. (2002). Deep vein thrombosis prophylaxis: the effectiveness and implications of using below-knee or thigh-length graduated compression stockings. *Journal of Vascular Nursing, 20(2),* 53–59.

Carney, B. L. (2006). Evolution of wrong site surgery prevention strategies. *AORN Journal, 83(5),* 1115–1118, 1121–1122.

Centers for Disease Control and Prevention. (1999). Guidelines for prevention of surgical site infection, 1999. Retrieved March 24, 2008, from www.cdc.gov/ncidod/dhqp/pdf/guidelines/SSI.pdf.

Correll, D. J., Bader, A. M., Hull, M. W., et al. (2006). Value of preoperative clinic visits in identifying issues with potential impact on operating room efficiency. *Anesthesiology, 105(6),* 1254–1259.

Davis, B. (2002). Perioperative care of patients with latex allergy. *AORN Journal, 72(1),* 47–54.

Digner, M. (2007). At your convenience: preoperative assessment by telephone. *Journal of Perioperative Practice, 17(7),* 294–301.

Duncan, A. (2008). Nursing management: intraoperative care. In D. Brown, & H. Edwards (Eds.). *Lewis's medical–surgical nursing: assessment and management of clinical problems* (2nd ed.) (pp. 393–409). Sydney: Elsevier.

Ferrando, A., Ivaldi, C., Buttiglier, A., et al. (2005). Guidelines for preoperative assessment: impact on clinical practice and cost. *International Journal for Quality in Health Care, 17(4),* 323–329.

Ferschl, M. B., Tung, A., Sweitzer, B. J., et al. (2005). Preoperative clinics visits reduce operating room cancellations and delays. *Anesthesiology, 103(4),* 855–859.

Finegan, B. A., Rashiq, S., McAlister, F. A., O'Connor, P. (2005). Selective ordering of preoperative investigations by anesthesiologists reduces the number and cost of tests. *Canadian Journal of Anesthesia, 52(6),* 575–580.

Garcia-Miguel, F. J., Serrano-Aguilar, P. G., Lopez-Bastida, J. (2003). Preoperative assessment. *Lancet, 362(9397),* 1749–1757.

Garretson, S. (2004). Benefits of preoperative information programmes. *Nursing Standard, 4(18),* 33–37.

Halaszynski, T. M., Juda, R., Silverman, D. G. (2004). Optimizing postoperative outcomes with efficient preoperative assessment and management. *Critical Care Medicine, 32(4 suppl.),* S76–S86.

Health and Disability Commissioner. (2007). Your rights when using a health or disability service in New Zealand and how to make a complaint. Retrieved November 10, 2007, from http://www.hdc.org.nz/complaints.

Heizenroth, P. A. (2003). Positioning the patient for surgery. In J. Rothrock (Ed.). *Alexander's care of the patient in surgery* (12th ed.) (pp. 159–186). St Louis: Mosby.

Hilditch, W. G., Asbury, A. J., Crawford, J. M. (2003). Preoperative screening: criteria for referring to anaesthetists. *Anaesthesia, 58,* 117–124.

Ho, C. (2007). An audit of the value of pre-operative electrocardiograms before surgery (general anaesthetic) in a day surgery unit. *Scottish Medical Journal, 52(2),* 28–30.

Hodgson, P. (2006). Implementing the New Zealand health strategy 2006. Wellington: NZ Ministry of Health, Wellington. Retrieved November 16, 2007, from http://www.picosearch.com/cgi-bin/ts.pl.

Joanna Briggs Institute. (2000). Best practice: knowledge retention from preoperative patient information. *Joanna Briggs Institute, 4(6),* 1–6.

Johansson, K., Nuutila, L., Virtanen, H., et al. (2005). Preoperative education for orthopaedic patients: systematic review. *Journal of Advanced Nursing, 50(2),* 212–223.

Johnson, R. K., & Mortimer, A. J. (2002). Routine preoperative blood testing: is it necessary? *Anaesthesia,* *57,* 914–917.

Joo, H. S., Wong, J., Naik, V. N., Savoldelli, G. L. (2005). The value of screening preoperative chest X-rays: a systematic review. *Canadian Journal of Anesthesia, 52(6),* 568–574.

Keglovitz, L., & Kraft, M. (2002). Evaluating the patient before anaesthesia. In W. E. Hurford, M. T. Bailin, J. K. Davison, et al. (Eds.). Clinical anesthesia procedures of the Massachusetts General Hospital (7th ed.) (pp. 3–15). Philadelphia: Lippincott, Wilkins & Williams.

Kinley, H., Czoski-Murray, C., George, S., et al. (2003). Effectiveness of appropriately trained nurses in preoperative assessment: randomised controlled equivalence/non-inferiority trial. *British Medical Journal, 325,* 1323–1326.

Kjønniksen, I., Anderson, B. M., Søndenaa, V. G., Segadal, L. (2002). Preoperative hair removal—a systematic literature review. *AORN Journal, 75(5),* 928–938, 940.

Kuri, M., Nakagawa, M., Tanaka, H., et al. (2005). Determination of the duration of preoperative smoking cessation to improve wound healing after head and neck surgery. *Anesthesiology, 102,* 92–96.

Lui, L., Dzankic, S., Leung, J. (2002). Preoperative electrocardiogram abnormalities do not predict postoperative cardiac complications in geriatric surgical patients. *Journal of American Geriatric Society, 50,* 1186–1191.

Moller, A., & Villebro, N. (2005). Interventions for preoperative smoking cessation. *Cochrane Database of Systematic Reviews, 3,* CD002294, 1–14.

Napoli, M. (2002). Preoperative fasting: rules changed. Retrieved November 16, 2007, from http://www.medicalconsumers.org/pages/newsletter_excerpts.html.

Moores, A., & Pace, N. A. (2003). The information given by patients prior to giving consent to anaesthesia. *Anaesthesia, 58,* 703–706.

Naismith, C. (2008). Nursing management: preoperative care. In D. Brown, & H. Edwards (Eds.). *Lewis's medical surgical nursing: assessment and management of clinical problems* (2nd ed.) (pp. 376–392). Sydney: Elsevier.

National Institute for Clinical Excellence. (2003). Preoperative tests: the use of routine preoperative tests for elective surgery. Retrieved November 16, 2007, from www.nice.org.uk.

Nursing Council of New Zealand. (2005). Guidelines for cultural safety, the Treaty of Waitangi and Māori health in nursing education and practice. Retrieved November 16, 2007, from http://www.nursingcouncil.org.nz/CulturalSafety.pdf.

NZ Ministry of Health. (2004). Clearing the smoke: a five year plan for tobacco control in New Zealand 2004–2009. Wellington: NZ Ministry of Health.

Oakley, M. (2005). Preoperative assessment. In R. Pudner (Ed.). *Nursing the surgical patient* (2nd ed.) (pp. 3–16). London: Elsevier.

Ormrod, G., & Casey, D. (2004). The educational preparation of nursing staff undertaking pre-assessment of surgical patients: a discussion of the issues. *Nurse Education Today, 24,* 256–262.

Pearson, A., Richardson, M., Peels, S., Cairns, M. (2004). The pre admission care of patients undergoing day surgery: a systematic review. *Health Care Reports, 2(1),* 1–20.

Perioperative Nurses College of New Zealand Nurses Organisation (PNCNZNO). (2005). Recommended standards, guidelines, and position statements for safe practice in the perioperative setting. Retrieved December 5, 2007, from http://www.nzno.org.nz/Site/Sections/Colleges/Perioperative/Standguide.aspx.

Queensland Health. (2005). Queensland health policy statement: ensuring intended surgery. Retrieved December 5, 2007, from http://www.health.qld.gov.au/patientsafety/eis/documents/26961.pdf.

Rai, M. R., & Pandit, J. J. (2003). Day of surgery cancellations after nurse-led pre-assessment in an elective surgical centre: the first 2 years. *Anaesthesia, 58,* 684–711.

Ramsden, I. M. (2002). Cultural safety and nursing education in Aotearoa and Te Waipounamu. Victoria University, Wellington, unpublished doctoral dissertation

Richardson-Tench, M. (2002). Unmasked! The discursive practice of the operating room nurse: a Foucauldian feminist analysis. Unpublished thesis. Melbourne: Monash University.

Richardson-Tench, M., Pearson, A., Cairns, M. (2005). The changing face of surgery: the use of systematic reviews to establish best practice guidelines for day surgery units. *British Journal of Perioperative Nursing, 15(8),* 240–248.

Seal, L. A., & Paul-Cheadle, D. (2004). A systems approach to preoperative surgical patient skin preparation. *American Journal of Infection Control, 32(2),* 57–62.

Shiffman, S., Rolf, C., Hellebusch, S., et al. (2002). Real-world efficacy of prescription and over-the-counter nicotine replacement therapy. *Addiction, 97,* 505–516.

Shiffman, S. (2007). Use of more nicotine lozenges leads to better success in quitting smoking. *Addiction, 102,* 809–814.

Solca, M. (2006). Evidence based preoperative evaluation. *Best Practice & Research Clinical Anaesthesiology, 20(2)*, 231–236.

Staunton, P., & Chiarella, M. (2008). *Nursing and the law* (6th ed.). Sydney: Elsevier.

Tanner, J., Woodings, D., Moncaster, K. (2006). Preoperative hair removal to reduce surgical site infection. *Cochrane Database of Systematic Reviews, 2*, CD004122.

The Joint Commission. (2003). Universal protocol for preventing wrong site, wrong procedure, wrong person surgery. Retrieved March 5, 2008, from http://www.jointcommission.org/NR/rdonlyres/E3C600EB-043B-4E86-B04E-CA4A89AD5433/0/universal_protocol.pdf.

Valleylab. (2003). Clinical information hotline. Electrosurgery safety update: patient return electrode warming. Retrieved November 16, 2007, from http://www.valleylab.com/education/hotline/pdfs/hotline_0303.pdf.

Valleylab. (2004). Clinical information hotline. General cautions and warnings for patient and operating room safety. Retrieved November 16, 2007, from http://www.valleylab.com/education/hotline/pdfs/hotline_0408.pdf .

Van Klei, W. A., Hennis, P. J., Moen, J., et al. (2004). The accuracy of trained nurses in preoperative health assessment: results of the open study. *Anaesthesia, 59*, 971–978.

Van Klei, W. A., Moons, K. G. M., Rutten, C. L. G., et al. (2002). The effect of outpatient preoperative evaluation of hospital inpatients on cancellation of surgery and length of hospital stay. *Anesthesia Analgesia, 94*, 644–649.

Wagner, D., Byrne, M., Kolcaba, K. (2006). Effects of comfort warming on perioperative patients. *AORN Journal, 84(3)*, 427–448.

Walsgrove, H. (2006). Putting education into practice for preoperative patient assessment. *Nursing Standard, 20(47)*, 35–39.

Warner, D. O. (2005a). Preoperative smoking cessation: the role of the primary care provider. *Mayo Clinic Proceedings, 80(2)*, 252–258.

Warner, D. O. (2005b). Preoperative smoking cessation: how long is long enough? *Anesthesiology, 102*, 883–884.

Webster, J., & Osborne, S. (2007). Preoperative bathing or showering with skin antiseptics to prevent surgical site infection. *Cochrane Database of Systematic Reviews, 2*, CD004985.

Wicker, P., & O'Neill, J. (2006). *Caring for the perioperative patient*. Oxford: Blackwell Publishing.

Wilkinson, D. (2007). Non-physician anaesthesia in the UK: a history. *Journal of Perioperative Practice, 17(4)*, 162–170.

Wilson, N. (2007). Review of the evidence for major population-level tobacco control interventions. Wellington: NZ Ministry of Health. Retrieved December 5, 2007, from http://www.moh.govt.nz/tobacco.

Yaun, H., Chung, F., Wong, D., Edward, R. (2005). Current preoperative testing in ambulatory surgery are widely disparate: a survey of CAS members. *Canadian Journal of Anesthesia, 52(7)*, 675–679.

FURTHER READING

ACORN. (2006). *ACORN standards for perioperative nursing*. Adelaide: Australian College of Operating Room Nurses.

Barnes, P. K., Emerson, P. A., Hajnal, S., et al. (2000). Influence of an anaesthetist on nurse-led, computer-based preoperative assessment. *Anaesthesia, 55*, 576–589.

Berry, M. (2007). Herbal medicines: considerations for the perioperative setting. *Day Surgery Australia, 6(2)*, 10–16.

de Chesnay, M., Wharton, R., Pamp, C. (2005). Cultural competence, resilience and advocacy. In M. de Chesnay (Ed.). *Caring for the vulnerable: perspectives in nursing theory, practice and research* (pp. 31–41). Sudbury, MA: Jones & Bartlett.

NZ Ministry of Health. (2004). Clearing the smoke: a five year plan for tobacco control in New Zealand 2004–2009. Retrieved November 16, 2007, from http://www.moh.govt.nz/tobacco.

NZ Ministry of Health. (2007). New Zealand smoking cessation guidelines. Retrieved November 16, 2007, from http://www.moh.govt.nz/tobacco.

Ziolkowski, L., & Strzyzewski, N. (2001). Perianesthesia assessment: foundation of care. *Journal of PeriAnesthesia Nursing, 16(6)*, 359–370.

CHAPTER 3

The perioperative environment

Michelle Loth and Liz Welstead

LEARNING OBJECTIVES

After reading this chapter, you should be able to:

- describe the design, layout and traffic patterns of the operating suite
- identify the environmental controls and cleaning requirements for the operating suite
- discuss the occupational health and safety issues, including radiation, electricity, fire, latex allergy, manual handling and sharps injury
- discuss the use of technology within the operating suite, including endoscopic equipment, electrosurgical unit and robotics.

KEY TERMS

electrosurgical unit

environmentally controlled unit

laser

latex allergy

operating suite design

robotics

smoke plume

traffic patterns

INTRODUCTION

The perioperative environment is a specially designed and regulated area that plays a significant role in patient safety during the surgical procedure. Incorporating special design features, such as positive pressure air conditioning, traffic patterns to restrict entry of contaminants from external sources of the hospital, easy-to-clean floor and wall surfaces, and electrical safety controls, all contribute to reduce the risk of infection to the surgical patient (Queensland Health, 2002). Safety features related to electrical equipment, radiation and laser further protect both patients and staff from hazards inherent in a highly technical environment.

This chapter explores the structural components of the operating suite and the impact that design features, including designated traffic patterns, control of temperature, humidity and ventilation systems, have on the safety of the patient. Occupational health and safety issues are explored, including those related to the use of electrosurgery, surgical plume, prevention of fire and explosion, latex allergy, occupational exposure, personal protective equipment and perioperative attire, radiation safety and safe chemical handling.

OPERATING SUITE DESIGN AND LAYOUT

The **operating suite design** and layout must accommodate the day-to-day workload and the corresponding fluctuations in staff and patient numbers (Centre for Health Assets Australasia [CHAA], 2006). The operating suite is an **environmentally controlled unit** consisting of many distinct functional areas. It may be adjacent to a preadmission area (or perioperative unit), through which patients for day surgery and those who will be admitted for longer stays are admitted.

When designing the operating suite, the decision regarding the number of operating rooms and recovery spaces is governed by many factors, including the number, type and complexity of surgical procedures to be undertaken and the number of postoperative beds available. There are several design models for the operating suite layout that achieve a balance between the environmental needs of the staff, infection control, operational flow and functional requirements (CHAA, 2006).

Every Australian state and territory and New Zealand have their own set of building codes, infection control guidelines and capital works guidelines to assist with hospital design when new hospitals are being planned or refurbishments are being undertaken (Carthey, 2006). Australasian Health Facility guidelines were released in 2006 to assist Australian and New Zealand health departments undertaking health facility projects to achieve the standards for building, space, equipment, fit out and furnishings, and are the minimum standard for design (Carthey, 2007).

Some of the planning models for the operating suite include the following:

- *Racetrack style.* In this model, the operating rooms are usually placed around a corridor containing equipment and supply areas (Fig 3-1). An outside 'racetrack' maybe used for the passage of dirty equipment and supplies to minimise any cross-contamination with clean areas (CHAA, 2006; Hauff, 2002).
- *Single corridor.* This model has a central corridor that divides the operating rooms and storage areas (Fig 3-2). This model, however, may not be appropriate if the corridor is not wide enough to allow the passage of clean and dirty supplies (CHAA, 2006; Hauff, 2002).
- *Small clusters.* This model clusters between two and four operating rooms with a shared sterile stock room (Fig 3-3). Disadvantages of this model include the additional costs associated with duplicating supplies in multiple sterile stock rooms (CHAA, 2006; Hauff, 2002).

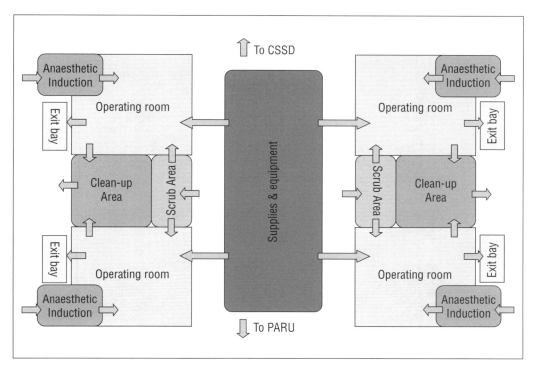

Figure 3-1 Racetrack model (CHAA, 2006; Phillips, 2007).

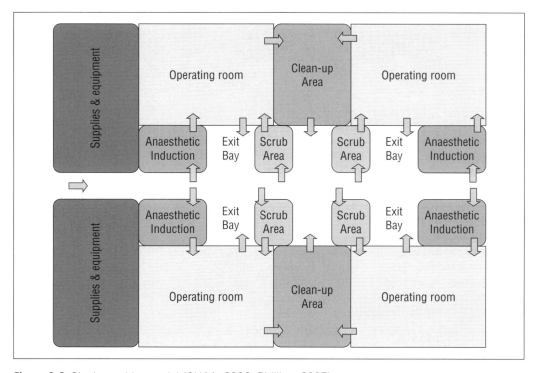

Figure 3-2 Single corridor model (CHAA, 2006; Phillips, 2007).

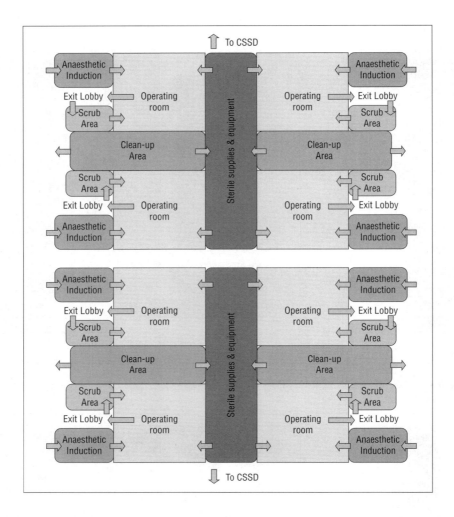

Figure 3-3 Small clusters model (CHAA, 2006).

The operating suite should have close or direct links with other units for convenience, patient safety and practicality (CHAA, 2006). These units include the:

- central sterilising supply department (CSSD)
- postanaesthesia recovery unit (PARU)
- emergency department
- intensive care unit (ICU)
- surgical wards
- delivery suite
- pathology
- blood bank
- medical imaging departments.

TRAFFIC PATTERNS

Traffic patterns are established to define movement throughout the operating suite for personnel, equipment, supplies and instrumentation, and to prevent contact from sources

	Patient	Staff	Supplies
Unrestricted	Emergency/ICU/wards/Admissions send patients to operating suite Operating room reception greet visitors & staff	Change rooms Tea rooms	Supplies received from stores Loan set delivery instrumentation for CSSD
Semi-restricted	Patients enter holding bay Induction rooms may be used	Staff gather necessary equipment and supplies for surgery	Cleaning ⟶ Sterilisation undertaken in CSSD Sterile items enter sterile stockroom Sterile supplies are gathered in preparation for operation.
Restricted	Patient enters operating room	Check operating room prior to list. Prepare sterile set-up Scrubbing, gowning & gloving Surgery performed	Set-up taken into the operating room for surgery (should be checked by nursing staff)
Semi-restricted	Patients enter PARU after surgery Discharged to ward or home	Terminal cleaning of operating room at end of list Environmental cleaning	Leftover sterile supplies returned to sterile stock room Instruments taken into clean-up room for transportation to CSSD Linen/waste/sharps disposal

Figure 3-4 Correct traffic flow in and out of the operating suite.

of potential contamination. Ideally, waste, contaminated supplies and soiled instruments should not travel down the same corridor as clean and sterile supplies. However, if this is necessary due to the suite's design, then measures must be undertaken to minimise any potential contamination of clean with dirty supplies (CHAA, 2006). Such a method could include using a sealed 'closed cart' system for transporting soiled and contaminated items to the sterilising department for decontamination.

OPERATING SUITE LAYOUT

The Australian College of Operating Room Nurses (ACORN) classifies the perioperative environment into four zones—transition, unrestricted, semi-restricted and restricted— which can be defined by the activities performed.

Transition area

Change rooms
Secure designated male and female change rooms with lockers and a daily supply of laundered perioperative attire must be provided for the authorised staff (ACORN, 2006b).

Unrestricted areas

Reception

The reception area is an unrestricted area that does not require those accessing it to wear perioperative attire. The reception area is a place for patients, families and staff to access information, such as operating suite schedules, location of waiting areas and case bookings.

Preoperative holding bay

In the unrestricted areas there is unlimited access to all personnel, who may wear either perioperative attire or street clothes. The preoperative holding bay is a waiting area for patients prior to surgery where admission procedures, such as patient identification checks, are carried out, all documentation is confirmed and the responsibility for the patient is handed over by the ward or perioperative unit staff to perioperative nurses. A nurse is usually assigned to work in this area to monitor the patients' condition and to help coordinate each operating room's schedule by calling for patients from the wards/perioperative unit in a timely manner to minimise delays (ACORN, 2006a).

Semi-restricted areas

The semi-restricted areas are limited to authorised personnel who are required to wear perioperative attire.

Anaesthetic rooms

Anaesthetic rooms are located directly next to the operating room and patients are transferred here from the holding bay when the anaesthetist is ready to prepare the patient for surgery. The anaesthetic nurse assigned to this area will take over the patient's care and assist the anaesthetist in preparing the patient for surgery by commencing intravenous infusions or inserting local or regional anaesthesia. General anaesthesia may be induced in the anaesthetic room or the patient may be transferred onto the operating table for induction, depending on protocol and the anaesthetist's preference.

Storage areas

Areas should be set aside within the operating suite to receive and decant bulk supplies before they are distributed to specialty storage areas within the suite. Consumables and specialised equipment, such as microscopes and laser machinery, must be stored in areas that are easily accessible from the operating rooms and anaesthetic bays.

Sterile stock room

Areas for storing wrapped, sterile supplies must be easily accessible from all operating rooms and may be contained in a central location. Sterile packages and trays are ideally stored on open wire shelving at least 250 mm above the floor and 440 mm from the ceiling. The open shelving allows dust to fall to the floor and permits cleaning to take place more effectively (ACORN, 2006f; Standards Australia, 2003, AS/NZS 4187).

To maximise storage space, many operating suites use mobile compactors. The sterile stock room must be kept cool and dry, with a temperature of 22–24°C and a relative humidity of 35–68% to prevent compromising the integrity of the sterile packages (ACORN 2006f). Sterile supplies need to be kept away from direct sunlight and, therefore, windows within this sterile stock area are not considered ideal (Standards Australia, 2003, AS/NZS 4187). The sterile stock room needs to be cleaned regularly and kept free of dust, vermin and insects (ACORN, 2006f).

Staff rooms

Because operating room staff wear perioperative attire, a staff room should be located within the operating suite where refreshments can be taken and staff can relax between procedures. Another area should also be designated a meeting/education room where staff meetings and in-service education can be conducted, and in which journals and textbooks, as well as access to the organisation's intranet and to the internet, are available to staff for ongoing education purposes.

Postanaesthesia recovery unit

The PARU can also be classified as a semi-restricted area; however, the wearing of perioperative attire is at the discretion of each hospital or facility (ACORN, 2006c). As well as perioperative staff, it needs to be accessible to medical and other staff wearing street clothes in the event of an emergency (Australian and New Zealand College of Anaesthetists, 2006).

In the PARU, patients who have undergone anaesthesia and/or surgery are provided care, so the PARU needs to be located close to the operating/procedure rooms. The layout and design of the PARU needs to allow for good observation of all patients simultaneously and especially from the staff station when required. Curtained cubicles may allow privacy for patients while still maintaining a wide space, as private rooms are inappropriate in the PARU (CHAA, 2006).

Sterilising department

The sterilising department's largest client will always be the operating suite and, therefore, it must be located within easy access to facilitate the passage of clean and dirty instruments between the two departments. Enclosed carts or containers with lids should be used to transport contaminated instruments to the sterilising department, and separate clean and dirty elevators should be used to transport instruments to and from the sterilising department if it is located on a different floor to the operating suite (CHAA, 2006).

The sterilising department layout must be clearly defined to distinguish the decontamination (dirty) and packaging/sterilising (clean) areas. Dirty instruments should be delivered directly into the cleaning or decontamination room for processing. All personnel must wear personal protective equipment while handling contaminated equipment, including protective ear wear as many instrument washers are noisy. After the instruments have been processed, they enter the clean side of the sterilising department, where specially trained staff check instruments, mark tray checklists, and package trays and instruments for sterilisation.

Restricted areas

Usually accessed from a semi-restricted area, the restricted areas include procedure and operating rooms, where staff must wear surgical attire and personal protective equipment (ACORN, 2006b).

Operating rooms

The minimum size recommended for a general operating room is 42 square metres, whereas a large operating room (usually designated for cardiac, neurosurgery, orthopaedic joint or transplantation surgery) is 52 square metres (CHAA, 2006).

Dedicated operating rooms

Some hospitals, particularly larger tertiary hospitals, dedicate operating rooms to specialty surgery (e.g. neurosurgery, orthopaedic surgery). This is beneficial as it allows specialised equipment, such as microscopes and special operating room tables, to remain within the operating room, reducing the potential for damage due to movement, although fixed equipment may limit the flexibility of the operating room in smaller suites (ACORN, 2006b; CHAA 2006).

Integrated operating rooms

Highly specialised, integrated operating rooms have been built in some tertiary level hospitals. These are referred to as integrated or interventional operating rooms, where all the highly technical equipment is connected together (integrated) for easy use and where the surgeon has complete control of much of it from within the sterile field. Such equipment can include the operating room lights, camera, light source and insufflator.

Interventional operating rooms (also called endovascular operating rooms) are a cross between the cardiac catheter unit (angioplasty suite) and a regular operating room. This provides a safe environment for the radiologist or surgeon to perform angioplasty procedures, with the additional security of an operating room in the event that an operation becomes necessary. The interventional operating room has many television screens strategically placed for surgeon comfort or to facilitate the viewing of multiple X-ray images simultaneously. An intraoperative X-ray machine ('C-arm') can be either mobile or table-mounted to facilitate angioplasty procedures. The C-arm can slide up

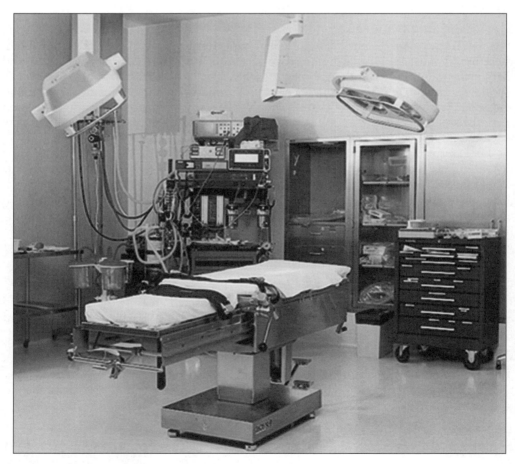

Figure 3-5 Typical operating room (Courtesy Greg McVicar).

and down the table to capture X-ray images anywhere along the length of the body. To accommodate the extra equipment and technology, the integrated operating room is usually double the size of a standard operating room, at about 80 square metres. With the increase in minimally invasive surgery, these highly specialised settings are likely to become the operating room of the future (Phillips, 2007).

Scrub areas

Scrub areas (or bays) provide sinks with running water and access to antiseptic solutions to accommodate several members of the surgical team undertaking the surgical scrub procedure simultaneously. To facilitate adherence to aseptic technique, these sinks need to be located directly outside the operating room to allow easy access to sterile gown and glove trolleys, which may be located in the scrub bay itself or within the operating room. To prevent slip injuries, the floor coverings in the scrub areas should be of a non-slip texture (CHAA, 2006).

DESIGN FEATURES OF THE OPERATING SUITE

Design considerations exist for the windows, ceilings, doors, floors and walls for the perioperative environment; they are necessitated by infection control practices and to accommodate environmental cleaning requirements.

Windows

Staff morale is always boosted by natural light, and having windows within the operating suite is recommended (ACORN, 2006b). However, it is not always practical to have windows in the operating room itself, where procedures such as minimally invasive surgery may require a darkened theatre to maximise the visual image on the screen. Also, when lasers are used, appropriate protective window coverings within the operating room must be provided (Queensland Health, 2002).

Ceilings, doors, floors and walls

Ceilings within the perioperative environment should be made of a non-reflective, non-porous material without cracks or open joins that permit the accumulation of dirt and are difficult to clean. Light fittings must be flush fitting and sealed to inhibit any dust or dirt entering the environment (CHAA, 2006). Swing-type doors for the operating room allow easy access for hands-free entry (Abreu & Potter, 2001). Consideration should be given to fitting the lower section of the door (from the floor edge up to 150 mm) with a thin layer of aluminium to protect it from constant battering and wetness due to frequent floor mopping. Floors are generally made of seamless vinyl that is impervious to moisture, easily cleaned, stain resistant, comfortable for long periods of standing and suitable for wheeled traffic (CHAA, 2006). Walls are also made of seamless vinyl and curved where they meet the floor to assist in effective cleaning. The colour should be neutral with a matt or satin finish to reduce glare, which can be disturbing to the surgical team (Gruendemann & Mangum, 2001). Tiles, once a popular wall covering, are no longer considered a suitable finish within an operating room due to the potential for cracking, which poses infection control risks (CHAA, 2006). Due to the high traffic of trolleys in the unit, damage to walls and doors is inevitable and, therefore, consideration should be given for wall and corner protection (CHAA, 2006).

OTHER FEATURES OF THE OPERATING SUITE

The operating suite utilises many features to create and maintain a safe, clean environment for patients. These measures include the ability to set parameters for temperature, humidity and ventilation systems.

Temperature

The temperature range within the operating suite should be 18–24°C. Individual operating rooms should have a temperature range of 20–22°C; this temperature range inhibits bacterial growth and is tolerated well by both staff and patients (Gruendemann & Mangum, 2001). However, the temperature may require adjusting to accommodate some types of surgery and/or the condition of individual patients. For example, burns or paediatric patients require higher ambient temperatures as these patients are highly susceptible to hypothermia. In contrast, some types of neurosurgical patients require a much cooler environment.

Humidity

The humidity in the operating room should be maintained at 50–60% to both inhibit bacterial growth and decrease risks associated with static electricity. Additionally, high humidity can increase fatigue among the surgical team and is thus best avoided (ACORN, 2006b; Rothrock, 2007).

Ventilation

The three types of air-conditioning systems used within the perioperative environment are listed below.

1. *Conventional system*. This system uses filtered, recirculated air with a minimum of four fresh air changes within an hour (ACORN, 2006b).
2. *Ultra clean air system*. This system uses a special filter, called a high-efficiency particulate air (HEPA) filter, to produce clean air. This filter removes particles over 0.3 μm in diameter with an efficiency of 99.97%. The filtered air should move in a unidirectional motion, with 20–40 air changes per hour (ACORN, 2006b).
3. *Laminar airflow*. This system uses HEPA filtered air in an enclosed area within the operating room. This is usually created by using movable partitions to establish a rectangular enclosure centred on the operating table. The air moves in uniform velocity in either a horizontal or vertical direction, and there are up to 400 air changes per hour. Types of surgical interventions that may benefit from laminar airflow include orthopaedic joint replacement surgery, cardiac surgery and organ transplantation (ACORN, 2006b; Phillips, 2007).

Air-conditioning systems within the operating suite use positive pressure, which pushes air down from within the operating suite and out into the external environment. Positive air pressure is greater in the operating room than the surrounding corridors and scrub areas, with the exception of the sterile stock room, which has the same air pressure as inside the operating room (Queensland Health, 2002). This positive pressure forces air from the operating room out into the corridors, resulting in the air in the outer corridors having a higher microbial count. For this reason, operating room doors *must* be kept closed at all times (other than the necessary passage of staff, supplies and the patient) to reduce the risk of airborne contaminants entering the surgical field. The microbial count within the individual operating room is usually at its peak during the time of the skin incision because this follows a period of maximum air disturbance created by staff gloving and gowning, patient draping, the movement of operating room staff and the frequent opening and closing of the operating room doors. Because the microbial count rises every time the operating room doors are opened, it is necessary to ensure all required supplies are readily at hand (within the operating room, generally) during the course of any surgical procedure (Phillips, 2007; Woodhead & Wicker, 2005).

ELECTRICAL SAFETY

The large amount of electrical equipment used in an operating suite places both staff and patients at potential risk of electrocution should equipment become faulty or be mishandled by staff. A range of safety features are incorporated into the design of operating suites to reduce the risk of electrocution. These include devices such as line isolation monitoring (LIM) panels and, within each operating room, residual current devices (RCD), which indicate faulty equipment or leakage of electrical current by initiating an audible alarm, along with activating warning lights on the LIM panel; associated circuit breakers subsequently interrupt supply for the RCD.

All electrical equipment must be checked by the hospital's biomedical engineering department prior to installation and, thereafter, at regular intervals to ensure they are functioning safely and meet national standards. Staff should check each piece of electrical equipment prior to use to ensure correct functioning, including inspection of electrical cords for any damage. Extension cords are not used within operating rooms due to the danger they pose to patients—of accidental dislodgement—and the occupational health and safety risk for staff, who may trip over the cords (Standards Australia, 2004a, AS/NZS 2500).

There are two main types of electrical shock against which staff and patients must be protected.

1. *Macroshock*. This is the most common type of electrical shock experienced. It occurs when the body becomes a conductor of electrical current if it touches or is attached to faulty equipment, when leakage of current occurs. A person experiencing macroshock may exhibit muscle contractions, breathing difficulties and extreme pain. Under normal circumstances the skin provides resistance to electrical current. However, during surgical procedures this natural protection may be breached by the application of electrocardiograph (ECG) monitoring pads and/or electroconductive gel; additionally, the patient may be unconscious and paralysed due to anaesthesia and unable to escape the shock. Ventricular fibrillation (visible on the ECG monitoring screen) may occur as a result of the shock, depending on which part of the body is in contact with the electrical current and the magnitude of the current. Line isolation monitors are the first line of defence against macroshock, and areas with this protection are termed 'body protected', using the symbol shown in Figure 3-6 (Standards Australia, 2004a, AS/NZS 2500).

2. *Microshock*. In certain procedures, such as those where arterial catheters, pacing wires or other devices have direct connection to the heart, there is danger of a microshock, which may cause a fatal ventricular fibrillation to occur. Only very small amounts of electrical current are needed to induce fibrillation when it is transmitted directly to myocardial tissue, and there may be no external signs that the patient has suffered microshock. The line isolation monitors that protect against macroshock require

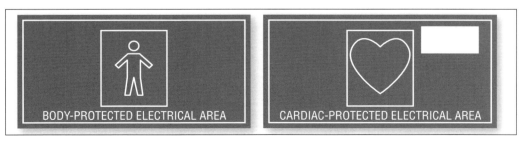

Figure 3-6 Signage used to denote body- and cardiac-protected electrical areas.

supplementing with special earthing devices, which alert staff to current leakage well below the level that would cause microshock (Standards Australia, 2004a, AS/NZS 2500). Areas that incorporate these special earthing devices are termed 'cardiac protected' and are identified using the symbol shown in Figure 3-6.

ELECTROSURGICAL EQUIPMENT

The **electrosurgical unit** (ESU), generally referred to as the diathermy machine, is a commonly used electrical device within the operating room. The ESU generates an electrical current at extremely high frequency, which cuts or coagulates tissue (as well as variations of the latter, such as tissue desiccation or fulguration) or 'diathermies it', thus generating a bloodless field.

There are two main types of diathermy—monopolar and bipolar—both of which have unique applications.

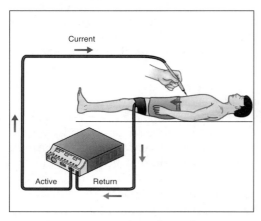

Figure 3-7 Monopolar electrosurgical circuit (Rothrock, 2007, p 221).

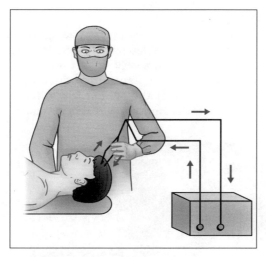

Figure 3-8 Bipolar electrosurgical circuit (Rothrock, 2007, p 221).

Monopolar diathermy

In *monopolar diathermy*, the current is usually applied to the tissue through the use of a small hand-held electrode, termed the 'active' electrode (Fig 3-7). This may be in the form of a 'diathermy' pencil, blade, forceps, needlepoint, loop or a ball depending on the surgery being performed. The surgeon activates the current by means of a switch on the 'pencil' to cut or coagulate tissue. The current then flows through the patient to the dispersive electrode pad, previously applied to the patient's body, and back to the ESU, thus completing the electrical circuit. The dispersive electrode is usually an adhesive pad that is covered with conductive gel, which is attached to a muscular area of the patient (e.g. thigh or buttocks); it is used to safely disperse the electrical current (Standards Australia, 2004a, AS/NZS 2500). This is further discussed below.

Bipolar diathermy

Bipolar diathermy uses a fine pair of forceps controlled by the surgeon via a foot pedal. It is mainly used for coagulation in plastic or paediatric surgery, where the vessels to be coagulated are minor (Standards Australia, 2004a, AS/NZS 2500). In this mode, the current from the ESU flows down one tyne of the forceps across the tissue that is grasped between the forceps and returns to the generator through the opposing tyne (Fig 3-8). This mode does not require a dispersive electrode pad ('patient plate').

Hazards of electrosurgery

In addition to the risk of electrocution, burns to the patient may result if the dispersive electrode pad has insufficient contact with the patient's skin. Depending on local policy, the dispersive electrode pad is applied to the patient either by a nurse or an orderly. If it is the latter person's responsibility, the circulating or instrument nurse must check the placement and also the condition of the patient's skin when the pad is removed at the conclusion of the procedure. Any damage to the patient's skin must be reported, documented and appropriate treatment instigated. When applying the dispersive electrode pad, the following safety points must be followed:

- the skin should be dry
- the area should be free of hair as this can affect the adherence of the pad, and shaving may be undertaken to ensure good contact
- well-vascularised tissue such as muscle (e.g. outer thigh or buttock) must be selected
- avoid bony protuberances—these do not provide a sufficient safe area of vascularised tissue
- pooling of fluids, such as antiseptic skin preparation solutions, in the area should be avoided
- an appropriate-sized pad must be used (i.e. an adult pad for an adult)
- the pad should be placed as close as possible to the site of surgery
- the pad should not be applied until after the patient is positioned, whenever possible, and carefully checked if a change of position occurs intraoperatively (Ball, 2007).

If the current finds an alternative pathway back to earth through wet drapes, via faulty leads, electrodes or cables, or via other contact of the patient's skin with metal (e.g. a hand touching the frame of the operating table), the patient may suffer burns. Burns to surgical or nursing staff may also occur if the current used finds an alternate pathway back to the ESU (e.g. through a hole in the glove of the person applying the active electrode, or in cases where the insulation on an endoscopic forceps is faulty). All ESUs have inbuilt alarm systems to disable faulty equipment and alert staff to situations where the dispersive electrode has become detached from the patient (Standards Australia, 2004a, AS/NZS 2500).

Another hazard of electrosurgery is the generation of smoke during tissue coagulation. The **smoke plume** has been shown to contain a number of dangerous toxins, carcinogens and viruses (Anderson, 2004). The surgical team in the immediate vicinity of the plume are at risk of inhaling surgical smoke for which the surgical mask provides little protection. Consideration should be given to the use of special smoke evacuation units, which suck the smoke via devices attached to the active electrode into an evacuation unit that is external to the sterile field. These units contain charcoal filters, which remove the toxic gases and odours (Ball, 2007). The wearing of well-fitting, high-filtration face masks by surgical personnel is also recommended during procedures where there is the likelihood of smoke being generated (e.g. orthopaedic or breast surgery) (Standards Australia, 2004b, AS/NZS 4173).

Related equipment

In recent years, ESUs have been developed that incorporate enhanced haemostatic features. Argon-enhanced electrosurgery combines argon gas with electrosurgery to improve the effectiveness of the coagulation mode by clearing blood more quickly from the surgical site and allowing the surgeon greater visibility. There is also less surgical smoke generated, making it a safer alternative to electrosurgery (Ball, 2007).

Another advancement in haemostasis is the use of ultrasonic technology, which uses high-frequency sound waves to cut and coagulate tissue (Johnson & Johnson Gateway, 2007). A transducer held by the surgeon converts electrical energy into mechanical vibration, which vaporises tissue in a very precise manner, resulting in less damage to surrounding tissue, no smoke, and none of the dangers associated with electrical currents as seen with electrosurgery (Ball, 2007).

LASER

The term **laser** is an acronym for 'light amplification by stimulated emission of radiation'. In simple terms, the type of light emitted by a laser differs from natural light because the latter is made up of many different colours, as can be demonstrated by the use of a prism, all colours being bent at different angles. Laser light, on the other hand, is all one colour, being all one wavelength, all bent at the same angle because of the way it is produced and given off. Depending upon the wavelength, different laser beams are absorbed by different media. The wavelength of many of these beams of laser light is not visible, which adds to the potential for injury (Standards Australia, 2004b, AS/NZS 4173).

Laser energy can be delivered in variations of either continuous or pulsed modes. The effects on tissue at which the laser beam is aimed include thermal, photodisruptive, electromechanical and photochemical effects. These effects may be deep or shallow, narrow or widespread, depending upon the way the beam is delivered, the wavelength of the beam and the qualities (including the colour) of the tissue onto which it is directed (Standards Australia, 2004b, AS/NZS 4173). The uses for laser are many and varied. For example, in ophthalmology, the neodymium:YAG (Nd:YAG) laser beam can rupture a clouded membrane in the eye; cosmetic surgeons may use the erbium:YAG laser to resurface the skin; an ear, nose and throat surgeon may use a carbon dioxide laser to remove a tumour from the vocal cords; and a urologist may use a holmium:YAG laser to ablate a ureteric calculi (Ball, 2007).

Hazards of laser

Lasers used in the perioperative environment are referred to as class 3b or class 4 medical lasers. These lasers have the potential to cause eye or skin damage if appropriate protection is not employed, and should therefore be used with extreme caution. Accidental deflection of the laser beam by polished instrumentation may cause injury, and broken fibres from fibreoptic cables can cause damage where they escape from protective casing. In every health care facility it is vital that only personnel who have undergone recognised training and are familiar with the features, operation and specific safety requirements of the machine in use operate the laser (Standards Australia, 2004b, AS/NZS 4173).

Because lasers are potentially so dangerous, strict adherence to prescribed practices and protocols are essential. For each laser there is a 'nominal ocular hazard area' (NOHA), which is the area in which the laser beam can potentially cause damage to the cornea, including through windows (when the wavelength is not absorbed by the window itself) and when the beam is accidentally misdirected. All personnel in the NOHA must wear the appropriate eye

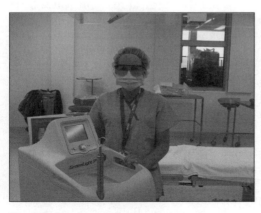

Figure 3-9 Laser safety goggles.

protection (Fig 3-9), and there must be warning signs on doors and windows, both of which are screened where necessary for the protection of other personnel.

Where laser procedures are performed with the use of fibreoptic cables, these should be carefully inspected prior to use and during handling to ensure individual fibres are not broken and therefore not emitting stray laser beams (Standards Australia, 2004b, AS/NZS 4173).

Laser surgery also generates smoke plume and similar safety precautions, such as those described for electrosurgery, should be taken (Ball, 2007).

TECHNOLOGY AND THE OPERATING SUITE

The worldwide boom in technology that has been witnessed over the past several decades has revolutionised the way surgical procedures are being carried out. Minimally invasive or 'keyhole' surgery was first introduced in the late 1980s and has now become the preferred option for many common operations that were once routinely performed as 'open' procedures (e.g. cholecystectomy, appendicectomy). Endoscopic technology is ever increasing, with most organs of the body accessible via a minimally invasive route. Advantages to the patient include reduced length of surgery and anaesthesia, shorter hospital stay and quicker return to normal life (Ball, 2007). While it is beyond the scope of this text to discuss all the latest technology, an overview is essential as this type of surgery presents new challenges, both for surgeons and perioperative nurses, to learn new skills and become involved in advancing technologies.

Robotics is perhaps the most advanced of the latest technologies and, even though it is only available in larger hospitals, has potential to further revolutionise minimally invasive surgery. Devices such as the da Vinci robot (Fig 3-10) use mechanical 'arms' to hold and manoeuvre endoscopic instruments and cameras more steadily than the human hand. The robotic devices are controlled by a surgeon sitting at a console away

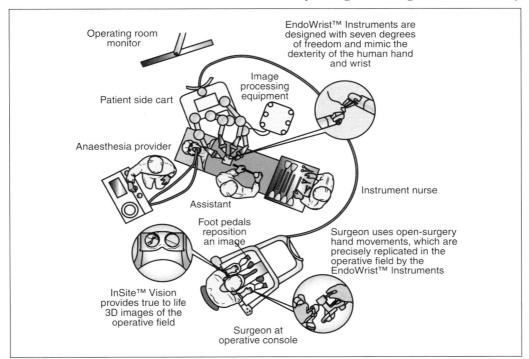

Figure 3-10 da Vinci robotic equipment (Phillips, 2007, p 654).

from the operating table, viewing the operative site through a three-dimensional (3D) viewer and manipulating the robotic instrumentation via precision hand-held controls. The advantages of undertaking surgery via this method are greater concentration levels for the surgeon, enhanced 3D visualisation of the surgical anatomy and greater precision as hand tremor is eliminated; in addition, the robotic arms have greater manoeuvrability than the human wrist (Ball, 2007).

Performing surgery using this modality has enormous potential, as a surgeon sitting at the console in one hospital can perform surgery on a patient in another hospital. It is thought that in the future this could have application for space exploration—the ultimate in remote surgery (Ball, 2007).

PREPARATION OF THE OPERATING ROOM

Prior to commencing work within the operating suite each day, the nurses assigned to the operating room must carry out a full check of the equipment and, by visual inspection, ensure items such as room and operating lights, trolleys, the operating table, ESU, suction equipment, linen skips and rubbish bags are present, in working order and are clean. All tables, trolleys and horizontal surfaces within the operating room are wiped over with neutral detergent to remove any dust that has settled overnight. The equipment within the theatre should be checked and, if any item is missing or faulty, corrective action should be taken before the patient enters the operating room.

The anaesthetic, circulating and instrument nurses should discuss any specific requirements for the patients on the operating list. Any additional equipment required for specific procedures (e.g. positioning equipment, microscopes) must be acquired and checked prior to commencement of surgery (ACORN, 2006a).

Room cleaning

In between each case, all rubbish and linen must be removed from the operating room and spot cleaning of any blood and body fluid spills undertaken with an approved hospital cleaning agent. Wiping trolleys and tables and cleaning contaminated furniture, equipment, floors, walls and lights also needs to be undertaken between each case. Any equipment that has been used during an operation and not required for subsequent procedures should be cleaned and returned to its storage area. These activities should be carried out by orderlies or other assistive personnel under the direction of the nursing staff.

Terminal cleaning

After the completion of the surgical procedures for the day, the operating room should be terminally cleaned. This includes a thorough cleaning of the equipment within the operating room itself, scrub areas and corridors in the immediate area that have been used during the day. All cleaning should be undertaken with an approved hospital cleaning agent, using lint-free cloths and mechanical friction to remove contamination and debris. Depending on individual local operational protocols, this cleaning is usually carried out by designated cleaning staff; however, it remains the responsibility of perioperative nurses to ensure that appropriate cleaning has taken place.

After the operating room and surrounding areas have been cleaned and tidied, the necessary restocking should be undertaken and all furniture and equipment placed in its usual position in anticipation for the next patient. This is particularly relevant for operating room readiness for emergency surgery (or disaster preparedness). In addition to cleaning between procedures and terminal cleaning, a strict schedule of periodic environmental cleaning is carried out according to hospital and infection control protocols (ACORN, 2006d).

WASTE MANAGEMENT

Correct segregation of waste is essential for infection control purposes and also in managing the volume and expense caused by the generation of clinical waste within the hospital. Staff can assist by being educated in waste management policies and consistent in placing waste in the most appropriate receptacle. Waste can be divided into:

- general—items that are not heavily soiled or saturated in blood or body fluids (e.g. paper, packaging, masks, gloves, dressings) (Queensland Health, 2007)
- clinical/contaminated—items saturated in blood or body fluids (e.g. used swabs and sponges, contents of suction canisters, amputated limbs, body tissue not required for pathology)
- recyclable—items that the hospital is able to either recycle on site or transport to contractors (e.g. plastic bottles, paper, instrument wraps)
- cytotoxic—items used in surgery involving the use of cytotoxic drugs.

OCCUPATIONAL HEALTH AND SAFETY

In addition to the hazards associated with the use of electricity, diathermy and laser, there are other hazards that are particular to the perioperative environment. Perioperative nurses must be aware of these risks for the protection of self, patients and other personnel.

Manual handling

The transfer and positioning of patients and the movement of equipment are activities with which all staff working within the operating suite will be involved and there is a need for awareness of the potential hazards that manual handling may pose. Mandatory education must be provided in manual handling techniques and injury prevention, for both patients and staff. Keeping a level of fitness and suppleness is recommended for all staff to prevent back and shoulder injuries, which are the most commonly suffered injuries by staff (Meijsen & Knibbe, 2007). Transferring and positioning patients are activities that must involve a team of people working in a coordinated manner to ensure the safety of all involved (NSW Health, 2005a). Devices to assist with the transfer of patients include slide sheets and boards (pat slides or rollers). In some hospitals, devices such as hover mats are also available, which are inflatable mattresses that are specially designed to transfer patients easily to and from the operating table with minimal manual handling requirements.

Prevention of fire or explosion

The risks of fire and explosion are high in the perioperative environment because oxygen and other flammable gases are in abundant supply due to anaesthesia requirements. There are many flammable materials available to fuel any fire, such as drapes, sponges and packaging, and the main ignition sources are electrosurgical or laser equipment. When alcoholic skin preparations are used, special care must be taken as they add an additional dangerous element, that of a known fire accelerant. This includes ensuring that the operative area is allowed to dry following application of the skin preparation solution and before the drapes are applied; and preventing solution soaking into hair or under pads (NSW Health, 2007). Although rare, the potential also exists for explosion when diathermy is used on hollow organs containing flammable gases, such as the bowel (SA Health Department, 2007; Standards Australia, 2004a, AS/NZS 2500).

Some strategies to reduce the risks to patients and staff are the use of moistened sponges around the operative site, venting the drapes during head and neck surgery or ophthalmic surgery to allow gases to escape the head area, and keeping the 'diathermy

> **Box 3-1** Fire in the operating room
>
> Although fires in the operating room are a rare event, they do still happen. In 2002 in New Zealand, a fire occurred during a caesarean section. The cause of the fire was directly related to the alcohol vapours that were released from the pooled skin preparation solution, and which had accumulated under the fire-retardant drapes. The correctly functioning ESU was the source of ignition. The patient received full thickness burns to 16% of her body. The severity of her injury was worsened by the intensity of the fire due to pooling of the alcoholic solution and its accelerant properties. No injury occurred to the staff present, whose quick actions prevented further injury to all present. The fetus was also unharmed.
>
> Waitemata District Health Board (2002)

pencil' in a quiver/holster to avoid accidental activation (Rothrock, 2007). Knowledge of fire evacuation policies is also vital and many operating suites conduct annual fire evacuation exercises.

Latex allergy

Natural rubber latex gloves are made from the milky sap from the *Hevea brasiliensis* tree. Because of the qualities of natural latex, it is used extensively in many industries, particularly health care, where it is most widely used as latex gloves. This is because the product is inexpensive, provides an excellent barrier that protects the patient and the wearer from exposure to potentially harmful infective agents, and provides good tactile properties for the wearer. When natural rubber latex is processed into gloves, many of the latex proteins are lost, and the remaining extractable proteins are those that are implicated in **latex allergy**.

In the 1980s and earlier, the protein content in the gloves was higher than today, and powder was applied to prevent the sides from sticking together and to facilitate easier donning. The proteins in the gloves adhered to the powder, which became airborne when the gloves were donned or removed. The proteins were then inhaled and spread through the air. The exposure of health care workers to latex proteins in this environment was, therefore, very high, and evidence suggests that there is a correlation between the use of latex products and latex allergy among health care professionals.

Powdered gloves are now rarely worn in health care environments, and advances are constantly being made to lower the protein levels and the subsequent allergen content of latex gloves and to find ways to make them easier to don without reducing the tactility of the product (NSW Health, 2005b; Reed, 2003; Yip, 2003). Latex allergy among patients and health care workers has also increased markedly since the introduction of (initially) universal, now standard precautions, which have resulted in the increased requirement to wear gloves for every patient contact.

Types of latex allergy

Allergic reactions to latex can be wide-ranging. There are three types of reactions:

1. *Irritant dermatitis*. This is the most commonly reported problem. It is a local, non-allergic skin reaction characterised by redness, dryness, scaling, blistering and cracking. Such changes may be caused by sweating, glove irritation or frequent hand washing. The use of cotton liners or non-latex gloves is recommended.
2. *Allergic contact dermatitis*. This is termed a type IV reaction and is a mediated immune response or delayed-type hypersensitivity to the chemical additives in gloves. It usually takes 6–48 hours to emerge after exposure and normally resolves when exposure ceases. It is recommended that sufferers wear non-latex gloves.

Box 3-2 Risk of developing a latex allergy

Have you experienced a severe reaction to avocado, bananas, kiwi fruit, or potatoes? If so, you are at greater risk of developing latex allergy. You are also more likely to suffer from a reaction if you suffer from conditions such as hay fever, hives or asthma or general atopia. You are more likely to develop a type I reaction if you have had repeated exposure of mucous membrane tissue to latex, such as frequent surgery, and as a health care worker if you frequently wear latex gloves or are exposed to the glove powder from powdered latex gloves.

Davis (2000)

---

3. *Immediate hypersensitivity to latex.* This is termed a type I reaction. It is the most serious response to contact with latex products or inhalation of latex proteins. Reactions are characterised by a range of symptoms, including itchy and runny eyes and nose, hives, angioedema (swelling), asthma, anaphylaxis and death (Australian Society of Clinical Immunology and Allergy [ASCIA], 2005; NSW Health, 2005b; Yip, 2003).

Prevention of latex allergy

There is no known cure for latex allergy and so prevention is the key. The most effective way to prevent latex allergy is to ensure that only powder-free or latex-free gloves are used to prevent further sensitisation (ASCIA, 2005). In addition, it may be helpful to ensure hands are washed after wearing latex gloves. Hands should be kept free of abrasions and sores wherever possible, and barrier protection should be employed using a water-based hand care product rather than oil-based hand care products. If symptoms of latex allergy do occur, then synthetic gloves must be used and all contact with items containing latex should be avoided (ASCIA, 2005). This is difficult for perioperative nurses and there have been instances where those with latex allergies have been required to find work in an alternative environment. Box 3-3 provides a case study of a rather disturbing and extreme latex reaction which has changed one Australian nurse's life dramatically.

Latex-sensitive patient precautions

Patients with latex sensitivity must be cared for in an environment free from contact with latex products. All operating suites should have designated 'latex-free' kits containing all the equipment necessary to care for a latex-sensitive patient. Requirements for caring for the latex-sensitive patient include:

- all perioperative staff wearing synthetic gloves and removing or changing any items of attire containing latex
- sourcing equipment that is latex-free
- posting signs denoting a latex-free environment on external doors
- using only non-latex items within the operating room
- protecting the patient from anything that may contain latex (e.g. arm boards and operating room tables that may contain latex are covered with linen) (ASCIA, 2005; NSW Health, 2005b).

Occupational exposure

Protection against exposure to infectious agents is discussed in Chapter 5. This section discusses protection against sharps injuries and exposure to chemical and radiation hazards.

Box 3-3 Allergic to work

One nurse's experience with latex allergy began soon after she commenced practice in the perioperative environment. Within 6 months she had developed allergic dermatitis on her hands. At first she did not think too much of it and wore non-latex gloves only when she had a rash. When she began to develop generalised itching and wheals over her body, she presumed she had developed an allergy to hospital-laundered clothes. She accepted a position that involved less clinical work, but even so she began to get severe headaches and extreme fatigue at work and also became quite irritable. The symptoms suddenly escalated one day, about 7 years after commencing work in the perioperative environment. A rash began on her hands and soon developed into generalised itching, her head ached and she became extremely irritable. Then she began to experience a tight, crushing feeling in her chest, a hoarse voice and then a very hot flush. Her colleagues reacted quickly and administered treatment and she was able to go home that night, although her life was never the same.

While the organisation for which she works and its senior nursing executive have been very supportive, she has experienced financial, professional, personal and emotional ramifications. In addition:

- she can no longer work in the operating room or any other clinical area
- she has had to retrain and is no longer able to work with friends and colleagues with whom she was happy and comfortable
- she cannot be exposed to anyone who is wearing latex, including in their clothes, or even balloons delivered to the office for a party—a trip to the dentist is potentially life-threatening!
- because of her escalating reactions, this intensely private person has had to share information about her medical condition, as she is unable to manage her reactions on her own. Her colleagues have already saved her life on two occasions.

Anonymous personal communication (2007)

Sharps injury

During perioperative procedures, potentially dangerous items are constantly being handled and passed between members of the surgical team. They include obvious items such as intravenous needles, suture needles and scalpel blades, but also less obvious items, such as retractors (e.g. cats paws and skin hooks) and even sharp body pieces, such as splintered bone.

The likelihood of sharps injury increases during highly invasive, long procedures, with team member fatigue and fast pace also adding to the risk. Procedures identified as high risk also include those where the

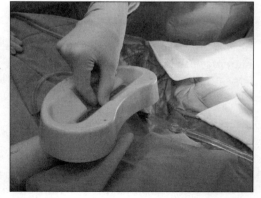

Figure 3-11 Correct method of passing a scalpel using a puncture-resistant container.

surgical team are operating in poorly visualised or confined spaces, such as the mouth or deep body cavities, and during some orthopaedic procedures (ACORN, 2006e; Girard, 2004; Silēn-Lipponen et al., 2005).

Some points to reduce the risk of injury include:

- paying special attention when passing/receiving sharp items and avoid rushing or being distracted
- organising the work area and determining with the surgeon a place where reusable sharp items are placed during surgical procedures
- using blunt needles (suture and drawing up) where possible
- no recapping or resheathing needles on the sterile field
- using retractors rather than hands to aid in visualising the operative site
- using a hands-free technique for passing sharp instruments, including a designated puncture-resistant container (kidney dish or flat tray) containing only one item at a time
- using a needle holder to remove sharps from applicators or handles rather than hands
- placing all disposable sharps in a designated sharps container as close to the point of use as possible and as soon as is practicable following use
- that the person who has used the sharp instrument is responsible for its safe disposal; at the end of a surgical procedure this responsibility falls upon the instrument nurse (ACORN, 2006e; Australian Department of Health and Ageing, 2004).

Radiation safety

There are two types of radiation—non-ionising and ionising. *Non-ionising radiation* is electromagnetic radiation and is emitted from electrical sources, such as power lines, from radiofrequency sources, such as mobile phones, and from the major ultraviolet source, the sun. *Ionising radiation* can be divided into two subgroups: non-harmful alpha, beta and neutron particles, with exposure through activities of normal living; and gamma rays and X-rays, which can penetrate deeper into tissue and can be harmful to humans. Metals such as lead are used to protect against these harmful rays (Australian Radiation Protection And Nuclear Safety Agency [ARPANSA], 2003).

Exposure to mechanical sources of ionising radiation that emit X-rays in the perioperative environment is often unavoidable, such as when image intensification (fluoroscopy) is used intraoperatively or when mobile radiography units are used to check the placement of internally placed appliances. Because the effects of ionising radiation are cumulative but at the same

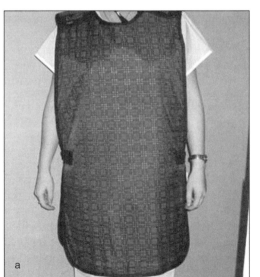
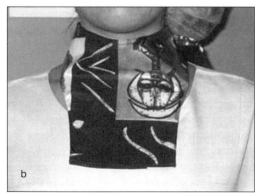

Figure 3-12 (a) X-ray gown and (b) thyroid protector.

time are not seen or felt, constant vigilance is required to ensure occupational exposure is kept to a minimum. The single most effective protection against exposure is avoidance (i.e. leaving the vicinity of the radiation source). If this is not possible, then standing behind mobile lead shields or using the equation—double the distance away from the source of radiation equals one-quarter of the exposure—applies (Phillips, 2007).

This may not be possible for some members of the surgical team and, when it is necessary to remain in the room, appropriate X-ray protective apparel that meets national standards, as described in Standards Australia AS/NZS 4543 (2000), must be worn, including protective gowns, thyroid shields, goggles and gloves. Whenever the gown is removed, it should be hung on special gown hangers or laid out flat, as any folds can crack the protective barrier and render it ineffective. Protective equipment must undergo regular checks to ensure its integrity has been maintained (Phillips, 2007). Staff regularly involved in patient screening may wear a dose meter badge that is regularly checked to identify if occupational exposure limits are exceeded (ARPANSA, 2003).

Where a member of staff is pregnant, the fetus should not be exposed to any more radiation than a member of the general public would be and the staff member should not be required to be in the operating room wherever possible (NOHSC, 2002).

Chemical safety

Many chemicals are used in the operating suite, including the detergents used to clean between cases, enzymatic cleaners used on instruments, high-grade disinfectants or chemical sterilising products, such as peracetic acid, and drugs, such as cytotoxic agents. Some basic principles always apply when handling chemical agents:

- Staff using chemicals should be aware of the requirements for safe use and handling, and also the treatment for accidental exposure, including where spill kits and other requirements are stored.
- Protective apparel must be worn. Depending on the chemical agent, this will include gloves and eye protection and sometimes long-sleeved impervious gowns and gauntlets. A number of chemicals emit vapours that may not be detectable by a normal sense of smell. Therefore, air concentrations should be monitored regularly and kept within prescribed limits, and exhaust fans, fume cabinets and exhaust ventilation units should be used.
- All chemicals should be stored, used and disposed of according to the manufacturer's recommendations and state/territory or national guidelines.
- Material Safety and Data Sheets (MSDS), which provide all relevant information about the chemical, should be available in all departments for easy reference (ACORN, 2006g).

CONCLUSION

The perioperative environment is a complex and challenging one, where a variety of activities and design measures aid in maintaining a clean and safe environment for the patient undergoing surgery and the staff who work in this area. These measures include a well-planned operating suite with designated traffic patterns, environmentally controlled conditions and cleaning schedules. Advancing technological and electrosurgical equipment and many hazardous substances that staff are exposed to in the operating suite can pose risks to patients and staff. Safety is paramount with the use of equipment, and staff require an understanding of how, when and why equipment is used to ensure safe practice. Finally, occupational health and safety issues for both the patient and the health care worker are essential elements for consideration in the perioperative environment.

CRITICAL THINKING EXERCISES

1. Operating suite layout

- How is your operating suite designed?
- Does your unit follow a clean-to-dirty traffic pattern?
- Draw a floor plan of your operating suite and shade the transition, unrestricted, semi-restricted and restricted areas in different colours.

2. Electrical safety

- Using the manufacturer's instructions, list any additional precautions you need to be aware of when applying a diathermy plate other than those mentioned in this text.
- What is the rationale for these precautions?

3. Technology of the operating suite

- Identify technologies used within your operating suite (e.g. laser, microscopes) and how these affect both the care of the patient and the work practices of perioperative nurses.

4. Occupational exposure

- Identify how staff and patients are protected from sharps injuries within the operating suite.
- How are sharps handled and disposed?

RESOURCES

Australasian Healthcare Facility Guidelines
    www.healthfacilityguidelines.com.au
Australasian Society of Clinical Immunology and Allergy
    www.allergy.org.au
Australian Department of Health and Ageing
    www.health.gov.au
Australian Radiation Protection and Nuclear Safety Agency
    www.arpansa.gov.au
NZNO National Division of Infection Control Nurses
    www.infectioncontrol.co.nz
Royal Children's Hospital, Melbourne, Biomedical Engineering
    www.rch.org.au/bme_rch/safety.cfm
Standards Australia
    www.standards.org.au

REFERENCES

Abreu, E., & Potter, D. (2001). Recommendations for renovating an operating theater at an emergency obstetric care facility. *International Journal of Gynecology & Obstetrics, 75,* 287–294.

ACORN. (2006a). *ACORN standards for perioperative nursing including nursing roles, guidelines, position statements and competency standards. G2. Management of the perioperative environment.* Adelaide: Australian College of Operating Room Nurses.

ACORN. (2006b). *ACORN standards for perioperative nursing including nursing roles, guidelines, position statements and competency standards. G3. Planning and design of the perioperative environment.* Adelaide: Australian College of Operating Room Nurses.

ACORN. (2006c). *ACORN standards for perioperative nursing including nursing roles, guidelines, position statements and competency standards. G4. Management of post anaesthesia recovery (PAR) unit.* Adelaide: Australian College of Operating Room Nurses.

ACORN. (2006d). *ACORN standards for perioperative nursing including nursing roles, guidelines, position statements and competency standards. S6. Environmental management.* Adelaide: Australian College of Operating Room Nurses.

ACORN. (2006e). *ACORN standards for perioperative nursing including nursing roles, guidelines, position statements and competency standards. S7. Infection prevention.* Adelaide: Australian College of Operating Room Nurses.

ACORN. (2006f). *ACORN standards for perioperative nursing including nursing roles, guidelines, position statements and competency standards. S16. Reprocessing of reusable items: cleaning, packaging, sterilisation and storage of sterile supplies.* Adelaide: Australian College of Operating Room Nurses.

ACORN. (2006g). *ACORN standards for perioperative nursing including nursing roles, guidelines, position statements and competency standards. S22. Use of high level disinfectant in the perioperative environment.* Adelaide: Australian College of Operating Room Nurses.

Anderson, K. (2004). Safe use of lasers in the operating room—what perioperative nurses should know. *AORN Journal, 79(1),* 171–172, 174, 176–182.

Australian and New Zealand College of Anaesthetists. (2006). *Professional documents of the Australian and New Zealand College of Anaesthetists. PS4. Recommendations for the post anaesthesia recovery room.* Retrieved October 10, 2007, from http://www.anzca.edu.au/infocentres/pdfdocs/PS4-2006.pdf 10.

Australian Department of Health and Ageing. (2004). Infection control guidelines for the prevention of transmission of infectious diseases in the health care setting. Retrieved October 27, 2007, from http://www.health.gov.au/internet/wcms/Publishing.nsf/Content/icg-guidelines-index.htm/$FILE/howto.pdf.

Australian Radiation Protection and Nuclear Safety Agency. (2003). Ionising radiation and health. Retrieved October 27, 2007, from http://www.arpansa.gov.au/radiationprotection/FactSheets/is_rad.cfm.

Australian Society of Clinical Immunology and Allergy. (2005). Guidelines for the hospital management of latex-allergic patients. Retrieved October 10, 2007, from www.allergy.org.au.

Ball, K. (2007). Surgical modalities. In J. C. Rothrock (Ed.). *Alexander's care of the patient in surgery* (13th ed.) (pp. 183–227). St Louis: Mosby.

Carthey, J. (2006). Australian e-guidelines for health facility design. In A. Dilani (Ed.). *Design and health IV. Future trends in healthcare design* (pp. 227–34). Stockholm: International Academy for Design & Health. Retrieved October 29, 2007, from http://www.fbe.unsw.edu.au/chaa/downloads/Papers_Presentations/2006_Carthey_AustralianE-Guidelines.pdf.

Carthey, J. (2007). Guiding quality design. *Hospital & Healthcare, March,* 21–3. Retrieved October 14, 2007, from http://www.fbe.unsw.edu.au/chaa/downloads/Papers_Presentations/2007_Carthey_Guiding QualityDesign.pdf.

Centre for Health Assets Australasia. (2006). Australasian healthcare facility guidelines. Retrieved October 10, 2007, from www.healthfacilityguidelines.com.au.

Davis, B. (2000). Perioperative care of patients with latex allergy. *AORN Journal, 72(1),* 47–53.

Girard, N. (2004). Countdown to safety. *AORN Journal, 79(3),* 575–576.

Gruendemann, B., & Mangum, S. (2001). *Infection control in the surgical settings.* Philadelphia: Elsevier.

Hauff, W. (2002). OR suite planning concepts. Retrieved October 15, 2007, from http://www.ordesignandconstruction.com/dp/concepts.htm.

Johnson & Johnson Gateway. (2007). Harmonic scalpel—technology overview. Retrieved October 26, 2007, from www.jnjgateway.com.

Lewis, S., Heitkemper, M., Dirksen, S., et al. (Eds.). (2007). *Medical-surgical nursing: assessment and management of clinical problems* (7th ed.). St Louis: Elsevier.

Meijsen, P., & Knibbe, H. (2007). Work-related musculoskeletal disorders of perioperative personnel in the Netherlands. *AORN Journal, 86(2),* 193–194, 196–198, 200–208.

NOHSC. (1995; republished March 2002). Recommendations for limiting exposure to ionizing radiation: 3022. Retrieved October 25, 2007, from www.ascc.gov.au.

NSW Health. (2005a). Manual handling incidents—NSW Public Health Services—policy/best practice guidelines prevention. Sydney: NSW Government, PD2005_224.

NSW Health. (2005b). Latex allergy—policy framework and guidelines for the prevention and management. Sydney: NSW Government, PD2005_490.

NSW Health. (2007). Alcohol-based skin preparations and fire in the operating theatre safety information. Sydney: NSW Government, SI:001/07.

Phillips, N. (Ed.). (2007). *Berry & Kohn's operating room technique* (11th ed.). St Louis: Mosby.

Queensland Health. (2002). Capital works guidelines building and refurbishment: infection control guidelines. Retrieved October 10, 2007, from http://www.health.qld.gov.au/cwamb/cwguide/Infection Guide.pdf.

Queensland Health. (2007). Waste management: waste segregation procedure. Retrieved October 24, 2007, from http://qheps.health.qld.gov.au/PHS/Documents/ehu/manual/31631.pdf.

Reed, D. (2003). Update on latex allergy among health care personnel. *AORN Journal, 78(3),* 409–412, 416–420, 422–426.

Rothrock, J. C. (Ed.). (2007). *Alexander's care of the patient in surgery* (13th ed.). St Louis: Mosby.

Royal Children's Hospital, Melbourne. (2008). Biomedical engineering—electrical safety. Retrieved January 2, 2007, from http://www.rch.org.au/bme_rch/safety.cfm.

SA Health Department. (2007). Surgical fire prevention and management. Guidance Notice no. GI 02/07. Adelaide: SA Health Department.

Shoup, A., Reilly, M., Kless, J. (2008). Nursing management: intraoperative care. In D. Brown, & H. Edwards (Eds.). *Lewis's medical–surgical nursing. Assessment and management of clinical problems* (2nd ed.) (p. 394). Sydney: Elsevier.

Silēn-Lipponen, M., Tossavainen, K., Turunen, H., Smith, A. (2005). Potential errors and their prevention in operating room teamwork as expressed by Finnish, British and American Nurses. *International Journal of Nursing Practice, 11,* 21–32.

Standards Australia. (2000). AS/NZS 4543 Protective devices against diagnostic medical X-radiation. Sydney: Standards Australia.

Standards Australia. (2003). AS/NZS 4187 Cleaning, disinfecting and sterilizing reusable medical and surgical instruments and equipment, and maintenance of associated environments in health care facilities. Sydney: Standards Australia.

Standards Australia. (2004a). AS/NZS 2500 Guide to the safe use of electricity in patient care. Sydney: Standards Australia.

Standards Australia. (2004b). AS/NZS 4173 Guide to the safe use of lasers in health care. Sydney: Standards Australia.

Waitemata District Health Board. (2002). Report into the operating fire incident. Retrieved October 25, 2007, from http://www.medsafe.govt.nz/downloads/alertWaitemata.pdf.

Woodhead, K., & Wicker, P. (2005). *A textbook of perioperative care.* Sydney: Elsevier.

Yip, E. (2003). Accommodating latex allergy concerns in surgical settings. *AORN Journal, 78(4),* 595–596, 598, 601–603.

FURTHER READING

Bayley, G., & McIndoe, A. (2004). Fires and explosion. *Anaesthesia & Intensive Care Medicine, 5(11),* 364–366.

Beesley, J., & Taylor, L. (2006). Reducing the risk of surgical fires: are you assessing the risk? *Journal of Perioperative Practice, 16(12),* 591–597.

Cunnington, J. (2006). Waste responsibility: or wasted opportunity. *Journal of Perioperative Practice, 16(10),* 476–480.

Francis, P. (2006). Evolution of robotics and implementing a perioperative robotics nurse specialist role. *AORN Journal, 83(3),* 630–632, 634–642, 644–646, 649–650.

Heath, J., Johanson, W., Blake, N. (2004). Healthy work environments: a validation of the literature. *Journal of Nursing Administration, 34,* 524–530.

Nelson, J., Biven, A., Shinn, A., et al. (2006). Microbial flora on operating room telephones. *AORN Journal, 83(3),* 607–608, 610–611, 613–617, 619–620, 622–626.

Scott, E., & Beswick, K. (2004a). Hazards of diathermy plume. Part 1. A literature review. *British Journal of Perioperative Nursing, 14(9),* 409–414.

Scott, E., & Beswick, K. (2004b). Hazards of diathermy plume. Part 2. Producing quantified data. *British Journal of Perioperative Nursing, 14(10),* 452–456.

4

Patient safety

Lois Hamlin, Marika Jenkins and Lisa Conlon

LEARNING OBJECTIVES

After reading this chapter, you should be able to:

• understand the anatomical and physiological concepts related to patient positioning
• explore the neurovascular and integumentary consequences associated with anaesthesia and surgery, and ways to manage them
• examine several core nursing interventions aimed at ensuring patient safety, including patient identification, 'time out' and the surgical count
• identify the nature and incidence of surgical adverse events and the perioperative nurse's role in preventing them
• discuss best practice when handling tissue specimens for pathology

---

KEY TERMS

inadvertent hypothermia
patient positioning
patient safety

patient transfer
surgical count
tissue specimen

tourniquet
venous thromboembolism

INTRODUCTION

Patient safety is a paramount consideration of all nurses, but nowhere is this a greater priority than in the perioperative environment. This is due to the vulnerability of the surgical patient and the nature of the environment itself. This chapter explores several key concepts and issues that are directly relevant to patient safety prior to (preoperatively), during (intraoperatively) and immediately following (postoperatively) anaesthesia and surgery. These include patient-specific issues, such as correct patient identification, appropriate preoperative patient assessment and correct patient positioning for the intended surgery. Pertinent anatomical and physiological aspects are also included, with nursing interventions aimed at keeping patients unharmed.

The perioperative environment and related technologies, such as the use of tourniquets, pose their own unique risks; these are explored, along with methods to eliminate, reduce or control them. The risk that surgery poses should not be underestimated, with adverse events occurring more commonly among surgical patients than other patient cohorts. Several of these originate in the perioperative environment.

PATIENT POSITIONING

To ensure the safety of the patient and surgical team members during patient transfer, a planned approach is needed, and one which takes into consideration patient assessment, the surgical position required and the transfer method to be used.

Patient transfer

Before **patient transfer** from a trolley or bed to the operating table (and vice versa) the following must be considered:

- patient history and comorbidities
- patient age and mobility
- skin integrity
- the surgical procedure to be undertaken
- the requirements of the surgeon, anaesthetists and others for access to the surgical site/airway
- the presence of drains, catheters, intravenous lines or other items/equipment
- the type and availability of transferring equipment
- available team members (Heizenroth, 2007).

These factors will influence the team's preparation and the equipment required to carry out the transfer. The patient's age and mobility have a bearing on the resources required; for example, a well, mobile patient may be able to move to the operating table unaided. In contrast, an elderly, frail or less mobile patient will require greater assistance from the surgical team and equipment. Particular care, planning and/or equipment is required to manage frail, elderly patients (those over 80 years of age) or obese patients, especially the morbidly obese (Phillips, 2007). The latter require specialised lifting equipment (e.g. 'hover mats') and purpose-designed operating tables and fittings to accommodate them safely intraoperatively, and to protect staff.

Care must be taken when transferring patients with intravenous (IV) cannula(s), IV infusions, drains, catheters or other items already in place. Their dislodgement can create discomfort (or worse) and replacing them is time-consuming. The planned procedure, patient condition, and staff and equipment availability will determine whether the initial transfer occurs while the patient is conscious or following induction of anaesthesia. Additionally, consideration must be given for patients who need repositioning intraoperatively (e.g. during bilateral hip replacement), as disorganised or unplanned movements during repositioning increase the risk of damage to the initial operative site, or can result in airway compromise.

Surgeon, anaesthetist and other staff requirements for patient access need to be considered. At all times, the anaesthetist must be able to ensure ventilatory adequacy, have IV access and address requirements for haemodynamic monitoring. The surgeon needs access to the surgical site and the instrument nurse needs to be able to maintain a sterile field throughout the procedure (Fell & Kirkbride, 2007). Consequently, the patient's position is often a compromise between competing demands for surgical access balanced against the patient's need for safety and protection (Hamlin, 2005a).

Transfer methods and rationales

All surgical team members have equal responsibility for maintaining patient safety during transfer. The anaesthetist, who has responsibility for the patient's airway, generally coordinates the lift (Heizenroth, 2007). The duty of the registered nurse (RN) is to assess the surgical environment and patient, and ensure that the most appropriate transfer equipment, positional aids and staff are available. During the transfer a team leader, usually (but not always) the anaesthetist, directs the team, including the patient if he or she is conscious. When the patient is anaesthetised and/or unconscious, this role will normally revert to the anaesthetist, as maintenance of a patent airway and ventilation are the main priorities (Fell & Kirkbride, 2007).

When conscious patients participate in the move, interventions needed to secure a safe transfer include:

* ensuring there is a minimal gap between the trolley and the operating table
* using the brakes on both the trolley and the operating table
* making sure the patient's gown is not caught in the trolley/bed side rails
* always placing a team member on the opposite side of the table to guide the patient.

Prior to and at each stage of the transfer of a fully conscious patient who is participating in the move, clear directions and explanations are necessary. The staff member instructing patients should direct patients to feel for the sides of the operating table as they move across, so they can be confident they are centrally located. The trolley or bed should not be moved away until the patient is securely positioned and confirms this. If the patient has reduced mobility and cannot move independently, then equipment such as patient slide boards, patient slide sheets or mechanical devices (e.g. hover mat) is needed. These devices enable patient transfer while reducing the risk of injury to staff members. A minimum of four staff members are generally required for the safe transfer of these patients, using the safety precautions described above.

When transferring unconscious or anaesthetised patients, the anaesthetist manages the patient's airway and supports the head. As the patient has no muscle control, limbs need safeguarding so they do not overhang the operating table, predisposing them to injury.

Arms are secured across patients' chest or by their side and legs are supported and moved in alignment with the body. These patients will have IV access and monitoring devices established and care must be taken not to obstruct or dislodge these.

Complications

Injuries associated with patient transfer include skin tears, joint dislocations, muscle and/or nerve damage, obstruction or dislodgement of IV infusion tubing or catheters, and patient falls (Phillips, 2007). Additionally, staff members risk injury. These incidents occur when:

- surgical team members are too few in number or are inexperienced
- the appropriate transferring devices and/or positional aids are absent, incorrectly used or are not used at all.

All surgical team members require manual handling training, as well as in-service education when new lifting equipment is commissioned. They must also be aware of the potential adverse events associated with transferring and positioning patients so that they can enact prevention strategies and lessen the risk of such events.

Patient positioning

Correct **patient positioning** is essential to performing a safe and unconstrained surgical procedure. The required position can place patients at risk of injury, particularly if the procedure is lengthy and/or requires general anaesthesia. Patients are positioned so that:

- there is optimum surgical access
- cardiovascular and respiratory functions are not compromised
- body alignment is maintained
- injury and falls are prevented (Hamlin, 2005a).

Patients are immobile during surgery and, because they are no longer able to change and control their body position, they are at an increased risk of developing decubitus ulcers, venous thromboembolism and pulmonary dysfunction (Fulbrook & Grealy, 2007). Additionally, unconscious, immobile patients cannot change an uncomfortable position or complain of discomfort or pain related to their position.

Anatomical and physiological considerations for patient positioning

A patient's tolerance of the stresses imposed by the surgical intervention depends significantly on the normal functioning of the vital systems, and each body system must be considered when planning the patient's position for surgery. The goals of positioning include the prevention of injury from pressure, crushing, stretching, pinching or obstruction (Phillips, 2007). The development of such injuries is influenced by the:

- position required for the procedure—all positions pose a risk, some more so than others
- patient's health status and physical condition—the very young and elderly patients present greater positional challenges (Phillips, 2007), as do obese patients (McChlery 2007), irrespective of any other underlying pathophysiology
- estimated length of time for the procedure and the associated immobility—the longer the surgery takes, the greater the risk (Phillips, 2007)
- type of operating table used and positioning aids required/available
- type of anaesthetic given
- planned surgical procedure (Fell & Kirkbride, 2007; Hamlin, 2005a; Heizenroth, 2007).

Integumentary system

The integumentary system can be injured as a result of the physical forces used to maintain the surgical position, as well as the way the patient is moved. These physical forces include pressure, shear and friction (Heizenroth, 2007).

Pressure

Pressure is the force placed on the patient's underlying tissues. In order to avoid injury, normal capillary interface pressure (23–32 mmHg) must be maintained (Phillips, 2007). Above these levels, blood flow and tissue perfusion become restricted (see Fig 4-1).

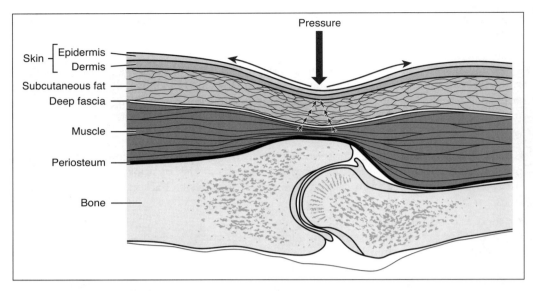

Figure 4-1 Effects of pressure on underlying tissue (Phillips, 2007, p 498).

Pressure can be created by the patient's own body weight as gravity presses it downwards. It can also be the weight of devices that are placed on or against the patient, such as instruments, drills or Mayo stands, or surgical team members leaning on the patient. Additionally, bed attachments or positioning aids can press against or pinch parts of the patient's body.

Shear

Shear is the movement of underlying tissue when the skeletal structure moves while the skin remains stationary. A parallel force creates shear. This occurs when, for example, the head of the operating table is lowered and the patient is placed in a head-down, supine position (Trendelenburg). As gravity pulls the skeleton down, the underlying tissues are stretched, folded or torn as they move with it. This can result in vascular occlusion as well as damaging the (static) skin (Heizenroth, 2007; Phillips, 2007).

Friction

Friction is the force produced when two surfaces rub against each other. Friction to the patient's skin occurs when the body is dragged across the operating table rather than lifted; this can abrade, burn or tear the patient's skin and encourage the development of decubitus ulcers (Hamlin, 2008).

The use of a pressure sore risk assessment tool preoperatively can assist in determining the degree of individual patient risk; however, there is limited evidence of the use of such tools (or other preoperative assessment activities) by perioperative nurses, although their use by ward staff may be indicated on the patient's preoperative checklist (Hurley & McAleavy, 2006).

Musculoskeletal system

During surgery and anaesthesia, normal protective reflexes (e.g. pain and pressure receptors) are depressed in the patient and muscle tone is lost as a result of the action of the pharmacological agents used. Consequently, patients are no longer able to respond normally if, during positioning and surgery, their muscles, tendons and/or ligaments are overstretched, twisted or strained, or body alignment is not maintained. Injury can also occur if dependent limbs fall over the edge of the operating table. It is advisable to use a body strap/safety belt to secure the patient to the operating table.

Nervous system

The action of anaesthetic agents, which cause a loss of sensation and protective reflexes, increases the likelihood of nerve injury occurring. In most cases these injuries occur due to the formation of lesions, secondary to damage incurred by undue pressure, stretching, twisting and pinching of nerves. The ulnar nerve is the nerve most frequently injured during the perioperative period (Rank, 2008). Table 4-1 outlines nerves that are commonly injured and the causes (Heizenroth, 2007).

Table 4-1 Peripheral nerves at risk of injury	
Nerve involved	**Cause of damage**
Brachial plexus	• Extending the arm beyond 90° angle, when an arm board is used • Pressure from shoulder braces (used in the Trendelenburg position) • Patient's body weight on the lower (dependent) arm when in lateral position • Arm unsecured and allowed to fall off the table • Splitting of the sternum during cardiac surgery • Over-rotation and lateral flexion of the patient's head (see Fig 4-2)
Median, radial and ulnar nerves	• Pressure on the medial aspect of the patient's arm when devices used to secure the arm are unpadded, or restraints are too tight • Patient's body weight on the lower (dependent) arm when in lateral position
Femoral nerve	• Inappropriate positioning of abdominal or vaginal retractors • Inappropriate positioning of the patient in the lithotomy position, resulting in over-stretching of the nerve (see Fig 4-3)
Sciatic nerve	• Hyperflexion of the hip joint, particularly when patient's legs are lifted incorrectly during surgery (see Fig 4-4)
Common peroneal nerve	• Pressure of the stirrups or leg-holding devices on the patient's calf when in lithotomy position (all variants) • Failure to place a pillow between the patient's legs when lateral position used • Incorrectly sized or inappropriate application of sequential compressive devices • Pressure from devices placed under the patient's knees (see Fig 4-5)

Heizenroth (2007)

Cardiovascular system

Anaesthetic agents can affect the cardiovascular system by causing peripheral vasodilation and subsequent pooling of blood in the extremities, resulting in hypotension (Heizenroth, 2007). Patient positioning can further affect this phenomenon; for example, a head-up, supine (reverse Trendelenburg) position will cause blood to pool in the lower extremities. Consequently, the movement of patients into and out of these positions must be measured and unhurried. Pregnant patients and those with large abdominal masses are particularly at risk of supine hypotensive syndrome (Fell & Kirkbride, 2007).

Adequate arterial circulation is necessary to perfuse tissue, and occlusion or pressure on peripheral vessels, such as might be caused by positioning devices or safety belts/straps, must be avoided (Phillips, 2007). For example, patients who are placed in the

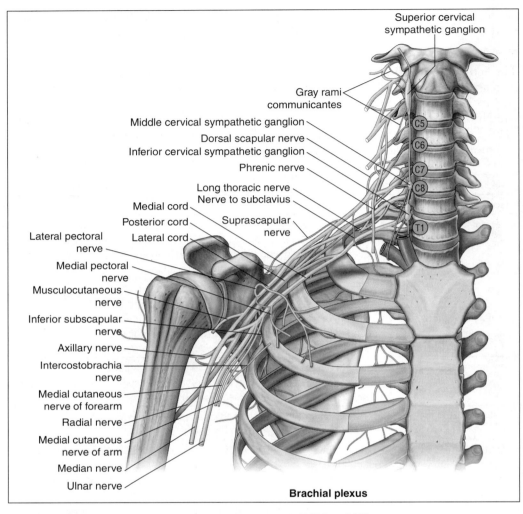

Figure 4-2 Brachial plexus on the right side (Drake et al., 2008, p 369).

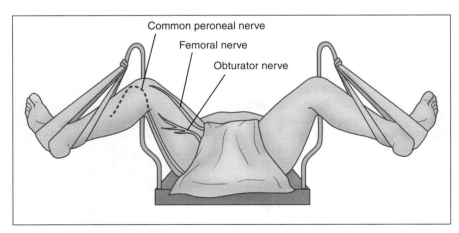

Figure 4-3 Nerves of the inner thigh (Rothrock, 2007, p 140).

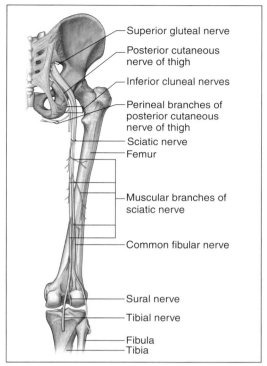

Figure 4-4 Right sciatic nerve (Drake et al., 2008, p 295).

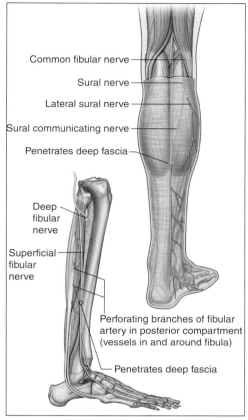

Figure 4-5 Right leg, lateral view (Drake et al., 2005, p 554).

lithotomy position are at risk of compartment syndrome in their lower limb(s), which occurs when perfusion pressure falls below tissue pressure in a closed anatomical space or compartment (Wilde, 2004). This can occur when patients are in this position for extended periods of time. Compartment syndrome develops via a combination of prolonged tissue ischaemia and subsequent reperfusion of muscle within a tight osseofascial compartment and, untreated, leads to necrosis and functional impairment (Dua et al., 2002).

Additionally, there is increased potential for thromboembolic episodes. Different positions, such as lithotomy, the time spent in these positions and the devices used to maintain them (e.g. safety belts, stirrups or other leg-holding devices) contribute to venostasis and the formation of thrombi.

Respiratory system

Respiratory function can also be compromised, particularly when a patient is positioned head-down, supine (Trendelenburg), which causes the abdominal viscera and organs to shift up towards the diaphragm, subsequently affecting inspiratory and expiratory tidal volumes. This is especially so for patients who are obese, pregnant or have pre-existing respiratory disease (Heizenroth, 2007). The prone position also impedes respiratory function. Ideally, patients should spend as little time as possible in these positions. Excessive pressure caused by positional aids or the placement of the patients' arms on the chest area should also be avoided (Heizenroth, 2007).

Surgical positions

There are several standard surgical positions, with a range of variations, and standard operating tables are designed to accommodate this range. Positions commonly used include:

- supine
- prone
- lateral
- lithotomy
- Trendelenburg and reverse Trendelenburg
- fracture table position
- Fowler's and semi-Fowler's position.

Supine position

In the supine position, patients lie on their back with their arms either secured at their sides or placed out on an arm board. This commonly used position provides access to the abdominal, peritoneal and cardiothoracic cavities, the extremities and the head and neck. Table 4-2 shows nursing interventions and rationales for this position.

Table 4-2 Supine position—nursing interventions and rationales	
Nursing intervention	**Rationale**
1. Padded operating table mattress—gel mattress or air support surface overlay.	1. Padding or special mattress overlays protect occiput, scapulae, olecranon, vertebrae, sacrum, coccyx and calcaneus from undue pressure.
2. Padding or gel pads placed on extensions or other positional aids as required (arm boards, J boards).	2. Protects ulnar nerve from pressure-induced damage.
3. Heels may require padding/sheepskin bootees, especially if the patient is elderly or malnourished.	3. Padding/bootees protect the heels from undue pressure.
4. Keep arm board(s) level with the operating table and at an angle of 90° (or less). Arm(s) must be loosely secured to the board.	4. Protects peripheral vasculature and nerves from damage, including the brachial plexus and ulnar nerve.
5. Legs remain uncrossed at the ankle.	5. Relieves undue pressure, decreasing risk of venous thrombosis.

Heizenroth (2007); Phillips (2007); Rank (2008)

Prone position

In the prone position, patients lie face down. This position is used when surgical access to the spine, rectum or dorsal areas of the extremities is required. It can be achieved on a standard operating table or it may require a specially designed table or table fittings (e.g. a laminectomy frame); the choice is determined by the particular surgical intervention.

The patient is anaesthetised in the supine position prior to transfer, and the airway is secured using a reinforced, flexible endotracheal tube (ETT), which will not kink. The ETT is secured with tape by the anaesthetist. The patient is then lifted and placed with the abdomen down on the operating table, and the face turned to one side. This transfer requires a minimum of four people to be executed safely, with one member of the team, usually the anaesthetist, supporting the patient's head and neck and safeguarding the airway at all times. The position requires additional padding (often in the form of multiple pillows or rolls on the operating table) to protect vulnerable areas, such as patient's ear and cheek on the dependent side, the breasts (females), genitalia (males), patellae and toes (see Fig 4-6). Table 4-3 shows nursing interventions and rationales for the prone position.

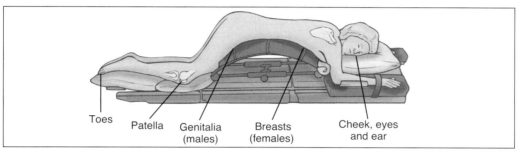

Toes   Patella   Genitalia   Breasts   Cheek, eyes
                   (males)   (females)   and ear

Figure 4-6 Prone position (Rothrock, 2007, p 154).

Table 4-3 Prone position—nursing interventions and rationales	
Nursing intervention	**Rationale**
1. Padded operating table mattress—gel mattress or pillows/rolls (or gel pad over laminectomy frame, if used).	1. Extra padding needed to protect vulnerable areas, such as the dependent cheek, ear, breasts (female), genitalia (males), patellae and toes.
2. Padding placed on extensions as required (arm boards, J boards). Arms should be secured loosely, palm down on padded arm boards and kept in natural alignment. They should not be allowed to hang over the edge of the operating table.	2. Arms are moved down and forward and placed on the arm board slowly and carefully to minimise the risk of damage to the brachial plexus. Arms hanging over the table edge can sustain damage to the radial nerve.
3. Eye ointment placed in both eyes, eyelids are then securely taped closed.	3. The eyes are vulnerable to corneal abrasion.

Heizenroth (2007); Phillips (2007); Rank (2008)

Lateral position

In the lateral position, which is used for procedures involving the chest, kidney or hip joint, the patient lies on the non-operative (dependent) side, with the operative side uppermost. It requires a selection of positional aids to secure the patient because there is a risk of the patient rolling forward or backwards intraoperatively or even falling off the table. The patient is anaesthetised in the supine position and then transferred or turned onto the dependent (non-operative) side. Positional aids include specially designed, padded arm rests (e.g. Carter Brain arm rest) to support the upper arm and keep it away from the operative area; table/safety straps and pliable bean bags are used to hold the patient securely to the operating table and maintain the position throughout surgery (Fig 4-7). Alternatively, padded table attachments (lateral supports or kidney braces), one at the patient's back and a larger one supporting the abdomen, can be used. Table 4-4 shows nursing interventions and rationales for the lateral position.

| **Table 4-4** Lateral position—nursing interventions and rationales ||
Nursing intervention	**Rationale**
1. Padded operating table mattress and padding placed on extensions as required (arm boards and arm supports) and pillow for head.	1. Protection of pressure points on the dependent side—the ear, shoulder, hip, ankle.
2. Pillow is placed between the patient's knees.	2. Knees will rub against each other, damaging the skin; additionally, undue pressure can damage the peroneal nerve.
3. Spine is kept in alignment by placing a pillow under the patient's head.	3. The spine is vulnerable to misalignment and twisting; this misalignment can place pressure on the dependent brachial plexus.
4. Patient needs securing by the use of either lateral supports (kidney braces) (padded) at the abdomen and back, or the use of devices such as bean bags or a Vac-Pac and a safety belt/table strap over the patient's upper thigh.	4. Prevents the patient from falling off the operating table. The use of these devices also ensures the patient does not move intraoperatively.
5. Ensure the patient's shoulder on the non-operative (dependent) side is not over-extended and the lower arm is protected, usually by securing it to an arm board. The upper arm is placed on a lateral arm support.	5. Prevents damage to the brachial plexus and ulnar nerve.
6. Kidney surgery requires access to the retroperitoneal area of the flank. In this case, the patient is positioned so that the lower iliac crest is below the lumbar break where the kidney bridge is located on operating table. The latter is subsequently elevated (slowly) and the operating table flexed to lower the patient's upper torso and legs.	6. Prevents the dependent flank area from compression and subsequent pooling of blood in the lower extremities.

Heizenroth (2007); Phillips (2007)

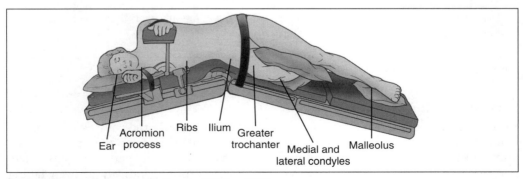

Acromion process · Ear · Ribs · Ilium · Greater trochanter · Medial and lateral condyles · Malleolus

Figure 4-7 Lateral position (Rothrock, 2007, p 156).

Lithotomy position

For patients undergoing gynaecological and urological surgery, the lithotomy position is required. This position involves the patient lying supine with their legs raised, abducted and secured in leg positioning devices (stirrups) to expose the perineal area. Depending on the surgical access required, the patient's legs can be held at various angles to the trunk—in a low, standard or high lithotomy position. These positions are maintained with the use of a range of stirrups, which are chosen after considering the type of surgery and proposed length of time for the procedure (Figs 4-8, 4-9). One of the most important precautions to consider while placing a patient in this position is the high risk of nerve damage and hip dislocation if the legs are not raised simultaneously, slowly and at the same angle and height at all times. Table 4-5 shows nursing interventions and rationales for the lithotomy position.

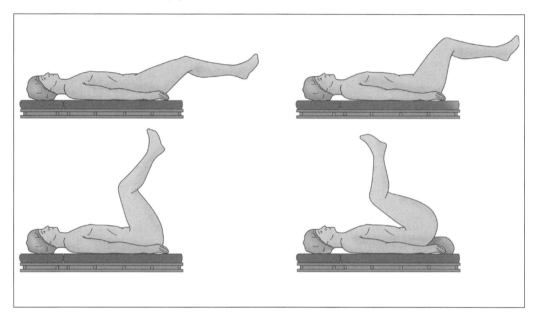

Figure 4-8 The four basic lithotomy positions (Rochrock, 2007, p 151).

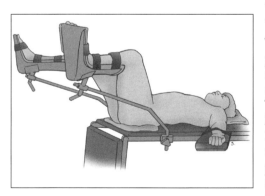

Figure 4-9 Lithotomy position using boot-type stirrups (Rothrock, 2007, p 151).

Trendelenburg position and reverse Trendelenburg position

These positions are variations of the supine position, with patients lying in a dorsal recumbent position (i.e. on their back). The operating table is tilted head down for the Trendelenburg position, which is used for lower abdominal or pelvic surgery (Fig 4-10). In the reverse Trendelenburg position, the patient is head-up, feet down, supine; this position is used for head and neck surgery and minimally invasive, upper abdominal procedures (Fig 4-11). An important factor to consider for these positions is the potential for shearing forces to occur. This

Table 4-5 Lithotomy position—nursing interventions and rationales

Nursing intervention	Rationale
1. Secure stirrups/leg-holding devices at an equal level and height.	1. Ensures stirrups do not dislodge during surgery, and that patient's hips and legs are kept in alignment.
2. Bring the patient's legs up into the stirrups simultaneously and slowly, keeping them at an equal height and angle at all times.	2. Maintains hip alignment and prevents dislocation of the hip joint and overstretching of the femoral nerve. Moving them slowly prevents blood pressure fluctuations.
3. The patient's buttocks should remain on the table at all times and not allowed to overhang.	3. Reduces the risk of lumbosacral strain and sciatic nerve damage.
4. Ensure the patient's fingers are not in the way of the stirrups when altering the height and position of the latter.	4. Fingers can be crushed in the stirrup joints.
5. Ensure the stirrup poles and foot rests are padded.	5. Padding decreases the risk of thrombus formation or compartment syndrome and protects the posterior tibial and common peroneal nerves.
6. Observe precautions for venous thrombosis during longer procedures.	6. Pressure on veins from the stirrups can increase the risk of thrombosis formation.

Heizenroth (2007); Phillips (2007); Rank (2008)

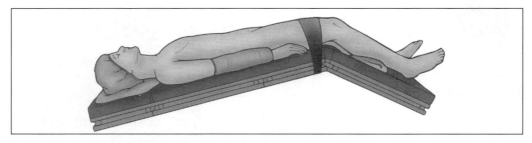

Figure 4-10 Trendelenburg position (Rothrock, 2007, p 149).

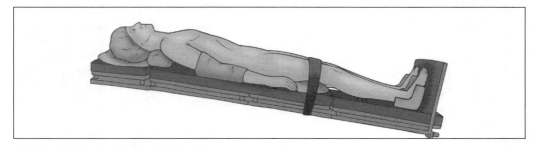

Figure 4-11 Reverse Trendelenburg position (Rothrock, 2007, p 150).

Table 4-6 Trendelenburg position—nursing interventions and rationales

Nursing intervention	Rationale
1. Observe the same precautions as for the supine position.	1. This is a supine position variation.
2. Break the table slightly, at the position of the knees.	2. Helps prevent the effects of shearing forces as it counteracts gravitation pull.
3. Observe respiratory function closely.	3. Severe angled tilts diminish the patient's lung capacity due to the pressure of the abdominal organs on the diaphragm, resulting in compression of the lung bases.
4. Observe lower extremity circulation.	4. May be diminished due to blood pooling in the head and upper torso.
5. Tilt patient in and out of the position slowly.	5. Avoids sudden blood pressure shifts.

Heizenroth (2007); Phillips (2007)

Table 4-7 Reverse Trendelenburg position—nursing interventions and rationales

Nursing intervention	Rationale
1. Observe the same precautions as for the supine position.	1. This is a supine position variation.
2. Tilt patient in and out of the position slowly.	2. Avoids sudden blood pressure shifts.
3. Ensure a padded foot rest is secured to the foot of operating table.	3. Prevents the patient slipping off the table.

Heizenroth (2007); Phillips (2007)

can be avoided by flexing the table at the position of the patient's knees, decreasing the gravitational pull towards the head in the Trendelenburg position. In the reverse Trendelenburg position, a padded table attachment can be fitted to the foot of the operating table on which the patient's feet rest. Tables 4-6 and 4-7 show nursing interventions and rationales for these positions.

Fracture table position

Some orthopaedic procedures require the use of a specialised fracture table. Indications for use include correcting fractured neck of femurs, as well as performing some femoral procedures, because the table permits rotation and manipulation of the operative limb. Patients are anaesthetised prior to transfer onto this table. They are placed supine on the fracture table with the pelvis stabilised against a well-padded perineal post to protect against genital injury (Fig 4-12). If needed, traction is achieved by restraining the injured limb in a well-padded, boot-like device that is part of the table's movable traction arm. The non-operative leg is placed on a support attachment and kept out of the way of the operative limb. The patient's arms are also secured away from the operative field. Nursing interventions associated with the supine position apply. Additionally, the distal lower extremity pulses should be assessed before, during and on case completion.

Fowler's/semi-Fowler's position

The patient placed in the Fowler's/semi-Fowler's position is secured in an upright (sitting) position. This position is used for surgery involving the ears, nose, shoulders, abdomen,

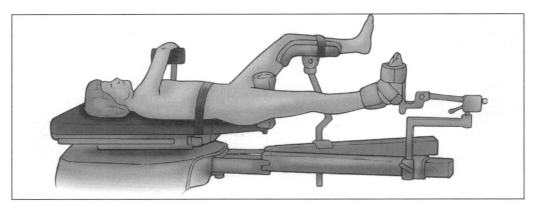

Figure 4-12 Fracture table position (Rothrock, 2007, p 150).

breasts and for some cranial procedures. In the latter case, the patient's head is held in a brace or supported with a head support attachment. Initially, the patient is placed in the supine position and, once anaesthetised, the table is manipulated so that the patient assumes a sitting position. The angle of this position (Fowler's or semi-Fowler's) will vary according to the type of surgery and access required. Arms must be secured so they do not fall by the side of the body. They can rest on a pillow on the lap. A padded footboard prevents foot drop. This position can cause pelvic pooling or venous stasis, resulting in cardiovascular instability, orthopaedic injury and tissue pressure injury/necrosis (Fell & Kirkbride, 2007). It can also cause an air embolus to enter the right atrium, necessitating immediate repositioning of the patient to a left lateral position, placement of the table into steep Trendelenburg and insertion of a central venous catheter to withdraw the air bubble (Phillips, 2007).

PREVENTION AND MANAGEMENT OF INADVERTENT HYPOTHERMIA

Inadvertent (or unplanned) **hypothermia** is a commonly reported complication in surgical patients (Bellamy, 2007; Bitner et al., 2007). It is defined as the unintentional drop of a patient's core body temperature to below 36°C during surgery (American Society of PeriAnesthesia Nurses, 2001; Welsh, 2002), although this figure is disputed. (*Note:* Planned hypothermia is an aspect of some cardiopulmonary and neurosurgical procedures.)

The development of a hypothermic state occurs due to the effect of anaesthetic agents on the metabolic rate and on hypothalamic function, resulting in a loss of normal physiological responses (e.g. shivering and vasoconstriction). Extrinsic factors, such as inadequately clothed surgical patients and a low ambient operating room temperature (which is normally 18–20°C), compound the risk, as does lengthy surgery, prolonged exposure of major abdominal/thoracic organs, and the use of cool IV and irrigating fluids (Hardman, 2007).

Patients who are at greater risk of developing inadvertent hypothermia include:

- those with underdeveloped or impaired thermoregulatory systems, for example, the elderly and neonates (Bitner et al., 2007)
- burns patients, in particular, those with full thickness burns to more than 10% of body surface area (BSA) or partial thickness burns (>25% BSA)
- immunocompromised patients who have depleted cellular level energy stores
- patients with small body mass (Rothrock, 2007)
- patients with conditions such as muscle atrophy, hyperthyroidism or hypothyroidism, arthritis, impaired metabolic rate or circulatory failure.

Hypothermia is categorised as mild (32–35°C), moderate (30–32°C) or severe hypothermia (<30°C), with various symptoms that transpire in each of these classifications (Bellamy, 2007; Saullo, 2007).

Complications

The consequences of inadvertent hypothermia, which are dependent on the change in core temperature, include:

*   decrease in cardiac output
*   reduced tissue oxygenation
*   metabolic acidosis
*   oliguria
*   altered platelet and clotting function
*   reduced hepatic blood flow and slower drug metabolism
*   postoperative shivering and increased oxygen consumption
*   myocardial ischaemia
*   increase length of stay in postanaesthesia recovery unit
*   increased risk of postoperative infection due to suppression of the immune system (Bitner et al., 2007; Hardman, 2007).

Management strategies

Hypothermia can be prevented if the appropriate strategies are employed. These include patient assessment, regular temperature monitoring of susceptible patients and, if necessary, active warming during the perioperative period. Some evidence suggests that preoperative (or pre-induction) active warming of patients prevents or decreases hypothermia (due to heat redistribution) and is easier to implement and more efficacious than intraoperative warming (Bitner et al., 2007; Kiekkas & Karga, 2005); however, this is disputed (Mahajan, 2007) and is not a widespread practice. Prior to the commencement of surgery the nurse should assess the patient, environment and procedure to be performed in order to establish appropriate preventive measures. These measures may include:

*   the use of active warming devices, such as forced air warming devices or warming mattresses
*   the use of fluid warmers for IV fluids
*   the warming of irrigation fluids used intraoperatively
*   using blankets and head wrapping
*   increasing the ambient room temperature and humidity, when feasible, for example, during neonatal or burns surgery (Rothrock, 2007).

TOURNIQUETS

Tourniquets are often used during surgery on limbs and digits to constrict their blood flow, resulting in a bloodless field at the distal surgical site. These devices may be mechanical (e.g. a blood pressure cuff), or electronic or pneumatic, which utilise a heavier, more secure type of blood pressure cuff, for use on the arms or legs (Phillips, 2007). Pneumatic tourniquets consist of an inflatable cuff connected via tubing to a pressure regulator, compressed gas supply and display unit. Simpler devices, such as rubber tubing or bands, are used on digits.

Recommendations for the safe use of tourniquets include the correct application of the cuff, use of the correct amount of pressure, accurate patient observation and documentation of use, and directions for cleaning and decontamination of cuffs. As there are several differing (and complex) types of tourniquets, specific manufacturer's recommendations should guide use, in conjunction with departmental policy and procedures.

The use of tourniquets is associated with significant risk (McEwen, 2007; O'Connor & Murphy, 2007). Tourniquets compress underlying soft tissue, as well as deprive the area of blood supply. Consequently, they have been linked to soft tissue injuries involving skin, muscle, nerves and vasculature; additionally, their use can have systemic sequelae (Tuncali et al., 2003). Complications include:

- nerve injury (reported most frequently) (McEwen, 2007; O'Connor & Murphy, 2007)
- post-tourniquet syndrome (sustained postoperative swelling of limb)
- compartment syndrome
- pressure sores and chemical burns
- digital necrosis
- toxic reactions
- fatal or near-fatal pulmonary embolism and deep vein thrombosis after deflation (McEwen, 2007; O'Connor & Murphy, 2007).

Tourniquet use

When selecting a cuff, the length and width should be individualised for each patient (AORN, 2007). This will depend on the shape and diameter of the extremity and the particular procedure the patient is undergoing (AORN, 2007). The widest cuff possible within any given length should be selected because wider cuffs occlude blood flow at lower pressures. The length of the cuff also needs to be considered; it should overlap by at least 7.5 cm but no more than 15 cm, as excessively long cuffs increase pressure on the underlying tissue and wrinkle the underlying skin. The choice of site of the cuff remains subject to debate (O'Connor & Murphy, 2007).

Prior to tourniquet inflation, an Esmarch's (rubber) bandage is wrapped around the operative limb to exsanguinate it. To avoid skin damage, soft, wrinkle-free padding is wrapped around the limb before applying the tourniquet cuff. To prevent skin preparation solutions from collecting under the cuff and causing skin maceration or burns, an impervious, U-shaped drape is placed around the cuff. The requisite cuff (or inflation) pressure varies, depending on the patient's limb occlusion pressure (LOP) (Table 4-8). Ideally, LOP is determined using a Doppler stethoscope (AORN, 2007; O'Connor & Murphy, 2007).

Table 4-8 Tourniquet inflation pressures (adults)

Limb occlusion pressure (LOP)	Pneumatic cuff pressure
<130 mmHg	Add 40 mmHg pressure
131–190 mmHg	Add 60 mmHg pressure
>190 mmHg	Add 80 mmHg pressure

For paediatric patients, adding 50 mmHg to LOP is recommended (AORN, 2007).

The use of pneumatic tourniquets is contraindicated in patients with vascular disease, impaired limb circulation, or in the presence of an arteriovenous access fistula because of the increased risk of injury and paralysis (McEwen, 2007). Complications from tourniquet use arise due to excessive cuff pressures and/or length of inflation time. However, there is an apparent paucity of evidence to determine safe time periods of tourniquet ischaemia; recommendations vary from 1 to 2 hours, with a 10–15 minute release of pressure before reinflation (AORN, 2007; McEwen, 2007). In general, upper limbs tolerate shorter periods of ischaemia compared to lower limbs (AORN, 2007).

Newer, automated tourniquets now incorporate pressure-control devices that measure the LOP. These devices stop inflating the cuff once the minimum pressure necessary to occlude the arterial blood flow, distal to the cuff, is reached. Non-automated tourniquets still require the operator of the unit to pre-set the inflation pressure. The use of rubber bands or tubing (e.g. a Penrose drain) on digits precludes the use of pressure monitoring devices. However, as with pneumatic tourniquets, the operative digit should be assessed before and after application, and tourniquet use documented.

The circulating nurse should assess the use of the pneumatic tourniquet regularly to:

- monitor the inflation pressure to detect fluctuations
- monitor and record the duration of inflation and inform the surgical team when the cuff has been inflated for 1 hour, and every 15 minutes thereafter (Phillips, 2007)
- document the use of tourniquet, including cuff location, name of the staff member who applied it, the tourniquet's serial number, devices used for skin protection, cuff pressure, and times of inflation and deflation
- assess skin integrity under the cuff before and after use.

ENSURING CORRECT PATIENT/SITE OF SURGERY

A safe environment for surgical patients requires a planned and systematic approach to perioperative care delivery. Such an approach requires the implementation of policies and procedures that define the actions of staff. A key aspect of surgical patient safety is to ensure that the right patient undergoes the intended surgical intervention. However, humans err, mistakes are made and patients undergo the wrong surgery, or the wrong site or side is operated on. Rogers et al. (2004) identified several common factors that are associated with these particular adverse events. These factors included emergency cases, procedures performed under time pressures, uncommonly seen patient characteristics, procedures being performed by multiple surgeons or numerous procedures being performed on the one patient concurrently. While the incidence and causes of these adverse events are discussed in detail in Chapter 11, it is sufficient to say here that what is known about these adverse events, notwithstanding that such knowledge is imperfect, has led to the collaborative development and implementation of a five-step protocol to reduce or eliminate the incidence of wrong patient/site/side surgeries. Table 4-9 describes the protocol.

Table 4-9 Protocol for ensuring correct patient, correct site, correct procedure	
Step 1	Check the consent form or procedure request form is correct
Step 2	Mark the site for the surgery or other invasive procedure
Step 3	Confirm identification with the patient
Step 4	Take team 'time out' in the operating room, treatment or examination area
Step 5	Ensure appropriate diagnostic images and implants are available

Australian Commission for Safety and Quality in HealthCare (2004)

'Time out' procedure

The confirmation of the patient and procedure happens at several stages of the patient's perioperative journey, with the final check occurring in the operating room immediately prior to surgery. The 'time out' procedure is initiated in the presence of the patient and involves all members of the surgical team, who must be present and must cease all other activities at this juncture. 'Time out' requires participating staff to verbally confirm the presence of the correct patient, the marking of the surgical site (when applicable), the planned procedure and the availability of surgical implant(s), if needed. Documentation of this procedure is necessary, although it differs between health care facilities. It is the individual nurse's responsibility to follow the facility's process for 'time out' and document this.

THE SURGICAL COUNT

The purpose of the **surgical count** is to ensure that all items used during a surgical procedure are removed and can be accounted for on completion of the procedure. This activity is performed to reduce the risk of injury to the surgical patient associated with the inadvertent retention of a surgical item (ACORN, 2006) and is considered the 'gold standard' to manage this risk (Gibbs, 2003). The count is the responsibility of the perioperative RN in charge of the case.

Perioperative nursing standards guide the conduct of a count (ACORN, 2006; Perioperative Nurses College [NZNO], 2003). These standards identify roles and responsibilities, spell out a detailed process for conducting a count and provide rationales. They also describe actions to take in emergency surgery or in the event of an incorrect surgical count being recorded. In Australia, the use of the Australian College of Operating Room Nurses' (ACORN) counting standard has been established in common law as the standard for the practice of counting (Staunton & Chiarella, 2008). However, counting is not always sufficient to prevent the inadvertent retention of surgical items (Gibbs, 2003; Gibbs & Auerbach, 2001; Hamlin, 2005b) and other ways to prevent this, which take a systems approach to error reduction, are being developed or trialled; for example, electronic tagging (Fabian, 2005) or the insertion of radiofrequency identification chips in surgical sponges and instruments. The latter has proven successful in pilot studies (Hamlin, 2005b; Macario et al., 2006).

The count

Even though there are minor differences in the published practice standards, the ACORN standard, S3: *Counting of accountable items used during surgery* (2006) or that published by the Perioperative Nurses College (NZNO) (2003) both provide a comprehensive approach to the surgical count.

Although not all surgical items must be counted per se, the RN in charge of the case is accountable for them. Those items that must be counted include:

- instruments recorded on the tray list
- absorbent items, including sponges, swabs, patties, cherries, peanuts, eye swabs (strolls), gauze strips, cotton wool balls and skin preparation swabs
- sharps, including needles, detachable blades, disposable scalpels and diathermy tips
- vascular items, comprising vessel loops ('ligaloops'), 'snuggers', cardiac snares, tapes, ligature reels, 'ligaboots' (rubber shods), clip cartridges and disposable bulldog clips
- disposable retraction instruments, for example, fish hooks and visceral retractors
- any additional items opened during the procedure.

Other items can be counted at the discretion of the RN in charge and/or the instrument nurse (ACORN, 2006).

General principles, and roles and responsibilities of staff

All facilities should formulate a policy that outlines a standardised approach to counting and ensure that their surgical teams comply with it.

- The circulating nurse and the instrument nurse have primary responsibility for the count and work collaboratively with other members of the surgical team to ensure all surgical items are retrieved on completion of surgery.
- The count is the responsibility of the RN in charge of the case, and the surgeon must allow sufficient time for its completion.
- The role of the surgeon is to carry out a manual and visual search of the operative field to ensure that all instruments and equipment are removed prior to completion of the surgical procedure.
- The circulating nurse documents the count in the patient's intraoperative nursing record.
- Disposable, accountable items used must be handled in a way that reduces the risk of the item being retained.

If an accountable item is opened by the anaesthetic team during the surgical procedure, it is the responsibility of that team member to inform the instrument nurse and/or circulating nurse, who must sight the item and document it on the count sheet.

Undertaking the surgical count

Prior to doing the count, the following actions are needed:

- Sponges, swabs, peanuts, cherries, patties and eye strolls are checked for uniformity and packaged in multiples of five.
- Items should be packaged so they cannot be separated during transfer to the sterile field prior to counting.
- Haemostat (artery) forceps are bundled in sets of five, whenever possible, for sterilising. It is acknowledged that some trays will contain a single haemostat forceps.
- Tray lists are used to identify all of the items in any given tray (ACORN, 2006).

The counting procedure

The counting procedure is as follows:

- Completion of a minimum of three counts of all accountable items (and any other items the instrument nurse determines should be counted) is recommended.
- A count is performed whenever accountable items are used during a surgical procedure.
- The count is carried out by two nurses, one of whom must be an RN, with both nurses counting aloud together.
- The initial count is performed immediately prior to the commencement of the surgical procedure. After the completion of the first count, all accountable items remain in the operating room until the completion of the surgery and the final count. The tray list is used to check that all instruments in the tray are accounted for prior to the commencement of the surgical procedure. This list is signed by the instrument nurse prior to the return of the tray for cleaning and resterilisation.
- All accountable items remain in their packing until counted. All items are then separated and counted. When counting swabs and sponges, each is opened so both nurses can see the X-ray detectable marker.
- If the count is interrupted, counting of that item is recommenced.
- Additional items added during the surgical procedure are counted and recorded.
- The second count is undertaken and recorded at the commencement of closure of the cavity or wound.
- A final count is performed and documented on commencement of the closure of the skin or an equivalent closure.

- The surgeon is informed of the outcome of each count.
- Additional counts can be undertaken at any time during the surgical procedure. Individual facility policies will provide guidance.
- A progressive 'counting away' technique is used.
- The surgeon is notified immediately of any discrepancy in the count and appropriate interventions are undertaken to rectify this situation (see section on 'incorrect count').
- The count sheet is signed by the two nurses responsible for the count.
- On completion of the surgical procedure, the surgeon also documents the outcome of the count in accordance with hospital/facility policy.
- The completed count sheet is included in the patient's medical record.
- All accountable items are removed from the operating room only at the end of the surgical procedure and prior to the commencement of the next surgical procedure (ACORN, 2006).

Limitations with the count standard/procedure

The key weaknesses of the counting standard are the prescriptive nature of the procedure, the lack of clarity about what constitutes an 'accountable' item and the Standard's failure to take into account current technologies and the use of plastics and other non-X-ray detectable items (Hamlin, 2005b). Nonetheless, until emerging technologies and other systematic ways to manage the risk of inadvertent retention of surgical items are developed, counting remains a key activity for perioperative nurses to ensure that no items are unaccounted for at the end of a case.

Incorrect count

According to Rothrock (2007), an incorrect count occurs when the items recorded on the count sheet do not match the actual number of items counted in the final count. If there is a discrepancy, the instrument nurse notifies the surgeon, anaesthetist and the nurse in charge of the operating suite. Such an eventuality requires an immediate search of the surgical environment, including the surgical wound, surgical field, drapes and linen, the floor and garbage receptacles. If the missing item is not located, an X-ray is obligatory prior to the patient leaving the operating room (unless contraindicated by the patient's condition) and the outcome documented. If the missing item is not located, the count sheet must reflect this. Additionally, a record of the incident, including actions taken to address it, is necessary in line with facility policy.

Research into the incidence of miscounts and incorrect counts has identified that some of these are errors of documentation (Butler et al., 2003). Documentation errors are associated with nursing staff changes intraoperatively and occur more frequently during elective cases. This research also uncovered some evidence of complacency among operating room staff regarding the count, which has been identified by others (Hamlin, 2005b).

Emergency situations

In an emergency and when the patient's condition is critical, normal counting procedures are waived and an X-ray is performed at the end of the surgical intervention (or when the patients' condition is sufficiently stable) (ACORN, 2006; Perioperative Nurses College [NZNO], 2003). This practice was appropriate when established decades ago (i.e. before the advent of micro-needles and micro-instrumentation); however, it continues in many operating rooms today (Jackson & Brady, 2008) notwithstanding the limitation of X-rays, which fail to identify many surgical items used in practice currently (Macilquham et al., 2003). The surgeon must be informed when a count is not completed and participate in actions to redress the consequences.

CARE AND HANDLING OF SPECIMENS

Many surgical procedures involve the collection of a specimen for pathology testing. The removal of a **tissue specimen** frequently necessitates an invasive process and it can be potentially devastating if mishandling/loss of the specimen occurs (Watson & Gregory Crum, 2005). Cases of specimen mishandling have resulted in misdiagnoses and, in some instances, patients have been required to undergo additional surgery to remove more tissue for pathology (Watson & Gregory Crum, 2005). In other cases, patients have received inappropriate or aggressive forms of treatment because it has not been possible to provide a satisfactory diagnosis with the remaining tissues (Watson & Gregory Crum, 2005). As a result, it is important to establish clear and unambiguous processes for the collection and transportation of specimens. Additionally, perioperative nurses need to be empowered to manage instances of tissue/specimen mishandling (e.g. if a surgeon drops a tissue sample) via a formal incident reporting system (Espin et al., 2007).

Recommended practices provide guidance for the handling, containment, identification, labelling and transporting of specimens within the perioperative environment and beyond. These are outlined in Table 4-10.

Table 4-10 Correct handling and transportation of specimens	
Recommended practices	**Process**
Ensure an accurate patient and specimen identification procedure is undertaken.	• Confirm labels to be used for specimen identification contain correct patient details. • Specimen identification should be commenced at the time of removal with verbal and written communication between surgeon and nursing staff. • Communication should involve a 'write down, read back' process. • Identification of the specimen should include site, type of tissue, diagnosis (if known) and any other relevant clinical information. • All specimens removed from the patient should be documented on the specimen container, perioperative nurse's report and pathology form.
Provide secure collection and handling of specimen without contamination.	• Specimens should be contained and then labelled as soon as possible after collection to prevent mishandling and identification errors. • Any use of preservative, or the need for fresh or frozen tissue sections, should be established with the surgeon prior to the commencement of the procedure and again at the time of collection. • Size of specimen and amount of required preservative solution should be considered when selecting the most appropriate container. • All containers need to be rigid, impervious, leak-proof and have tight-fitting lids. • Staff should use personal protective equipment.

(contd)

Table 4-10 Correct handling and transportation of specimens *(contd)*

Recommended practices	Process
Provide accurate labelling of the specimen container.	• Patient identification labels should be securely attached to the specimen container. • All labels should be placed on the container and not the lid. This will ensure the correct details are not lost when the lid is removed in the pathology department. • The container also needs to be labelled in pen with specimen type, site, and date and time of the collection.
Establish accurate communication and documentation of the collection and chain of custody.	• Health facilities should establish methods to document the collection of pathology specimens. • Log books are commonly used to document specimens that are taken from the operating suite to the pathology department. Information in these logs should include type of specimen, patient identification details, diagnosis, studies required, date and time of collection, surgeon's name and contact details, and the name of the nurse who prepared the specimen for transport. • Whenever possible, printed documentation, such as patient identification labels, should be used. • When details are handwritten, they should be clear and legible. • All documentation logged should establish a clear chain of custody from time of specimen removal to arrival in the pathology department.
Ensure safe and appropriate transportation of specimen to pathology laboratory.	• All specimens collected in the operating suite should be documented in the log book. • This log book may contain a place for the signature of the pathology technician, who takes custody of the specimen. • Staff need to check that all documentation and labels on the specimen containers are fully completed prior to sending them to the pathology department.

AORN (2006)

While guidelines such as these are useful, they must be used in conjunction with other practices, such as those associated with infection control and the use of personal protective equipment, and the management of specimens subjected to regular audit.

PREVENTION AND MANAGEMENT OF VENOUS THROMBOEMBOLISM

The development of venous thrombosis and subsequent pulmonary embolus (PE) make up two components of the condition of **venous thromboembolism** (VTE). VTE is a mostly preventable surgical complication, yet remains a significant cause of postoperative morbidity and mortality (White, 2003). The factors postulated by Virchow (Mahajan, 2007) as contributing to venous thrombi (and therefore PE) are:

• changes in the composition of blood (hypercoagulability)
• damage to walls of blood vessels
• venous stasis.

Patients at increased risk of developing VTE are:

- the elderly
- those undergoing major surgery, especially pelvic procedures
- orthopaedic patients, especially those undergoing reconstructive surgery
- smokers
- the obese
- those with a history of thromboembolism
- trauma victims
- those with metabolic disorders, malignancy or blood dyscrasias
- those on oral contraceptive pill and hormone replacement medications (Mahajan, 2007; Parnaby, 2004; Turpie et al., 2002).

Intraoperative risks for the development of VTE include:

- the length of surgery
- venous compression
- hypovolaemia
- hypotension
- hypothermia.

Use of a tourniquet may also contribute to VTE (Buggy, 2007; Heizenroth, 2007; McEwen, 2007; Philips, 2007).

Between 70% and 90% of patients with VTE are asymptomatic (Cantrell et al., 2007; Mahajan, 2007). The symptoms that may develop are summarised in Table 4-11. A greater risk to the patient occurs if a thrombus breaks off and travels via the venous system to the right ventricle, and from there to the pulmonary artery or one of its branches, resulting in a PE, which can be life-threatening. Most PE originate in the lower limb or pelvic veins (Mahajan, 2007).

Table 4-11 Signs and symptoms of VTE	
Deep vein thrombosis	**Pulmonary embolism***
Calf tenderness and pain, especially on dorsiflexion (positive Homan's sign)	Tachycardia
Swelling and warmth of the affected limb	Dyspnoea
Low-grade fever	Chest pain
Skin colour changes (erythema)	Hypotension
	Hypoxaemia
	Acute decrease in end-tidal carbon dioxide concentration
	Cardiovascular collapse/sudden death

*Intraoperative and postoperative complication.

Cantrell et al. (2007); Mahajan (2007)

Management

Both pharmacological and non-pharmacological therapies and actions can be used to prevent VTE. These are outlined in Table 4-12.

Pre-emptive management of at-risk patients or immediate treatment of a deep vein thrombosis (DVT) may prevent the subsequent development of PE. However, appropriate, local VTE risk-assessment guidelines are essential so that prophylactic measures are used in the correct at-risk group but are avoided in low-risk groups (Illingworth & Timmons, 2007).

Table 4-12 Prevention of VTE

Phases	Management	
	Pharmacological	*Non-pharmacological*
Preoperative	• Cease oral contraceptive medication at least 6 weeks prior to elective surgery. • Cease complementary/ alternative therapies, such as garlic, evening primrose oil, ginseng. • Prophylactic anticoagulation in susceptible patients (e.g. those undergoing lengthy, pelvic surgery).	• Application of correctly fitted anti-embolytic (or graduated compression) stockings (GCS). • Patient education and practice of deep breathing and limb exercises, and the correct use of GCS.
Intraoperative	• Prophylactic anticoagulation with low-molecular-weight heparin.	• Application of sequential compression devices. • Correct positioning of the patient and careful use of positional aids.
Postoperative	• Continue anticoagulation subcutaneously or orally (for longer term use, e.g. warfarin).	• Early ambulation. • Continued use of GCS. • Continuation of deep breathing and leg exercises, especially if prolonged bed rest is anticipated. • Ensure adequate hydration.

Bryant & Knights (2007); Heizenroth (2007); Mahajan (2007); Phillips (2007)

CONCLUSION

This chapter has provided information pertinent to patient safety within the perioperative setting. It has outlined basic anatomical and physiological considerations related to patient transfer and positioning, the potential sequelae for incorrectly positioned patients and the interventions necessary to avoid them. Common complications related to surgery, such as inadvertent (unplanned) hypothermia and venous thromboembolism, and the measures used to prevent or ameliorate them, have been explored, and their limitations in practice noted. This chapter has also examined the policies, procedures and standards that underpin correct site surgery and the surgical count, and presented some of the research that highlights the weaknesses of them. Nonetheless, these practices and their underpinning standards provide guidance for perioperative nursing care, and they evolve continuously. Best practice related to the care and handling of tissue specimens has been addressed, along with caring for patients when tourniquets are used to facilitate surgery.

Although trite, it is true that no health care professional sets out to do harm; however, humans err, mistakes are made and patients experience adverse events. The sections covered in this chapter have provided rationales for the interventions commonly used to prevent these adverse events and ensure the patient is provided with the safest possible care.

CRITICAL THINKING EXERCISES

1. Patient transfer

You are the circulating nurse working in an orthopaedic operating room. Your patient has been wheeled into the operating room by the anaesthetist and you are preparing to transfer her onto the operating table.

- Discuss the interventions (with rationales) that you need to use to complete this transfer safely for the patient and the team.

2. Pressure area care

Your patient is undergoing a laminectomy and has been anaesthetised and placed in the prone position on a laminectomy frame on the operating table.

- Discuss the risks associated with this position, and the pressure-reduction and other strategies to avoid them.

3. Inadvertent (unplanned) hypothermia

You are allocated the role of anaesthetist nurse for a hemicolectomy procedure on a 72-year-old female. Two hours into the procedure, you notice that the patient's temperature has dropped from a baseline of 36.5°C to 35°C.

- What would your response be to this situation?
- How could this have been prevented?

4. The surgical count

You have recently commenced working in a busy perioperative suite as a new graduate registered nurse. You have been allocated to the role of circulating nurse for a busy gynaecological surgical list.

- How often are you required to complete a surgical count during each case?
- Why and at what stages of the surgical procedure do you carry out these counts?
- Identify and discuss with a colleague two reasons why a count may be incorrect.

RESOURCES

American Association of Nurse Anesthetists
    www.aana.com
American Society of periAnesthesia Nurses
    www.aspan.org
Anesthesiology
    www.anesthesiology.org
Association for Perioperative Practice
    www.afpp.org.uk
Association of periOperative Registered Nurses
    www.aorn.org
Australian College of Operating Room Nurses
    www.acorn.org.au
Australian and New Zealand College of Anaesthetists
    www.anzca.edu.au
International Federation of Nurse Anesthetists
    www.ifna-int.org
International Federation of Perioperative Nurses
    www.ifpn.org.uk

Operating Room Nurses Association of Canada
www.ornac.ca
ORNursesDownUnder
http://www.angelfire.com/nd/ornursesdownunder
Patient Safety Institute
www.ptsafety.org
Perioperative Nurses College of the New Zealand Nurses Organisation
www.pnc.org.nz
Preoperative education
http://www.aorn.org/patient
Preop Surgery Centre
www.preop.com

REFERENCES

ACORN. (2006). *ACORN standards for perioperative nursing including nursing roles, guidelines, position statements and competency standards.* Adelaide: Australian College of Operating Room Nurses.

American Society of PeriAnesthesia Nurses. (2001). Patient temperature: an introduction to the clinical guideline for the prevention of unplanned perioperative hypothermia. *Journal of PeriAnesthesia Nursing, 15(3),* 151–155.

AORN. (2006). *Standards, recommended practices and guidelines. Recommended practices for handling specimens in the perioperative practice setting.* Denver, CO: Association for periOperative Registered Nurses.

AORN. (2007). *Standards, recommended practices and guidelines. Recommended practices for the use of the pneumatic tourniquet in the perioperative practice setting.* Denver, CO: Association for periOperative Registered Nurses.

Australian Commission for Safety and Quality in HealthCare. (2004). Charting the safety and quality of healthcare in Australia. Retrieved November 16, 2007, from http://www.safetyandquality.org/internet/safety/publishing.nsf/Content/F1AB7CD29C037EFBCA25716F00033691/$File/chartbk.pdf.

Bellamy, C. (2007). Inadvertent hypothermia in the operating theatre: an examination. *Journal of Perioperative Practice, 17(1),* 18–25.

Bitner, J., Hilde, L., Hall, K., Duvendack, T. (2007). A team approach to the prevention of unplanned postoperative hypothermia. *AORN Journal, 85(5),* 921–929.

Buggy, D. (2007). Metabolism, the stress response to surgery and perioperative thermoregulation. In A. Aitkenhead, G. Smith, D. Rowbotham (Eds.). *Textbook of anaesthesia* (5th ed.) (pp. 400–415). Edinburgh: Churchill Livingstone.

Butler, M., Boxer, E., Sutherland-Fraser, S. (2003). The factors that contribute to count and documentation errors in counting: a pilot study. *ACORN Journal, 15(1),* 10–14.

Bryant, B., & Knights, K. (2007). *Pharmacology for health professionals* (2nd ed.). Sydney: Elsevier.

Cantrell, S., Ward, K., Van Wicklin, S. (2007). Translating research on venous thromboembolism into practice. *AORN Journal, 86(4),* 590–604.

Drake, R., Vogl, W., Mitchell, A. (2005). *Gray's anatomy for students.* Philadelphia: Elsevier.

Drake, R., Vogl, W., Mitchell, A., et al. (2008). *Gray's atlas of anatomy.* Philadelphia: Elsevier.

Dua, R., Bankes, M., Dowd, G., Lewis, A. (2002). Compartment syndrome following pelvic surgery in the lithotomy position. *Annals of the Royal College of Surgeons of England, 84(3),* 170–171.

Espin, S., Regehr, G., Levinson, W., et al. (2007). Factors influencing perioperative nurses' error reporting preferences. *AORN Journal, 83(3),* 527–543.

Fabian, C. (2005). Electronic tagging of surgical sponges to prevent their accidental retention. *Surgery, 137(3),* 298–301.

Fell, D., & Kirkbride, D. (2007). The practical conduct of anaesthesia. In A. Aitkenhead, G. Smith, D. Rowbotham (Eds.). *Textbook of anaesthesia* (5th ed.) (pp. 297–314). Edinburgh: Churchill Livingstone.

Fulbrook, P., & Grealy, B. (2007). Essential nursing care of the critically ill patient. In D. Elliot, L. Aiken, W. Chaboyer (Eds.). *ACCCN's critical care nursing* (pp. 187–214). Sydney: Elsevier.

Gibbs, V. (2003). Retained surgical sponge. Agency for Healthcare Research and Quality, Morbidity & Mortality Rounds on the Web. Retrieved April 8, 2008, from http://www.webmm.ahrq.gov/cases.aspx.

Gibbs, V., & Auerbach, A. (2001). The retained surgical sponge. In K. Shojania, B. Duncan, K. McDonald, R. Wachter (Eds.). *Making healthcare safer: a critical analysis of patient safety practices* (pp. 255–257). Rockville, MD: Agency for Healthcare Research and Quality. Retrieved April 8, 2008, from http://www.ahrq.gov/clinic/ptsafety/chap22.htm.

Hamlin, L. (2005a). Perioperative concepts and nursing management. In M. Farrell (Ed.). *Smeltzer and Bare's medical–surgical nursing* (pp. 400–465). Sydney: Lippincott, Williams & Wilkins.

Hamlin, L. (2005b). Setting the standard: the role of the Australian College of Operating Room Nurses. University of Technology, Sydney, unpublished doctoral thesis

Hamlin, L. (2008). *Perioperative nursing*. In V. Wilson, S. Hillege, J. French (Eds.). *Taylor's fundamentals of nursing* (7th ed.) (in press). Sydney: Lippincott, Williams & Wilkins.

Hardman, J. (2007). Complications of anaesthesia. In A. Aitkenhead, G. Smith, D. Rowbotham (Eds.). *Textbook of anaesthesia* (5th ed.) (pp. 367–399). Edinburgh: Churchill Livingstone.

Heizenroth, J. (2007). Positioning the patient for surgery. In J. Rothrock, & D. McEwen (Eds.). *Alexander's care of the patient in surgery* (13th ed.) (pp. 130–157). St Louis: Mosby.

Hurley, C., & McAleavy, J. (2006). Preoperative assessment and intraoperative care planning. *Journal of Perioperative Practice, 16(1),* 187–914.

Illingworth, C., & Timmons, S. (2007). An audit of intermittent pneumatic compression (IPC) in the prophylaxis of asymptomatic deep vein thrombosis (DVT). *Journal of Perioperative Practice, 17(11),* 522–528.

Jackson, S., & Brady, S. (2008). Counting difficulties: retained instruments, sponges and needles. *AORN Journal, 87(2),* 315–321.

Kiekkas, P., & Karga, M. (2005). Prewarming preventing intraoperative hypothermia. *British Journal of Perioperative Nursing, 15(10),* 444–451.

Macario, A., Morris, D., Morris, S. (2006). Initial clinical evaluation of a handheld device for detecting retained surgical gauze sponges using radiofrequency identification technology. *Archives of Surgery, 141,* 659–662.

Macilquham, M., Riley, R., Grossberg, P. (2003). Identifying lost surgical needles using radiographic techniques. *AORN Journal, 78(1),* 73–78.

Mahajan, R. (2007). Postoperative care. In A. Aitkenhead, G Smith, D Rowbotham (Eds.). *Textbook of anaesthesia.* (5th ed.) (pp. 484–509). Edinburgh: Churchill Livingstone.

McChlery, S. (2007). The perioperative care of a super morbidly obese pregnant woman: a case study. *Journal of Perioperative Practice, 17(11),* 530–534.

McEwen, J. (2007). Complications and preventative measures. Retrieved March 4, 2008, from http://www.tourniquet.org.

O'Connor, C., & Murphy, S. (2007). Pneumatic tourniquet use in the perioperative environment. *Journal of Perioperative Practice, 17(8),* 391–397.

Parnaby, C. (2004). A new anti-embolism stocking. *Journal of Perioperative Practice, 14(7),* 302–307.

Perioperative Nurses College (NZNO). (2003). Standards and guidelines for safe practice. Retrieved January 13, 2008, from http://www.pnc.org.nz/Site/Sections/Colleges/Perioperative/About.aspx.

Phillips, N. (2007). *Berry & Kohn's operating room technique* (11th ed.). St Louis: Mosby.

Rank, D. (2008). Patient positioning an OR team effort. *OR Nurse, 2(1),* 21–23.

Rogers, M. L., Cook, R. I., Bower, R., et al. (2004). Barriers to implementing wrong site surgery guidelines: a cognitive work analysis. *IEEE Transactions on Systems, Man, and Cybernetics, 34(6),* 757–763.

Rothrock, J. (2007). Patient and environmental safety. In J. Rothrock, & D. McEwen (Eds.). *Alexander's care of the patient in surgery* (13th ed.) (pp. 15–42). St Louis: Mosby.

Saullo, D. (2007). Trauma surgery. In J. Rothrock, & D. McEwen (Eds.). *Alexander's care of the patient in surgery* (13th ed.) (pp. 1165–1197). St Louis: Mosby.

Staunton, P., & Chiarella, M. (2008). *Nursing and the law* (6th ed.). Sydney: Elsevier.

Tuncali, B., Karci, A., Bacakoglu, A. K., et al. (2003). Controlled hypotension and minimal inflation pressure: a new approach for pneumatic tourniquet application in upper limb surgery. *Anesthesia and Analgesia, 97,* 1529–1532.

Turpie, G. G., Chin, B. S. P., Lip, Y. H. (2002). ABC of antithrombotic therapy. Venous thromboembolism treatment strategies. *British Medical Journal, 325,* 948–950.

Watson, D. S., & Gregory Crum, B. S. (2005). Improving specimen practices to reduce errors. *AORN Journal, 82(6),* 1051–1054.

Welsh, T. (2002). A common sense approach to hypothermia. *American Association of Nurse Anesthetists Journal, 70(3),* 227–231.

White, R. (2003). The epidemiology of venous thromboembolism. *Circulation, 17(suppl 1),* 14–18.

Wilde, S. (2004). Compartment syndrome: the silent danger related to patient positioning and surgery. *British Journal of Perioperative Nursing, 14(12),* 546–554.

FURTHER READING

Aitkenhead, A. R., Smith, G., Rowbotham, D. J. (Eds.). (2007). *Textbook of anaesthesia* (5th ed.). Edinburgh: Churchill Livingstone.

AORN. (2007). Recommended practices for the prevention of unplanned perioperative hypothermia. *AORN Journal, 85(5),* 972–988.

Brown, J., & Feather, D. (2005). Surgical equipment and materials left in patients. *British Journal of Perioperative Nursing, 15(6),* 259–265.

Caprini, J. (2005). Risk factors for venous thromboembolism. *American Journal of Medicine—Continuing Medical Education Series,* 1–10.

Drain, C. B. (2008). *Perianesthesia nursing a critical care approach* (5th ed.). St Louis: Saunders.

Kehl-Pruett, W. (2006). Deep vein thrombosis in hospitalized patients: a review of evidence-based guidelines for prevention. *Dimensions of Critical Care Nursing, 25(2),* 53–61.

Martin, J., & Warner, M. (1997). *Positioning in anesthesia and surgery* (3rd ed.). Philadelphia: Saunders.

Miller, R. (2004). *Miller's anesthesia* (6th ed.). Philadelphia: Churchill Livingstone.

Tetro, A. M., & Rudan, J. F. (2001). The effects of a pneumatic tourniquet on blood loss in total knee arthroplasty. *Canadian Journal of Surgery, 44(1),* 33–38.

Van Wicklin, S., Ward, K., Cantrell, S. (2006). Implementing a research utilization plan for prevention of deep vein thrombosis. *AORN Journal, 83(6),* 1353–1368.

CHAPTER 5

Asepsis and infection control

Menna Davies, Leonie Robertson and Narelle Sommerfeld

LEARNING OBJECTIVES

After reading this chapter, you should be able to:

- differentiate between microorganisms and their pathogenicity
- discuss the human body's mechanisms of defence against infection
- explore the measures used to minimise transmission of pathogens, including environmental controls, and the use of standard and additional precautions
- identify the principles and practices of asepsis, aseptic technique and surgical conscience
- describe the practices of scrubbing, gowning and gloving, skin preparation and draping of the surgical patient
- discuss the methods of sterilisation and disinfection.

KEY TERMS

additional precautions

asepsis

aseptic technique

endogenous

exogenous

microorganism

nosocomial infection

personal protective equipment

standard precautions

sterile field

surgical conscience

surgical site infection

INTRODUCTION

This chapter presents fundamental aspects of infection control and the application of the principles of asepsis, which are the cornerstone of perioperative nursing practice. The infective process is discussed, along with modes of transmission and how the body combats pathogenic microorganisms. Environmental controls enacted to reduce the spread of infection, along with standard and additional precautions, are described and their practical application discussed. The principles of asepsis, the practical application of aseptic technique and the concept of surgical conscience are examined; also addressed is the surgical scrub, and the methods of prepping and draping the surgical patient and creating a sterile field. Infection control as an adverse event and bioterrorism are briefly explored. Methods of sterilisation and disinfection complete this chapter.

CLASSIFICATION AND TYPES OF MICROORGANISMS

In order to understand the infective process and the measures taken to prevent transmission of **microorganisms**, it is necessary to review aspects of microbiology. It is beyond the scope of this text to explore microbiology in depth but a brief examination of the particular organisms of concern, in relation to the care of surgical patients, is presented. Two main classifications of microorganisms are described by Burton and Engelkirk (2000):

1. cellular (e.g. bacteria, algae, protozoa and fungi)
2. acellular (e.g. viruses and prions).

Microorganisms of special interest to perioperative nurses include several types of bacteria, fungi, viruses and prions, which are outlined below; this does not include all microorganisms that may be found in the hospital setting.

Bacteria

Bacteria are simple, unicellular organisms containing internal structures, such as a nucleus, cytoplasm, plasmids and ribosomes (Lee & Bishop, 2006). Even though there are thousands of bacteria, very few cause disease/infection. Bacteria are extremely adaptable and survive and grow in various environments, often multiplying rapidly. For example, a single *Escherichia coli* bacterium can reproduce itself in 20 minutes and give rise to over a million bacterial cells in about 10 hours (Lee & Bishop, 2006).

Bacteria are the commonest cause of **surgical site infections** (SSIs), with staphylococci and streptococci being responsible for many of these (Lee & Bishop, 2006; Nicolette, 2007). Most bacteria found in the perioperative environment are shed from the skin of personnel (Nicolette, 2007); hand washing is the most efficacious way of countering their spread.

Gram-positive cocci

Staphylococci

Staphylococci (e.g. *Staphylococcus aureus* and *Staphylococcus epidermidis*) are round or spherical-shaped Gram-positive bacteria, and are part of the normal flora found on the skin and mucous membrane of the nasopharynx, urethra and vagina. They can exist in these areas without any adverse effect on the host and those that live on the skin are termed 'transient' organisms. Staphylococci can survive for long periods in the air, dust, bedding and clothing, making cleanliness of the perioperative environment paramount (Phillips, 2007). These bacteria are transmitted from the hands of the host to another person, where they can subsequently have significant negative effects. For example, they can enter the wound of a surgical patient and cause a wound infection or worse, because of their ability to develop resistance to antibiotics quickly (Lee & Bishop, 2006). Exotoxins secreted by *S. aureus* can cause toxic shock syndrome which, if left untreated, can be fatal (Lee & Bishop, 2006; Phillips, 2007). Staphylococci are strongly associated with healthcare-associated (nosocomial) infection (HAI).

Streptococci

Streptococci are responsible for a wide range of diseases and infections. These include throat and wound infections, pneumonia, septicaemia and necrotising fasciitis. *Streptococcus pyogenes* is frequently implicated in SSIs. Streptococci tend to be more virulent than staphylococci; however, they are much more likely than the latter to be sensitive to penicillin (Nicolette, 2007). Streptococci can be a normal resident of the upper airway, vagina and anus (Lee & Bishop, 2006; Nicolette, 2007) and are spread via direct and indirect contact, causing infection and illness in susceptible populations.

Enterococci

Enterococci are bacteria normally found in the gastrointestinal tract and female genital tract. They cause infections, such as SSI and septicaemia, when they are transmitted via the hands or contaminated equipment to susceptible, high-risk patients, including surgical patients (Nicolette, 2007). They are becoming an increasingly significant hospital pathogen because strains of enterococci have developed resistance to the antimicrobial drug vancomycin, which is the last resort treatment for methicillin-resistant staphylococcal infections (MRSA) (Lee & Bishop, 2006).

Gram-positive rods

Clostridia are Gram-positive anaerobic bacteria that produce toxins that cause serious illness, such as tetanus (*Clostridium tetani*) and gangrene (*Clostridium perfringens*). They have the ability to produce endospores, which enables them to encapsulate themselves in a special protein coat, giving them the ability to survive under adverse conditions (Lee & Bishop, 2006). Endospores can survive for many years and are highly resistant to drying and heat (Phillips, 2007). When conditions improve, the endospore germinates into a new bacterial cell. Sterilisation techniques must be able to destroy bacterial spores; these are discussed later in the chapter. *Clostridium difficile*, another example of this genus, can cause serious infection within the large intestine, especially in patients on long-term antibiotic therapy (Lee & Bishop, 2006; NZ Ministry of Health, 2007).

Fungi

There are two major types of fungi—yeast and moulds—and many are beneficial to humans; for example, moulds are a source of antibiotics (Lee & Bishop, 2007). They are often termed 'nature's original recyclers' because they secrete enzymes that decompose dead plant and animal matter, turning them into absorbable nutrients. Although of less significance within the perioperative setting, some fungal strains, such as *Candida albicans*, cause localised infections in the mouth and reproductive tract, which have the potential to become systemic infections. Fungi have been isolated in the nail beds of nurses who wear acrylic nails, even following normal surgical scrub techniques (NSW Health, 2007b). This has led to policies prohibiting acrylic nails within the operating suite due to the danger of transmitting fungal infections to patients (Australian Department of Health and Ageing, 2004).

Viruses

Unlike bacteria, viruses do not have a cellular structure and do not fit the classification for a living cell because they cannot reproduce or carry out any metabolic reactions. However, like some bacteria, they cause significant infections. Viruses replicate by invading a host cell and using the host cell's DNA, protein and other nutrients to survive and reproduce. In the process, they damage or destroy the host cell. The reproductive process concludes when the host cell bursts (cell lysis), spreading new viruses to nearby cells, where the process is repeated (Lee & Bishop, 2006). This process stimulates an antibody response in the infected person.

Hepatitis is one of the most common viruses and there are five identified strains (hepatitis A through to hepatitis E). The strains of most concern to perioperative nurses are hepatitis B and C as these, together with human immunodeficiency virus (HIV), can be transmitted through contact with blood and body fluids during invasive procedures. This may be through exposure to a sharps injury or via splashes into unprotected eyes or mucous membranes.

Prions

Prions are small infectious particles consisting of protein only with no nucleic acid. They are implicated in unusual neurodegenerative disorders, including bovine spongiform encephalopathy (BSE) or 'mad cow disease' and, in humans, Creutzfeldt-Jakob disease (CJD) (Lee & Bishop, 2006). The mechanism of infection that causes CJD is still unclear, although it is thought that prions have the ability to convert normal protein molecules into dangerous ones (Burton & Engelkirk, 2000). Prions are unusually resistant to conventional chemical and physical sterilising methods, and special protocols for managing instruments that have been used on infected or potentially infected patients are discussed later in this chapter (Nicolette, 2007). Table 5-1 summaries the common microorganisms found in the perioperative environment.

Table 5-1 Common microorganisms found in the perioperative environment

Microorganism	Usual environment	Mode of transmission
Staphylococci	Skin, hair Upper respiratory tract	Direct contact Airborne
Escherichia coli	Intestinal tract Urinary tract	Faeces, urine Direct contact
Streptococci	Oronasopharynx Skin, perianal area	Airborne Direct contact
Mycobacterium tuberculosis	Respiratory tract Urinary tract	Airborne, droplet Direct contact
Pseudomonas	Urinary tract Intestinal tract Water	Direct contact Urine, faeces Water
Serratia marcescens	Urinary tract Respiratory tract	Direct contact Water
Clostridium	Intestinal tract	Direct contact
Fungi	Dust, soil Inanimate objects	Airborne Direct contact
Hepatitis virus	Blood Body fluids	Blood-borne Direct contact

Phillips (2007)

Development of resistance to antimicrobial drugs

The emergence of strains of pathogens that are resistant to currently available antimicrobial drugs represents a significant threat to surgical patients. Those of concern in the perioperative environment include methicillin-resistant *S. aureus* (MRSA), which is also resistant to other categories of antimicrobials. MRSA has become a serious concern among hospitalised patients and can be fatal in those who are susceptible (Phillips, 2007). *S. aureus* is frequently implicated in SSIs (Lee & Bishop, 2006). Other microorganisms that have become resistant to antimicrobial drugs include vancomycin-resistant enterococci (VRE) and multi-drug resistant tuberculosis (TB), which is transmitted by droplets from infected individuals or improperly cleaned bronchoscopes and anaesthetic equipment. The prohibitive costs of developing new antimicrobial drugs have led to a greater emphasis on appropriate prescribing practices and more stringent infection control measures to limit the spread of resistant organisms in hospitals (Lee & Bishop, 2006; NZ Ministry of Health, 2007).

PROCESS OF INFECTION

The process of infection can be likened to the links in a chain—break any of the links and infection can be prevented (Nicolette, 2007). There are six links in the chain of infection:

1. infectious agent
2. reservoir
3. portal of entry
4. transmission
5. portal of exit
6. susceptible host.

Infectious agent

An infection results from microorganisms invading and multiplying in the host. Pathogenic microorganisms in the form of bacteria, viruses and fungi are the causative agents in wound and systemic infections suffered by patients.

Reservoir

The microorganisms responsible for the majority of HAI (**nosocomial infections**) originate either from the patient's own body flora (**endogenous** infections) or **exogenous** (external) sources, such as other patients, staff or equipment. Some microorganisms exist harmlessly on patients' skin, in hair follicles, sweat glands (staphylococci) or within the bowel as normal flora (*E. coli*). However, when these microorganisms enter another area of the body, they can cause infection (e.g. *E. coli* can cause bladder infections and *S. aureus* causes SSIs). Both transient and resident microorganisms are found on the skin (Tanner et al., 2007) and these can be transferred by direct contact between patients, health care workers, visitors and equipment, or by transfer to other body sites within the same patient, where infection can subsequently develop. Transient microorganisms are easily removed by good hand hygiene.

Portal of entry

The body has natural barriers to prevent the entry of microorganisms, including the skin, mucous membranes and their various secretions, such as tears, mucous and acid produced by the stomach. However, these defences can be breached in a number of ways:

1. *Inhalation.* Dust and water droplets that carry microorganisms can be transferred by people and enter the patient via the respiratory system (e.g. TB, influenza).

2. *Inoculation.* Microorganisms can enter the skin when the skin is breached through a sharps injury, trauma or a planned surgical incision.
3. *Ingestion.* Microorganisms can enter the intestinal tract through contaminated water or food.

Transmission

The transmission of microorganisms cannot occur unassisted. In the hospital setting, the most common mode of transmission is through people; this is mainly via the hands of health care workers, other patients or visitors directly touching the patient or through the use of contaminated objects (Gilmour, 2005). Vigilance in hand hygiene and the use of **aseptic technique** are the most efficient methods of preventing the transmission of microorganisms. Understanding the routes and sources of transmission is vital if this link in the chain is to be broken.

Portal of exit

For microorganisms to continue infecting other hosts, they must have a means of leaving the body. This may be via blood or other body fluids, faeces or droplets from the respiratory tract (Gilmour, 2005).

Susceptible host

Patients undergoing surgery become susceptible hosts when their skin barrier is breached by a surgical incision. Their immune system is also compromised, further increasing their susceptibility to infection. Other risk factors that increase susceptibility include those:

- who are very young or elderly
- with poor nutritional status
- with the presence of underlying conditions, such diabetes, vascular disease, or chronic renal or liver failure
- who are immunocompromised (e.g. patients receiving chemotherapy) (Gilmour, 2005).

Figure 5-1 demonstrates how implementing prevention strategies can break a link in the chain of transmission and safeguard the patient.

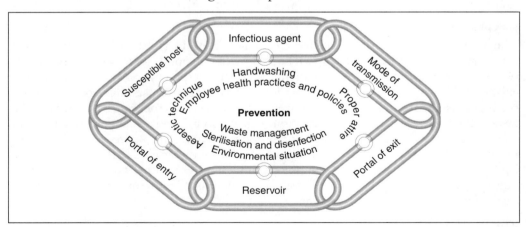

Figure 5-1 Prevention strategies that break the chain of infection (Woodhead & Wicker, 2005, p 86).

NORMAL BODY DEFENCES

Whether or not a person develops an infection as a result of invasion by microorganisms will depend on the susceptibility of that person (the host) and the virulence of the microorganism. It will also depend on the body's ability to defend itself against the invading pathogens.

External barriers

External barriers include the skin, mucous membranes and their respective secretions; these are the body's first line of defence in preventing infection. The epidermal layer of the skin contains a protein, keratin, which provides substantial resistance to bacterial enzymes and toxins. The dermal layer of skin contains sebum-secreting sebaceous glands, which lower the pH of the skin, inhibiting the growth of some bacteria and fungi (Lee & Bishop, 2006). Mucous membranes heal quickly despite much wear and tear, and their sticky, mucous secretions trap foreign particles and microorganisms.

Breaching the skin with a planned surgical incision bypasses this defence, increasing the risk of invasion by pathogenic organisms.

Inflammatory response

The onset of inflammation is a non-specific defence. It is the body's response to tissue damage and is evoked following any injury (e.g. physical, chemical, radiation) or invasion by microorganisms. The function of inflammation is to clear the injured site of cellular debris and any pathogens present, and to enable tissue repair to commence (Phillips, 2007). Once the inflammatory response is evoked, several biochemical mediators are released, localised vasodilation occurs and plasma fluid (containing leucocytes and proteins) moves into the injured area. This causes the four outward signs of inflammation, namely, redness, heat, swelling and pain (Lee & Bishop, 2006). If the inflammatory response does not eliminate all organisms or foreign material, healing of the injury is delayed and chronic inflammation can be result, which can persist for weeks or even months (Lee & Bishop, 2006).

Immune response

The immune response, the third line of protection, is a specific body defence. Immunity is the capacity of the body's immune system to defend itself successfully against potentially infectious agents. Immunity is acquired in two ways. Firstly, *active immunity* is acquired when the body has been exposed to or suffered an infection; this is 'naturally acquired' immunity. Artificially acquired active immunity results from immunisation, such as with vaccines (e.g. diphtheria) given in childhood. *Passive immunity* may be natural and occurs when antibodies are transferred from a person with immunity to another who does not have immunity (e.g. from mother to fetus across the placental barrier) (Lee & Bishop, 2006), or artificial and can be conferred with injections of immune globulins. For example, hepatitis B immunoglobulin injections may be given to a health care worker following a sharps injury and potential exposure to hepatitis B virus. Unlike active immunity, passive immunity is relatively short-lived (Lee & Bishop, 2006).

INFECTION AS AN ADVERSE EVENT

Infection is one of the most frequent adverse events associated with surgical procedures and/or interventions (Wicker & O'Neill, 2006). The cost of HAIs can be measured in terms of increased morbidity and mortality, increased length of stay in hospital and an increase in both human and clinical resources (Pittet, 2005). Worldwide, HAIs and the present threat from multiresistant organisms (MROs) are said to be responsible for the death of up to 1400 people daily; this constitutes one of medicine's greatest challenges (Best & Neuhauser, 2004). Such is the significance of MROs that health departments are now developing and implementing MRO-specific policies (NSW Health, 2007a; NZ Ministry of Health, 2007). Surgical patients have a three-fold greater risk of HAI compared to other patients (Australian Department of Health and Ageing, 2004). Despite compelling evidence about the effectiveness of hand washing in reducing the spread of infection within health care facilities, compliance remains problematic. Increasingly, attention must be paid to all of the practices described here because they are either effective or they reduce reliance on antibiotic therapies.

BIOTERRORISM

Finally, microorganisms are a key component of biological warfare, which has become a very real threat (Nicolette, 2007). The US Centers for Disease Control (CDC) has identified anthrax and smallpox as the two most likely biological weapons with the ability to be spread quickly and easily within large populations. The resultant panic and disruption to the social fabric requires all health professionals to be aware of local procedures when dealing with a potential pandemic (Nicolette, 2007). Although it is unlikely that perioperative nurses will care for surgical patients with these diseases, in the event of a national crisis, they may well be called upon as part of the emergency preparedness plan.

INFECTION CONTROL

Successful infection control practices focus on prevention; this involves identifying hazards and classifying associated risks (Australian Department of Health and Ageing, 2004). In turn, this requires health care facilities to develop infection control risk management plans, ideally within a clinical governance framework, to minimise the risk of preventable nosocomial infections (NSW Health, 2007a). Elements of successful infection control include quality and risk management policies, effective work practices and procedures, and adequate physical facilities and operational controls (Australian Department of Health and Ageing, 2004; Nicolette, 2007; NZ Ministry of Health, 2007). Major risk factors can be found within the perioperative setting , so additional and specific requirements to prevent infection are needed (Australian Department of Health and Ageing, 2004). These are addressed below.

Environmental controls

Chapter 3 looked at all aspects of the perioperative environment, noting that many operating suite design features are necessary for good infection control. These include the concept of the four zones of the perioperative environment. Personnel entering the semi-restricted and restricted zones of the operating suite must be correctly dressed in perioperative attire in order to minimise the entry of microorganisms found on the outside (street) clothing of personnel.

Attire

Correct perioperative attire (Fig 5-2) includes the following:

- Loose fitting, tightly woven cotton pants and top or dress. These minimise the friction and chafing caused by tight-fitting clothing, which subsequently causes the dispersal of epithelial skin cells into the environment.
- Caps or scarves are worn to cover the hair completely and beards require balaclava-type head wear. The hair is a significant source of microorganisms (Gruendemann & Mangum, 2001).
- Street clothes should not be worn underneath perioperative attire as they are heavily contaminated.
- Perioperative attire should be changed on leaving and re-entering the suite.
- Perioperative attire is changed daily and whenever it is visibly wet, soiled or

contaminated. It requires commercial laundering and must not be taken home for laundering (ACORN, 2006).

- Long-sleeved gown with cuffed wrists or the use of a 'warm-up' jacket is recommended to prevent the dispersal of epithelial skin cells from the arms.
- Warm-up jackets are worn buttoned up and gowns fastened at the back to prevent flapping and possible contamination of the sterile field.
- Closed-toe, well-fitting shoes, which are easy to clean, and made of material that is impervious to fluids and penetration by sharp items are necessary in the operating suite (Australian Department of Health and Ageing, 2004). The use of shoe coverings for infection control reasons is not warranted, as no cause-and-effect relationship has ever been demonstrated between footwear and SSIs; further, there is an increased risk of cross-infection when the wearer touches the coverings to remove them (Santos et al., 2005). It is highly recommended that a pair of shoes are designated for wear in the operating suite only (Santos et al., 2005) to avoid transmission of microorganisms to and from the home environment.
- Perioperative nursing standards related to the wearing of jewellery within the operating suite indicate that it should be limited to plain ear studs, a wedding band and thin chain necklace (which can be enclosed within the perioperative attire) (ACORN, 2006). Nails should be kept short, 0.5 cm in length. All nail polish should be removed as cracked nail polish harbours microorganisms. False nails and nail extensions can harbour fungal infections, which may be transmitted to the patient, and are best avoided (ACORN, 2006; NSW Health, 2007b).

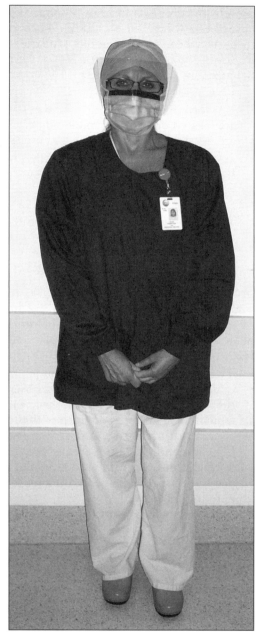

Figure 5-2 Correct perioperative attire.

Face masks

The wearing of fluid-resistant face masks is an important part of perioperative attire. The tradition of wearing masks was based on the unfounded assumption that their use protected patients, although there is limited evidence to support this (Lipp & Edwards, 2002). However, there is now sufficient evidence to warrant the use of face masks to prevent the droplet spread of oropharyngeal flora during insertion of spinal or epidural anaesthesia (Siegel et al., 2007). Their continued use is also predicated on the need to protect health care workers (Australian Department of Health and Ageing, 2004; Phillips, 2007; Siegel et al., 2007). Within the perioperative setting, the following practices are recommended.

Face masks:

- are worn in the operating suite wherever open sterile supplies or scrubbed personnel are located or as per hospital policy
- are worn to cover both nose and mouth, and tied securely at the back of the head
- are changed frequently and handled by the ties only to avoid contact with the area that has covered the nose and mouth; hands should be washed after removing the mask
- should not be left around the neck or stored in a pocket
- are an essential part of personal protective equipment; fluid-resistant masks, which meet appropriate Australian and New Zealand standards, protect the wearer from potential splashes during operative or invasive procedures (Australian Department of Health and Ageing, 2004; Siegel et al., 2007).

Moving around the operating room

Too much activity within the operating room provides opportunities for the transmission of microorganisms (Lee, 2005). In order to reduce unnecessary movement, forward planning is needed; for example, place all the requirements for a case in the operating room prior to commencement. Other considerations include the following:

- There should be minimal personnel in any operating room.
- It is important that all personnel observe guidelines limiting their movement within the operating room. This is necessary to minimise the creation of air currents, which circulate microorganisms that can subsequently land in the surgical wound, contaminating it (Lee, 2005; Phillips, 2007).
- Opening and closing operating room doors creates more air currents and alters the normally positive airflow within the operating room itself, further increasing the possibility of airborne contaminants, sourced from personnel, supplies and equipment, entering the wound.
- Talking should be kept to a minimum to lessen droplet spread (ACORN, 2006).

Infection control practices

Consistent with international standards and practices, a two-tiered approach to infection control is endorsed in Australia and New Zealand. Standard precautions are used for all patients regardless of their diagnosis or presumed infection status. Additional (or transmission-based) precautions are applicable only to the care of specified patients (Australian Department of Health and Ageing, 2004; NSW Health, 2007a).

Standard precautions

Standard precautions are designed to reduce the transmission of microorganisms from both recognised and unrecognised sources. They involve safe work practices and protective barriers (Siegel et al., 2007). Standard precautions protect patients and health care workers, and they apply to:

- blood (including dried blood)
- all body substances, secretions and excretions (excluding sweat), regardless of whether or not they contain visible blood
- non-intact skin and mucous membranes (including the eyes).

Hand hygiene is the single most important practice to reduce transmission of infectious agents in health care settings (NSW Health, 2007b). Hands must be washed after contact with the patient, after removing gloves and between tasks that involve contact with potentially contaminated equipment. Antimicrobial agents, such as chlorhexidine and waterless alcohol-based hand rubs, are available for routine hand hygiene.

Other facets of standard precautions include the use of **personal protective equipment** (PPE), which must be worn during activities when there is a risk of contact with blood or body fluids. PPE consists of the following items:

- Non-sterile gloves—these provide an effective barrier when touching contaminated equipment, blood and body fluids. Gloves should be removed after completing the task, hands washed and a fresh set of gloves donned before engaging in further activities involving potentially contaminated items. Circulating nurses must remove gloves prior to opening sterile supplies and they should not be worn if, during procedures, extra items are required from sterile stockrooms.
- Non-sterile gowns are available to protect the operating suite attire during patient care activities. They must be removed immediately following use.
- Face masks and eye protection in the form of face shields, goggles or visors must be worn to protect the mucous membrane of the eyes, nose and mouth during activities when there is the likelihood of sprays or splashes of blood or body fluid (Siegel et al., 2007).

Standard precautions not only rely on the use of PPE, they involve techniques that minimise the risk of transmission of blood-borne diseases. Within the operating room, these include:

- the use of puncture-resistant containers (or a neutral zone) within the sterile field when transferring sharps (e.g. scalpels, sutures and other sharp equipment) from instrument nurse to surgeon

---

Box 5-1 The father of infection control

In May 1847 in Vienna, Ignaz Phillip Semmelweis (1818–65) provided evidence of the significance of hand washing to prevent the spread of puerperal sepsis. Semmelweis, an obstetrician, observed that the maternal mortality rate in women attended by doctors was 20%, which was four to five times greater than in women attended only by midwives.

Semmelweis identified that midwives did not attend the anatomical laboratories where autopsies were carried out. Following the death of a colleague who accidentally cut his finger during an autopsy and died a few days later, it was discovered at autopsy that he had died from the same causative microorganism responsible for puerperal sepsis. This finding moved Semmelweis to immediately implement a rigorous hand washing policy using 4% chlorinated lime solution prior to the examination of women in labour. The results almost immediately lowered maternal mortality rates and a full year after the implementation of Semmelweis' hand washing policy the mortality rate from puerperal sepsis had dropped to 1.2%.

However, these results were not published for another 14 years and, although Semmelweis had many who supported his findings, there were those who opposed the idea of the doctor being the cause of the spread of puerperal sepsis. Semmelweis was not recognised for his findings until after his death.

Although the antiseptic practices of Semmelweis were ultimately adopted by the medical community throughout the world, he was never given the recognition during his lifetime that he so richly deserved (Grant et al., 2005).

- the use of magnetic needle mats to store and dispose of needles
- surgeons using designated instruments for retracting tissue, rather than hands, to prevent accidental sharps injury
- increased use of disposable stapling equipment to minimise the risks involved in using hand-held sutures to anastomose tissue
- good communication between surgical team members to ensure sharp items are not left lying unattended within the sterile field (Goldman, 2008)
- surgical team members wearing two sets of gloves—'double gloving'—to minimise sharps injury, as wearing a second pair of gloves has been shown to provide added protection against puncturing the inner gloves (Tanner & Parkinson, 2006).

Additional precautions

Additional (or transmission-based) **precautions** are the second line of approach to infection control. These precautions are applied when the mode of transmission of pathogenic microorganisms is airborne, via droplet or contact, or a combination of these routes. They are applied in conjunction with standard precautions.

Airborne precautions

Airborne transmission of microorganisms involves their spread via minute particles that can remain suspended in the air for extended periods or disseminated in dust particles. Examples of airborne-transmitted diseases are TB and chickenpox. Precautions against these infections require the use of close-fitting, particulate filter, personal respiratory protection devices or a P2 mask capable of filtering particles as small as 0.3 μm (Australian Department of Health and Ageing, 2004; Nicolette, 2007).

Droplet precautions

Droplet transmission involves larger particles generated when a person sneezes or coughs. Droplets are not as robust or long-lived as airborne particles. Examples of diseases transmitted by droplet are influenza and meningococcal infection. The P2 masks are effective in preventing transmission of droplet infections. It is recommended that patients with airborne or droplet infections wear a P2 or equivalent mask when being transported within the hospital to reduce the risk of infecting other people (Australian Department of Health and Ageing, 2004).

Contact precautions

Contact precautions are intended to prevent the transmission of infectious agents, including epidemiologically important microorganisms, which are spread by direct or indirect contact with the patient or a patient's environment (Siegel et al., 2007). They are applied to patients known to be infected with various epidemiologically significant organisms, including multiresistant organisms (e.g. MRSA, VRE), and when caring for patients with *C. difficile* infections (Siegel et al., 2007). As these organisms may be present on the patient's skin, clothing, bed clothes and equipment, health care workers must wear aprons or gowns, gloves, protective eye wear and masks when participating in patient care activities. All items of protective equipment must be disposed of once contact with the patient is completed and hands thoroughly washed. Whenever feasible, these patients should be isolated during their period of hospitalisation (Nicolette, 2007).

Adherence with these precautions decreases the transmission of infectious agents in health care settings (Siegel et al., 2007). However, several observational studies have shown limited adherence to recommended practices by health care workers (Castella et al., 2006; Siegel et al., 2007). Adherence to good infection control practices requires a work environment where there is commitment to safety on the part of management, which includes education, worker participation in safety programs and the provision of appropriate protective equipment (Griffin, 2005; Siegel et al., 2007).

ASEPSIS

Asepsis can be defined as the absence of pathogenic microorganisms on living tissue (Gilmour, 2005; Nicolette, 2007). The aim of aseptic practices is to eliminate infectious organisms in an effort to minimise contamination of the wound and prevent other infections, and thus aid in an uneventful postoperative recovery (Nicolette, 2007). Aseptic principles and practice are based on available scientific evidence and logical thought, although some are ritualistic and lack scientific rigour to support their use. However, infection control statistics generally support the application of aseptic principles and, until empiric evidence demonstrates otherwise, their use is widely supported (Nicolette, 2007; Siegel et al., 2007). Aseptic practices guide perioperative nurses' actions, for example, when opening sterile supplies, moving in and around the sterile field or setting up sterile instrument trolleys. In some instances, the principles provide arbitrary boundaries only, but they do assist the perioperative nurse to determine where sterile areas start and end, thus contributing to safe practice.

The sterile field

The patient is the centre of the **sterile field**, which comprises personnel wearing sterile attire, and those areas of the patient, operating table, instrument trolleys and other furniture that are covered in sterile drapes (Hamlin, 2008). Application of the principles and practices of aseptic technique, which are necessary to create and maintain a sterile field, rely on the perioperative nurse and other members of the surgical team exercising a surgical conscience (Phillips, 2007).

Surgical conscience

A **surgical conscience** is defined as an individual's professional honesty and inner morality system, which allows no compromise in practice. When there is a breach in accepted behaviours or aseptic technique, the incident must be corrected immediately, regardless of personal consequences or embarrassment. The placing of the patients' well-being above personal/professional embarrassment demonstrates good surgical conscience (Phillips, 2007).

Principles of asepsis

The principles of asepsis include the following:

- all personnel within the sterile field must wear a sterile gown and gloves and touch only sterile items
- unsterile personnel must only touch unsterile items
- sterile drapes must be used to create a sterile field around the proposed operative site
- items used within a sterile field must be sterile
- only the horizontal surfaces of tables draped with sterile drapes are considered sterile; any item that hangs below table top level is considered unsterile
- all items introduced onto a sterile field must be opened, dispensed and transferred by methods that maintain their sterility and integrity
- the sterile field must be monitored at all times and never left unattended
- all personnel moving around a sterile field should do so in a manner that maintains the integrity of the sterile field
- unsterile personnel should not lean across a sterile field or try to walk between two sterile fields (Nicolette, 2007; Phillips, 2007).

Putting these principles into practice can be daunting for the beginning perioperative nurse. However, practice under supervision will ensure that skills and dexterity are developed. Some practical hints for opening and presenting sterile items to the sterile field are:

- do not lean over the sterile field while dispensing items
- if in doubt of the sterility of an item, consider it contaminated and discard
- remain a safe distance (at least 30 cm) away from the sterile field
- the sterile article is opened without the hands touching the inside wrapper so that it is not contaminated
- open the wrapper furthest away first and the nearest wrapper last
- secure all open wrapper edges to avoid contamination
- items are either 'flipped' onto a sterile field or taken by a scrubbed person
- articles dropped are no longer considered sterile and must be discarded; after picking articles up off the floor, hands should be washed (ACORN, 2006; Nicolette, 2007; Phillips, 2007).

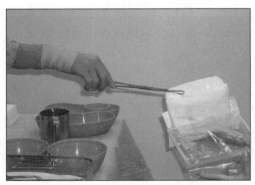

Figure 5-3 Circulating nurse presenting sterile item to the instrument nurse.

Microorganisms do not move around by themselves—they are transported by people, or air currents which contain dust. Discipline in controlling and monitoring one's own behaviours is an essential component of perioperative practice.

Opening sterile supplies

The circulating nurse provides a link between the sterile field and the sterile supplies required for a surgical procedure. This requires the ability to open and transfer sterile items safely onto the sterile field. Prior to opening sterile items, circulating nurses must wash their hands and carry out the following:

- Examine the external sterility indicator —this will indicate that the item has been through a sterilisation processes.
- Check the expiry date—although an event (e.g. dropping a sterile item) rather than time is the determining factor, some companies will place an expiry date on items.
- Check that the item is securely sealed and its packaging is intact—if not, discard it.
- Assess for water marks or any dampness—their presence indicates strikethrough has occurred, and the item can no longer be considered sterile.

If any doubt exists about the sterility or integrity of the package, it should be discarded. Items that have a peel-back seal

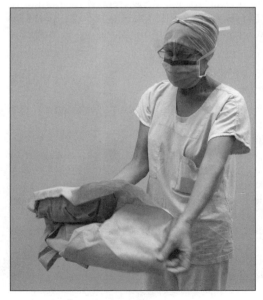

Figure 5-4 Unwrapping a sterile item.

(e.g. swabs or sutures) may be suitable for 'flipping' onto the sterile field (depending on individual hospital policy). This practice involves using a sterile bowl, on a separate stand away from the sterile instrument trolley(s), into which small sterile items can be 'flipped' (Hamlin, 2008). Flipping items directly onto sterile instrument trolleys should be avoided as it may hinder the instrument nurse in setting up the instruments. Worse still, if an item is contaminated during the flipping process, the whole sterile field is contaminated, not just the bowl, which is easily replaced. Whether a package can be safely transferred by flipping will depend on the item and the experience of the circulating nurse. If in doubt, the item should be opened and presented to the instrument nurse, who can use a sponge-holding forceps to take the item safely.

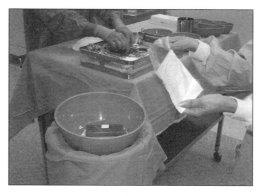

Figure 5-5 Flipping a sterile item into a sterile bowl.

Pouring liquids onto a sterile field

Any fluids added to the sterile field must first be checked by the instrument nurse to ensure that they are the correct fluid and not out of date. Points to remember are:

1. Do not reach over the sterile field.
2. Pour liquid carefully to prevent splashing onto the sterile field.
3. Pour the total contents of the container. Do not recap and reuse, as contamination could occur when recapping.
4. Do not allow any drips from the side of the bottle to fall onto the sterile field (Phillips, 2007).

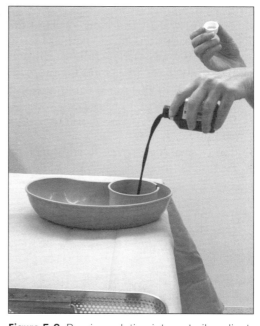

Figure 5-6 Pouring solution into a sterile galipot.

The surgical scrub

Before surgeons and instrument nurse(s) can prepare or enter a sterile field, they must perform a surgical scrub, followed by the donning of a sterile gown and gloves according to local hospital policy.

The practice of surgical scrubbing is an attempt to reduce SSIs. Although skin cannot be sterilised, it can be made surgically clean by undertaking a surgical scrub (Gruendemann & Mangum, 2001; Tanner et al., 2007). The scrubbing of the nails, hands and forearms with antiseptic solution reduces dirt and contamination, and transient and resident microorganisms, and minimises regrowth of the latter throughout the surgery.

Before the surgical scrub personnel should:

• be dressed in perioperative attire
• remove rings and confine/remove all other visible jewellery, such as earrings and neck chains

- wear PPE
- perform a close inspection of the hands, paying close attention to any breaks in the skin.
- open a sterile gown pack and add sterile gloves to it.

The antimicrobial scrub solution used may well be dictated by hospital policy and/or personal choice; however, alcohol-based products are generally considered the most efficacious (NSW Health, 2007b; Siegel et al., 2007; Tanner et al., 2007). These solutions are in common usage in Europe and are likely to be in widespread use in Australasia in the near future. Currently, aqueous solutions, such as povidone-iodine and chlorhexidine, are the most commonly used antimicrobial scrub solutions in use. The evidence from comparisons of aqueous scrub solutions with alcohol rubs, which contain additional active ingredients, is mixed and a systematic review by Tanner et al. (2008) revealed no difference between alcohol rubs that contain additional active ingredients and aqueous scrubs in reducing SSIs. There is evidence from studies in favour of both forms of hand antisepsis.

Both Australian and New Zealand professional perioperative organisations provide detailed descriptions of the surgical scrub and each operating suite should display the technique for all staff to follow. Although the actual technique may differ between countries, the basic principles for surgical scrubbing are:

1. First scrub of the day is 5 minutes in length and includes use of sterile scrub brush and nail cleaner.
2. Subsequent scrubs are 3 minutes (Australian Department of Health and Ageing, 2004).
3. Turn tap on to an even flow to prevent splashing.
4. Antiseptic solution applied to hands and arms should remain in contact with the skin according to manufacturer's instructions.
5. Prepare a sterile scrubbing brush, maintaining sterility until it is required.
6. When applying solution, work from hands to the elbow, using a circular motion to move up the arms, and do not return to the hands,
7. When rinsing hands and arms, water should flow from cleanest areas (the hands) to less clean areas (elbow) (i.e. always keep hands above the elbow) (Fig 5-7).
8. After completing the surgical scrub, the hands are held above the waist and are dried using a sterile towel, before donning a sterile gown.

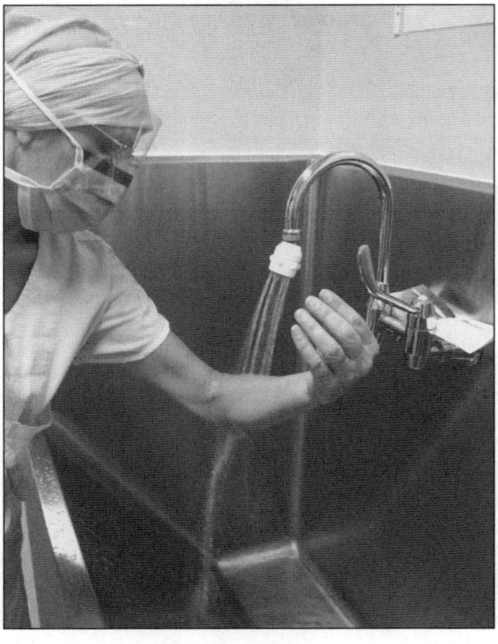

Figure 5-7 Rinsing hands and arms—water should flow from hands to the elbow.

Gowning

Sterile gowns are worn to provide a barrier to prevent the transfer of microorganisms to the patient during the surgical procedure. Their manufacture must meet relevant Australian and New Zealand standards for both disposable, resposable (i.e. limited reuse gowns) and reusable gowns to ensure barrier qualities. Reusable and disposable sterile gowns are folded differently and, therefore, the technique for donning may vary.

The main principles for gowning are (Fig 5-8):

- minimal handling during donning procedure
- extending both arms into sleeves simultaneously
- not extending arms through the gown cuffs—this allows for closed gloving
- keeping hands bent at the elbows and above the waist
- allowing an unsterile person to secure gown ties at the back.

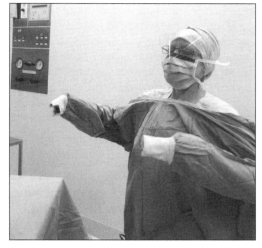

Figure 5-8 Donning a reusable linen gown.

Gloving

Closed gloving is the recommended method to don gloves as it reduces the risk of contamination of the sterile gloves by the bare hands. Double gloving is a recommended practice as it reduces the risk of sharps penetration (Australian Department of Health and Ageing, 2004; Tanner & Parkinson, 2006).

With the hands remaining inside the cuffs, remove one glove from the packet with one hand and with the palm of the other hand uppermost, the glove is placed onto the cuff with the fingers of the glove pointing towards the wrist, the thumb down and with the folded edge of the glove flush against the edge of the cuff of the gown.

With both hands working inside the gown sleeves, the thumbs hold onto the edge of the glove cuffs. Using one motion, the glove is stretched out and over the hand and the gown cuff is inserted into the glove. Both the glove and the gown are then grasped, manoeuvring the hand through the cuff into the glove (Fig 5-9). The procedure is repeated for the other hand.

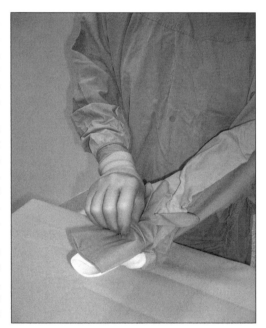

Figure 5-9 Demonstration of closed method of gloving.

The second pair of gloves are then donned by sliding each gloved hand into the second pair.

Once both pairs of gloves are donned, there is one final action taken to complete gowning. On the front of the gown are two ties, which require assistance to be tied to complete the gowning process. Disposable gowns have a paper tag attached to the ties, which can be handed to either a sterile or unsterile colleague. Having handed over the tag, the scrubbed person turns around and reclaims the tie, subsequently tying both ties together. If an unsterile colleague has assisted, care must be taken *not* to touch the paper tag she or he has handled. Reusable gowns do not usually have a sterile tag and the safest method of turning the gown is to hand the right hand tie to another scrubbed person and then complete the turn. The effect of this manoeuvre is to close the back panel of the sterile gown. It does not mean the back is sterile, but provides all-round protection to the wearer. Once gowned and gloved, the areas considered sterile are from the tips of the fingers to the elbows and from nipple to waist. It is acknowledged that these are arbitrary boundaries (Hamlin, 2008).

Assisted (open) gloving

Assisted gloving is the method whereby one scrubbed person gloves another scrubbed person; this may occur should the wearer contaminate a glove intraoperatively. Closed gloving cannot be achieved because the cuffs should not be pulled back over the hands as they are now unsterile. Therefore, the safest method of donning a replacement glove is for another sterile member of the team to assist with the gloving.

If both gown and gloves become contaminated, both must be removed and the donning procedure is carried out as previously described. Once gowned and gloved (Fig 5-10), the scrubbed person must stay close to the sterile field and not move out of the operating room into semi-restricted or unrestricted areas as this will increase the risk of cross-infection.

At the conclusion of the procedure, the surgical team must discard gowns, gloves and masks in contaminated waste containers within the operating room. This is done in a manner that 'contains and confines' contaminated items. For example, to avoid contamination of bare hands, the gown is removed first, rolled up so the inner surface is on the outside, and placed in the contaminated linen basket (if a reusable gown) or the contaminated waste bin (if a disposable gown). This is followed by the removal of the gloves. The hands should be washed following removal of the gown and gloves.

Skin preparation of the patient

The aim of preoperative skin preparation is to remove soil and transient and resident microorganisms from the patient's skin using an antimicrobial agent. Preoperative skin cleansing mechanically removes, chemically kills and inhibits contaminating and colonising skin flora (Lipp, 2005). This is believed to contribute to reducing the risk of wound contamination and SSIs (ACORN, 2006; Lipp, 2005). However, a systematic review of the use of skin antiseptics has failed to establish conclusively the effectiveness of preoperative skin preparations and which type of solution is most effective (Edwards et al., 2004). Thus, until evidence becomes available it is wise to continue to use skin antiseptics preoperatively (Lipp, 2005).

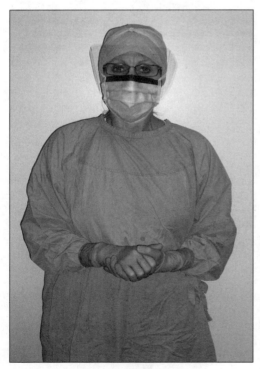

Figure 5-10 Nurse wearing sterile gown and gloves.

Commonly used antimicrobial agents include povidone-iodine 10% (with or without alcohol), chlorhexidine 0.5% with alcohol, and chlorhexidine and cetrimide.

Although there is no evidence that hair removal reduces SSIs among patients who have had hair removed prior to surgery (Tanner et al., 2006), it is still practised. If hair removal is required on clinical grounds, then it is recommended that clippers are used, rather than shaving with a razor, to prepare the operative site (Australian Department of Health and Ageing, 2004). Clipping has been found to be safer and less likely to produce nicks in the skin, which could lead to wound infections.

Following positioning of the patient, cleansing (often referred to as 'prepping') of the patient's skin with antimicrobial solution is completed, taking into account any allergies that the patient may have, the type of procedure to be carried out and the surgeon's preference. Preparation of the operative site is carried out either by the surgeon or instrument nurse using a broad-spectrum antimicrobial solution and gauze swabs, observing aseptic technique. Antiseptic skin cleansing commences from the cleanest area, usually the proposed operative site, and proceeds in concentric circles or squares outwards to the least clean areas. The prepared area should be wide enough to allow extension of the incision if required. Areas that have a high microbial count (e.g. groin, umbilicus, body orifices, open wounds or stomas) should be prepared last using a separate swab. The preparation of these areas is carried out in reverse, that is, the cleaner, peripheral areas are cleansed first prior to cleansing the more heavily contaminated areas, even though these may be the operative site. The surgical principle is to work from the cleanest to the least clean area (Nicolette, 2007; Phillips, 2007).

The antimicrobial solution should not be allowed to pool under the patient as this can cause skin maceration. Adequate time should be allowed for the antiseptic solution to dry before the drapes are applied. This is particularly important when using alcohol-based preparation solutions as the vapours from the alcohol must be allowed to evaporate before drapes are applied in order to reduce the risk of ignition and fire when electrosurgery is used (ACORN, 2006; Nicolette, 2007).

Draping the patient

To create a sterile field within which surgery can be carried out, sterile drapes are strategically placed on the patient in a manner that exposes only the operative site and isolates it from surrounding areas. Within this defined sterile field, the surgical procedure takes place and all those involved must be dressed in sterile gowns, gloves and personal protective attire. The drapes covering the patient's body provide an area on which instruments and equipment, such as suction tubing and the active diathermy electrode (hand piece), can be placed.

Reusable linen or synthetic single-use drapes used in the creation of the sterile field should be made of materials that inhibit the migration of microbial particles and moisture. Drapes may be available as single items or they may be packaged in predetermined configurations for specific surgical procedures. They are folded in such a manner as to facilitate easy opening and placement on the patient. Reusable drapes are held in place with towel clips or sutures, whereas single-use drapes have an adhesive section to secure them in place without slippage. An additional, transparent adhesive drape may be placed over the operative site to further isolate surrounding skin from the incision. The adhesive drape may also be impregnated with antimicrobial solution to minimise wound contamination.

Points to consider when handling drapes are as follows:

- Handle drapes as little as possible, as excessive movement can cause air currents and dispersal of dust particles.

- Hold the drapes above waist level and, once in place, do not move them. If a drape requires repositioning, it should be discarded and a new one used.
- Drape the incision site first and work towards the periphery, draping from sterile to unsterile.
- Protect the gloved hands from contamination by 'cuffing' the drape over them during placement (Nicolette, 2007).

Strikethrough

Gowns and drapes act as barriers to prevent the transmission of microorganisms from non-sterile to sterile areas. If moisture penetrates the gowns or drapes, it permits the passage of microorganisms from a non-sterile surface to a sterile surface; this is termed 'strikethrough'. The ability to prevent strikethrough is a critical factor in maintaining a sterile field and is achieved by the use of waterproof drapes and gowns (or by the use of plastic aprons under gowns made of permeable material). However, if strikethrough occurs on either gown or drapes, they must be replaced (NSW Health, 2007b).

On completion of the surgical procedure and following the application of a wound dressing, the drapes are removed immediately using a 'contain and confine' approach as described for the removal of gowns and gloves.

INSTRUMENT CLEANING, DECONTAMINATION AND STERILISATION

All reusable instruments and equipment used on a patient during a surgical procedure or investigative process must be decontaminated, cleaned, inspected, packaged and sterilised or disinfected before reuse to reduce the risk of cross-infection. Spaulding first proposed a system of classifying infection risk and appropriate processing methods in 1968 (Phillips, 2007), as shown in Table 5-2.

Table 5-2 Spaulding's classification of medical devices by infectious risk

Classification	Type of procedure	Level of decontamination required
Critical	Invasive device that enters tissue that is usually sterile or enters the vascular system (e.g. surgical instruments, biopsy forceps)	Requires sterilisation
Semi-critical	Device contacts intact mucous membrane but does not penetrate sterile tissue (e.g. flexible endoscopes)	Requires high-level disinfection (sterilisation preferred where practicable)
Non-critical	Device only contacts intact skin (e.g. stethoscope, sphygmomanometer cuff)	Can be processed by cleaning (and low-level disinfection where necessary)

Woodhead & Wicker (2005)

The standards for decontamination, cleaning and sterilising reusable instruments and equipment are detailed in the relevant Australian and New Zealand standards (Standards Australia, 2003, AS/NZS 4187). This Standard provides a detailed description to assist staff in sterilising departments and the operating suite.

Decontamination and cleaning

The first step in the process of instrument/equipment reuse is that of decontamination. Decontamination is a process by which physical or chemical agents are used to clean inanimate objects or surfaces (Phillips, 2007). Before items can be sterilised, they must be thoroughly cleaned of all organic material; they must also have the least microbial load (bioburden) achievable. Failure to remove this material prevents the sterilising agent coming into contact with all surfaces of the item and results in failure to achieve sterilisation.

The cleaning process begins in the operating room during the procedure with the instrument nurse wiping used instruments with a sterile sponge dampened with sterile water to keep them free of blood and tissue debris. Particular attention should be given to the tips and the joints of the instruments to prevent the build-up of blood and tissue on the instruments, which may hinder their effective use by the surgeon. This also helps reduce the bioburden. Instruments with lumens should be flushed through with sterile water to prevent blockage. Heavily contaminated instruments can be cleaned in a splash bowl containing sterile water (Dunscombe, 2007). Sterile normal saline should not be used for cleaning as it is corrosive and can damage the instruments. At the conclusion of the procedure, reusable instruments and equipment are returned to the sterilising department, where manual and mechanical cleaning takes place (Gruendemann & Mangum, 2001).

One of the initial steps in cleaning metal instruments is immersing them in a water bath containing enzymatic cleaning detergent through which high-frequency ultrasound vibrations are transmitted. The vibrations produce pressure changes in the water, creating tiny air bubbles, which implode around the instruments, dislodging the organic material in a process called cavitation (Hurrell, 2005). This method is especially effective in cleaning instruments that have grooved jaws, where organic material can be difficult to remove by manual cleaning. Therefore, instruments such as scissors and clamps must be fully opened to allow the cavitation process to reach all areas of the instrument. Delicate instruments should not be placed in the ultrasonic cleaner with larger, heavier items as they may be damaged by the latter during processing. Following ultrasonic cleaning, instruments are placed in automated mechanical washers, which use detergents and jet sprays of water to further thoroughly clean, rinse and dry the instruments. Drying the instruments is an important part of the decontamination process as wet instruments will quickly become colonised with microorganisms.

Specialised instruments and equipment such as endoscopes, drills and delicate instruments are processed separately as they have individual cleaning requirements. Endoscopes have air, water and biopsy channels, which require special brushes to be inserted along the length of the channel to ensure thorough cleaning. Most drills cannot be immersed in water and require cleaning with special brushes and air jets to dry the component parts. Fine instruments, such as those used in ophthalmic surgery, generally require manual cleaning following ultrasonic decontamination (Hurrell, 2005).

Inspection, assembly and packaging

Inspection

Following mechanical washing and drying, all instruments are visually inspected by the trained sterilising department staff to ensure that there is no damage or defects and that the item is functioning correctly (i.e. scissors are sharp, the jaws of clamps are properly aligned). To sterilise an item that is not functioning correctly could place the patient at risk should it fail during surgery (Hurrell, 2005).

Assembly

Surgical instruments can be assembled in trays or be individually packaged. All operating suites will have a range of instrument trays to cater for the procedures they commonly perform (e.g. laparotomy, hysterectomy, orthopaedic trays). There will also be a general tray of instruments to which individual items may be added, depending on the procedure. All trays are standardised and will contain a specified number and type of instruments identified on a tray list, which is packaged and sterilised with the tray. The tray list is used for checking the contents preoperatively and postoperatively by the instrument and circulating nurses to ensure no items are inadvertently left inside the patient.

Packaging

The aim of packaging the instruments and equipment is to protect the sterilised items against contamination until they are opened ready for use in a surgical procedure. A variety of packaging materials are available and their choice depends on the item to be packaged and the sterilising process to be used. The packaging material must be:

- permeable to air and sterilising agents
- resistant to penetration by microorganisms
- resistant to punctures and tears
- free from toxic ingredients and dyes
- compatible with the sterilising agent and sterilising conditions (Gruendemann & Mangum, 2001).

Packaging materials can be reusable textiles (e.g. linen) or they can be specialised synthetic, single-use, spun bond polymer (Gruendemann & Mangum, 2001). Single-use, self-sealing pouches made of specialised paper or plastic have also been designed for individual items. Metal instruments, endoscopes and drills can be packaged in trays or containers that are made of moulded plastic or metal with perforations to allow penetration by the sterilising agent.

Once assembled, the tray/container is wrapped, usually in two layers of packaging material (this may vary depending on the material and local policy), and folded in a manner that allows subsequent opening using aseptic technique. A label identifying the tray is placed on the external surface. Depending on the sterilising agent to be used, the wrapping material will be sealed using a specialised indicator tape, which will change colour during the sterilising process. This becomes a visual check that the item has undergone the sterilisation process and is checked by the circulating nurse prior to opening the item. The change in colour of the external indicator tape alone does not guarantee sterility of the item. Other sterilising parameters must be met before sterility is assured and these are discussed below. However, if the indicator tape is found not to have changed colour, the item must be considered unsterile and not used.

STERILISATION

Sterilisation is defined as 'the complete elimination or destruction of all forms of microbial life' (Nicolette, 2007). All items introduced into the sterile field must be sterile in order to minimise the risk of surgical site (or other) infection and to promote an uneventful recovery. A number of different methods are used to sterilise items used during the surgical procedure. Their use is based on the physical properties of the item to be sterilised. For example, metal instruments, plastic disposable items, cotton swabs and linen drapes all require a different sterilisation method. Table 5-3 outlines the methods of sterilisation.

Table 5-3 The methods of sterilisation

Method	Process	Action	Examples of items	Wrapping material	Biological indicators
Steam using autoclaves	Steam under pressure	Destroys cellular protein	Stainless steel Linen Moulded plastic	Linen Cotton/polyester Paper Cellulose/synthetic wrap Heat-stable pouches	*Geobacillus stearothermophilus*
Dry heat	Hot air oven	Oxidises cellular protein	Powders, oils	Metal canisters Aluminium foil Glass tubes, bottles	*Bacillus subtilis niger*
Ethylene oxide	100% ethylene oxide gas	Alkylation: chemical interference, which inactivates reproductive process	Laparoscopes Cardiac catheters	Paper pouches Perforated rigid containers	*Bacillus subtilis niger*
Gamma radiation	Cobalt-60 isotope	Destroys cellular DNA	Sponges Surgical gloves Petroleum gauze	Paper Plastic Cellulose	*Bacillus pumilus*
Gas plasma (Sterrad)	Low temperature hydrogen peroxide vapour	Disrupts cellular activity	Telescopes Drills Cameras	Linen Cellulose/synthetic wrap	*Bacillus subtilis niger*
Peracetic acid (Steris)	Low temperature liquid peracetic acid 35%	Disrupts cellular activity	Flexible endoscopes (e.g. gastroscopes)	Unwrapped in specialised rigid tray within sterilising processor	*Geobacillus stearothermophilus*

Gardner & Peel (2001); Nicolette, 2007; Standards Australia (2003, AS/NZS 4187)

Methods of sterilisation

For the purposes of sterilisation, instruments and equipment can be categorised into two groups:

1. heat, moisture or pressure resistant—these require low temperature sterilisation
2. heat, moisture or pressure stable—these items can be exposed to high temperature (Gruendemann & Mangum, 2001).

Steam

Saturated steam under pressure is one of the most effective and commonly used methods of sterilisation. It is an inexpensive method and can be used on items capable of withstanding high temperatures (121–134°C), such as metal instruments and bowls. Steam sterilisation takes place in specially designed sterilisers, often called 'autoclaves', into which trays and individual items are carefully arranged to allow all surfaces to come into contact with the saturated steam. The autoclaves are preprogrammed to reach and maintain a specific temperature, pressure and time ratio depending on the type of load being sterilised (i.e. settings will differ for metal ware compared to linen or mixed loads).

The autoclave chamber is sealed and the sterilisation process begins with the creation of a vacuum inside the autoclave chamber, which is achieved by sucking out all the air. Following removal of all the air, steam under pressure is introduced into the chamber and the temperature will rise to the preprogrammed setting. This is known as the 'penetration time'. When the required temperature and pressure is reached, the actual sterilisation of the items will begin. This is known as the 'holding time', which is approximately 15 minutes. When the holding time is completed, the steam is withdrawn and the load will be left to dry, using the residual heat in the metal walls. In the final stage of the process, filtered air is introduced, which returns the chamber to normal atmospheric pressure.

The steam sterilising process is designed to sterilise large loads of instruments within a central sterilising department, the end result of which is a wrapped, sterile item.

'Flash' sterilisation

A 'flash' steriliser is a smaller unit that uses steam but without the drying cycle of the models used in the central sterilising department. The cycle is rapid (hence the term 'flash'), usually only several minutes, and the item emerges wet.

Flash sterilisers are designed for the management of single items. Operating rooms may have one or two flash sterilisers, permitting the sterilisation of reusable items for immediate use (Standards Australia, 2003, AS/NZS 4187). Their use is not endorsed for regular sterilisation due to their inability to dry items, which can easily become contaminated during subsequent transport to the operative field, which may be some distance away. Flash sterilisation is generally limited to use in emergencies for single items that may have been accidentally contaminated during surgery and for which a replacement cannot be located. The use of flash sterilisation demands adequate decontamination/cleaning of instruments, and daily performance monitoring of steriliser cycles to ensure efficacy of the sterilisation process (Standards Australia, 2003, AS/NZS 4187).

Dry heat

Dry heat sterilisation in the form of hot air ovens was once the only method by which powders, oils and glass could be sterilised. Today, these items are more likely to be supplied by commercial companies who use gamma radiation as a sterilisation method.

This method is more economical as large volumes of the items can be sterilised. Dry heat is a slow, expensive method of sterilisation using a temperature range of 160–180°C, depending on the item and exposure time required (Gardner & Peel, 2001).

Ethylene oxide gas

Ethylene oxide (ETO) gas is a low-temperature (36–60°C) chemical method of sterilisation that is suitable for items that cannot be exposed to the high temperatures associated with steam or to dry heat. ETO is a highly toxic agent and exposure can cause severe toxic reactions, such as nausea, vomiting and respiratory difficulties, in health care workers. Therefore, strict occupational health and safety controls exist to protect operators of ETO sterilisers.

ETO is very effective in sterilising items such as rubber, silicone and polyethylene products, especially those with narrow lumens, and telescopes and drills. Items for sterilising are wrapped in single-use packaging or pouches and placed in an ETO steriliser, where the temperature and humidity are controlled before the ETO gas is introduced. The time taken to sterilise items can be up to 2 hours and, as ETO is absorbed into the items, there must be a further 2–12 hours' aeration time to ensure that the ETO has been completely eliminated from the items before it can be used (Gruendemann & Mangum, 2001; Nicolette, 2007; Standards Australia, 2003, AS/NZS 4187).

Gas plasma

The gas plasma method uses hydrogen peroxide vapour and plasma to create a state under which items such as cameras, telescopes and drills can be sterilised under low-temperature conditions. This method has, in many instances, superseded ETO because it is a less toxic and more rapid form of sterilisation. Gas plasma involves the introduction of hydrogen peroxide vapour into a closed vacuum chamber through which radiofrequency waves are introduced, creating an electromagnetic field and conditions that kill microorganisms. The cycle time is approximately 30–60 minutes, depending on the model of steriliser, and the by-products are oxygen and water, thus making it substantially more environmentally sound than ETO (Nicolette, 2007).

Peracetic acid

Peracetic acid is a low-temperature, liquid chemical method of sterilisation that is suited for use with endoscopes that cannot be sterilised using high temperatures. Commercially produced processing systems are increasingly used within operating rooms where flexible endoscopes (e.g. gastroscopes) are used frequently and require sterilisation close to the time of use. The active ingredient is peracetic acid 35%, which is highly corrosive and, therefore, is used in combination with an anticorrosive agent. The processing unit is fully computerised and is the size of a small suitcase, with a lid and an internal tray especially configured to fit a flexible endoscope. A connection kit fits onto the exposed ends of the internal lumen system to ensure the sterilising agent passes through each lumen. Once the lid is closed and the processor activated, the active peracetic acid mixes with water and is fed over and through the endoscope for a period of 12 minutes, followed by four rinse cycles, which use filtered water to flush the peracetic acid away. The whole cycle takes approximately 30 minutes and the result is a wet, sterile scope ready for immediate use.

As with all items, thorough cleaning of the endoscope must occur prior to sterilisation, using specialised brushes and enzymatic cleaning agents to ensure that all lumens are free of debris and bioburden (Nicolette, 2007). The end product of peracetic acid is environmentally safe acetic acid and water.

Gamma radiation

Many commercially packaged products that are unsuitable for sterilisation by chemical or heat processes are sterilised by irradiation using the isotope cobalt-60, which produces gamma rays. Gamma rays can penetrate large cartons of items, making this an economical method for large medical companies to sterilise items such as ointments, sponges, plastic drapes and surgical gloves. This method is suitable for commercial application only.

Creutzfeldt-Jakob disease

The causative prions of CJD are highly resistant to conventional decontamination and sterilisation methods. Special protocols are required to manage instruments if they have been used on patients known or thought to be at risk of carrying the disease. Ideally, disposable instruments should be used, but this may not prove to be practical. Many institutions quarantine reusable instruments used on suspected CJD patients until test results from the patients have been obtained. Negative results will mean that routine decontamination and sterilisation processes can be followed. Positive results will require instruments to be reprocessed using combinations of germicidal solutions for mechanical cleaning followed by steam sterilisation at temperatures and pressures in excess of those routinely required for steam sterilisation (Nicolette, 2007). The management of equipment exposed to CJD prions is still evolving as further research is carried out on this highly infective, but fortunately rare, disease.

Monitoring sterilisation processes

All sterilising methods must undergo validation processes to ensure that items are sterile and may be safely used on patients. The validation process refers to documented procedures for obtaining, recording and interpreting results needing to show that a process will consistently produce a sterile item. This commences with the commissioning of new sterilising equipment and ongoing performance qualifications comprising microbiological and physical parameters (Gardner & Peel, 2001).

Physical

Regular maintenance, monitoring and testing takes place of all sterilisers to ensure that they are functioning correctly in accordance with Standards Australia (2003, AS/NZS 4187). All sterilisers have external gauges, thermometers, timers and computer printouts to monitor their functions. Internal sensors can provide information about temperature, pressure and humidity for every load. Documentation of these parameters is performed to provide permanent records so as to provide retrospective proof that all loads have passed through the sterilisation process satisfactorily.

Chemical

External indicators appear on the outside of each package and these change colour when the item has passed through a sterilisation process. These may be incorporated into the wrapping material, as in pouches, or as a separate tape or spots attached to the outside of the wrapped item. Different types of external indicators are required for each type of sterilisation method. The external indicators do not demonstrate that the item is sterile but do provide important visual indicators that the item has undergone a sterilising process.

An internal chemical indicator strip, known as an integrator, is placed inside with the items to assess the complete penetration of steam or chemical vapours. If the sterilisation parameters have been met, the strip will change colour, and this will be verified at the point of use by the instrument nurse prior to using the instruments. If the integrator strip has not changed colour, the items must not be used as sterilisation may not have occurred.

Biological

Biological indicators are standardised preparations of bacterial spores that are included as part of the routine testing processes of sterilisers to demonstrate whether sterilisation conditions have been met. Biological indicators are inoculated with a known concentration of spore preparations, which will be different, depending on the sterilisation process. For example, the spores used to test steam sterilisation conditions are those of *Geobacillus stearothermophilis*. Following exposure to the sterilisation process, the indicators will be examined to ascertain if the spores have been destroyed, which indicates that this testing parameter has been met.

No one testing parameter alone will verify that sterilisation conditions have been met. Sterilisation is achieved when all the physical, chemical and biological parameters have been met (Gardner & Peel, 2001; Standards Australia, 2003, AS/NZS 4187).

Tracking and traceability

The ability to track instruments and trace patients is an integral component of safety and risk management processes. Written and computerised records are maintained within the sterilising department to provide retrospective proof that an item has satisfactorily passed through a sterilisation process. These records are important should an outbreak of infection occur where investigations demonstrate that there may have been a breakdown in the sterilisation process. Patients who have undergone procedures during the period in question and may have been infected need to be traced and their infectious status investigated. Tracking systems rely on trays of instruments having barcodes and being scanned during decontamination and reprocessing, with the data stored on computer for future reference (Hurrell, 2005).

However, a more effective tracking system is one that is able to track an individual instrument back to a specific patient. Currently few such systems exist; however, with advances in technology, sophisticated instrument tracking systems will become more widespread in the future.

Disinfection

Disinfection is described as a process of destroying all pathogenic organisms except spores from inanimate objects (Nicolette, 2007). The process can be used on items identified as semi-critical or non-critical (see Table 5-2). Disinfection involves the use of liquid chemical disinfectants, which can be classified as high, intermediate or low level depending on their killing capabilities.

- High level—glutaraldehyde: can destroy all microorganisms except spores; may be used to disinfect endoscopes.
- Intermediate level—phenolics (carbolic acid): can destroy tubercle bacilli and most viruses and fungi; mainly used on floors and furniture.
- Low level—chlorine compounds (bleach): can destroy some viruses and fungi; mainly used on floors and surfaces as will corrode metal instruments.

As with items for sterilisation, effective decontamination of the items or surfaces using enzymatic cleaners, detergents and water must occur prior to disinfection (Nicolette, 2007). Staff should wear personal protective attire when using disinfecting agents as contact can produce adverse skin or respiratory effects. Material Safety Data Sheets (MSDS) containing information on each chemical, its use, possible adverse effects and first aid and spill management should be available within the operating suite.

CONCLUSION

In conclusion, it is important to note that HAIs are considered an accurate indicator of the quality of patient care. The focus of this chapter has been on assisting perioperative nurses to understand and implement a range of practices and strategies that are aimed at preventing or minimising infection in the surgical patient. Perioperative nurses must work in collaboration with other members of the health care team to monitor infection control practices constantly to ensure quality care for patients.

CRITICAL THINKING EXERCISES

1. Perioperative attire

It is your first day in the operating suite and you are directed to the change room to change into perioperative attire.
- Why are you required to change into perioperative attire?
- Describe the attire you will wear.

2. Sterilisation procedures

- Locate your sterile stockroom and collect examples of items that have been sterilised by the methods described in this chapter. Note how sterility is indicated and the type of packaging used.

3. Aseptic technique

You have been asked to circulate for a procedure and to open the sterile supplies required.
- Describe the principles and practices of asepsis you will follow when opening the sterile equipment.

4. The surgical scrub

You are about to perform a surgical scrub.
- Describe the procedure you will follow when scrubbing, gowning and gloving.
- Identify the personal protective equipment you will wear.

RESOURCES

Agents of bioterrorism
    http://www.usamriid.army.mil/publicationspage.html
    www.bt.cdc.gov
Commonwealth of Australia Infection Control Policy
    http://www.health.gov.au/internet/wcms/publishing.nsf/Content/icg-guidelines-
        index.htm
Creutzfeldt-Jakob disease (CJD)
    http://www.cdc.gov/ncidod/dvrd/cjd/
    http://www.cdc.gov/ncidod/dvrd/vcjd/index.htm.
    http://www.hpa.org.uk/infections/topics_az/cjd/information_documents.htm
Multi-drug resistant organisms (MDRO)
    http://www.cdc.gov/ncidod/dhqp/pdf/ar/mdroGuideline2006.pd
Perioperative Nurses College of New Zealand Nurses Organisation
    http://www.pnc.org.nz/Site/Sections/Colleges/Perioperative/

Severe acute respiratory syndrome (SARS)
   www.who.int/csr/sarsarchive/2003_05_07a/en/
   www.cdc.gov/ncidod/sars
The Cochrane Collaboration
   http://www.cochrane.org/index.htm

REFERENCES

ACORN. (2006). *Standards for perioperative nursing, including nursing roles, guidelines, position statements, competency standards. S11. Perioperative attire.* Adelaide: Australian College of Operating Room Nurses.

Australian Department of Health and Ageing. (2004). Infection control guidelines for the prevention of transmission of infectious diseases in the health care setting. Retrieved September 14, 2007, from http://www.icg.health.gov.au.

Best, M., & Newhauser, D. (2004). Ignaz Semmelweis and the birth of infection control. *Quality Safety Health Care, 13*, 233–234.

Burton, G., & Engelkirk, P. (2000). *Microbiology for the health sciences.* Sydney: Lippincott Williams & Wilkins.

Castella, A., Charrier, L., Di Legami, V., et al. (2006). Surgical site infection surveillance: analysis of adherence to recommendations for routine infection control practices. *Infection Control and Hospital Epidemiology, 27(8)*, 835–840.

Dunscombe, A. (2007). Sutures, needles and instruments. In J. Rothrock, D. McEwen (Eds.). *Alexander's care of the patient in surgery* (13th ed.) (pp. 158–182). St Louis: Mosby.

Edwards, P., Lipp, A., Holmes, A. (2004). Preoperative skin antiseptics for preventing surgical wound infections after clean surgery. *Cochrane Database of Systematic Reviews, 3*, CD003949.

Gardner, J. F., & Peel, M. M. (2001). *Sterilization, disinfection and infection control* (3rd ed.). Sydney: Elsevier.

Gilmour, D. (2005). Infection control principles. In K. Woodhead, & P. Wicker (Eds.). *Textbook of perioperative care* (pp. 81–96). Edinburgh: Churchill Livingstone.

Goldman, M. (2008). *Pocket guide to the operating room* (3rd ed.). Philadelphia: F A Davis.

Grant, G., Grant, A., Lockwood, C., Simpson, C. J. (2005). Semmelweis, and transformational change. *American College of Obstetricians and Gynecologists, 106(2)*, 384–387.

Griffin, F. (2005). Best-practice protocols: preventing surgical site infection. *Nursing Management, 36(11)*, 22–26.

Gruendemann, B., & Mangum, S. (2001). *Infection prevention in surgical settings.* St Louis: Mosby.

Hamlin, L. (2008). Operating theatre practice. In S. Hughes, & A. Mardell (Eds.). *Handbook of perioperative nursing.* Oxford: Oxford University Press.

Hurrell, D. (2005). Decontamination of reusable medical devices. In K. Woodhead, & P. Wicker (Eds.). *Textbook of perioperative care* (pp. 97–118). Edinburgh: Churchill Livingstone.

Lee, G., & Bishop, P. (2006). *Microbiology and infection control for health professionals* (3rd ed.). Sydney: Pearson Prentice Hall.

Lee, J. (2005). Air, hair, knees, nose. *Infection Control and Hospital Epidemiology, 26(12)*, 900–902.

Lipp, A. (2005). An evaluation of preoperative skin antiseptics. *British Journal of Perioperative Nursing, 15(1)*, 12–19.

Lipp, A., & Edwards, P. (2002). Disposable surgical face masks: a systematic review. *Journal of Advanced Perioperative Care, 1(2)*, 41–46.

NSW Health. (2007a). Infection control policy: prevention and management of multi-resistant organisms (MRO). PD2007_084. Sydney: NSW Health.

NSW Health. (2007b). Infection control policy. Policy directives. PD2007_036. Sydney: NSW Health.

NZ Ministry of Health. (2007). Guidelines for the control of multi-drug resistant organisms in New Zealand. Wellington: NZMOH. Retrieved February 13, 2008, from http://www.moh.govt.nz/moh.nsf/pagesmh/3345.

Nicolette, L. (2007). Infection prevention and control in the perioperative setting. In J. Rothrock, & D. McEwen (Eds.). *Alexander's care of the patient in surgery* (13th ed.) (pp. 44–99). St Louis: Mosby.

Phillips, N. (2007). *Berry & Kohn's operating theatre technique* (11th ed.). St Louis: Mosby.

Pittet, D. (2005). Infection control and quality health care in the new millennium. *American Journal of Infection Control, 33(5)*, 258–267.

Santos, A., Lacerda, R., Graziano, K. (2005). Evidence of control and prevention of surgical site infection by shoe covers and private shoes: a systematic literature review. *Revista Latino—Americana de Enfermagen, 13(1)*, 86–92.

Siegel, J., Rhinehart, E., Jackson, M., et al. (2007). Guidelines for isolation precautions: preventing transmission of infectious agents in healthcare settings 2007. Retrieved March 14, 2008, from http://www.cdc.gov/ncidod/dhqp/pdf/guidelines/Isolation2007.pdf.

Standards Australia. (2003). AS/NZS 4187 Cleaning, disinfecting and sterilizing reusable medical and surgical instruments and equipment, and maintenance of associated environments in health care facilities. Sydney: Standards Australia.

Tanner, J., Blunsden, C., Fakis, A. (2007). National survey of hand antisepsis practices. *Journal of Perioperative Practice, 17(1)*, 27–37.

Tanner, J., & Parkinson, H. (2006). Double gloving to reduce surgical cross-infection. *Cochrane Database of Systematic Reviews, 3*, CD003087.

Tanner, J., Swarbrook, S., Stuart, J. (2008). Surgical hand antisepsis to reduce surgical site infection (review). *Cochrane Database of Systematic Reviews, 1*, CD004288.

Tanner, J., Woodings, D., Moncaster, K. (2006). Preoperative hair removal to reduce surgical site infection. *Cochrane Database of Systematic Reviews, 2*, CD004122.

Wicker, P., & O'Neil, J. (2006). *Caring for the perioperative patient*. Edinburgh: Churchill Livingstone.

Woodhead, K., & Wicker, P. (2005). *Textbook of perioperative care*. Edinburgh: Churchill Livingstone.

FURTHER READING

Botwinick, L., Bisognanom M., Haraden, C. (2006). Leadership guide to patient safety. Institute for Healthcare Improvement. Retrieved April 3, 2008, from www.ihi.org.

Gillespie, S., & Bamford, K. (2003). *Medical microbiology and infection at a glance* (2nd ed.). Malden, MA: Blackwell Publishing.

Haydon, D., Cleaveland, S., Taylor, L., Laurenson, M. (2002). Identifying reservoirs of infection: a conceptual and practical challenge. *Emerging Infections Diseases, 8(12)*. Retrieved April 3, 2008, from http://www.cdc.gov/ncidod/eid/vol8no12/01-0317.htm.

Health Protection Surveillance Centre. (2001). Strategy for the control of antimicrobial resistance in Ireland (SARI). Retrieved April 8, 2008, from http://www.ndsc.ie/hpsc/A-Z/MicrobiologyAntimicrobialResistance/StrategyforthecontrolofAntimicrobialResistanceinIrelandSARI.

Laine, J., & Aaarnio, P. (2004). Glove perforation in orthopaedic and trauma surgery. *Journal of Bone and Joint Surgery, 86(6)*, 898–900.

NSW Therapeutics Advisory Group. (2003). Drug utilisation. Retrieved April 8, 2008, from http://www.ciap.health.nsw.gov.au/nswtag/drug_utilisation.html 8.

NSW Therapeutic Advisory Group. (2007). Indicators for quality use of medicines in Australian hospitals. Retrieved April 8, 2008, from http://www.ciap.health.nsw.gov.au/nswtag.

Roxburgh, M., Gall, P., Leek, K. (2006). A cover up? Potential risks of wearing theatre clothing outside theatre. *Journal of Perioperative Practice, 16(1)*, 30–41.

Stringer, B., & Haines, T. (2006). Hands free technique: preventing occupational exposure during surgery. *Journal of Perioperative Practice, 16(10)*, 495–500.

Tanner, J. (2006). Surgical glove: perforation and protection. *Journal of Perioperative Practice, 16(3)*, 148–152.

Anaesthesia

Toni Gwynn-Jones and Julie Walters

LEARNING OBJECTIVES

After reading this chapter, you should be able to:

- discuss the physiological changes that occur during anaesthesia
- describe the different modalities of anaesthesia
- identify the drugs commonly used in anaesthesia
- identify equipment used for airway management
- identify patient monitoring required during anaesthesia
- discuss the fluid and electrolyte requirements of a patient undergoing anaesthesia
- describe complications that arise during anaesthesia and their management.

KEY TERMS

airway management	general anaesthesia	regional anaesthesia
epidural anaesthesia	haemodynamic monitoring	spinal anaesthesia
fluid and electrolyte balance	local anaesthesia	

INTRODUCTION

General anaesthesia dates back to William T Morton, an American dentist who was credited as being the first to use ether as a surgical anaesthetic in 1846. This discovery revolutionised surgery, making it possible for more complex procedures to be undertaken because patients could now be rendered unconscious with anaesthesia. Since then, anaesthesia has seen many advances and anaesthetists are now able to use a wide range of drugs, techniques and sophisticated equipment to provide patients with safe and pain-free surgery.

This chapter presents the concepts of the perianaesthesia care of the patient, including the different types of anaesthesia, drugs used and management of the patient's airway, together with the monitoring used during the perianaesthesia period. Complications and their management are discussed and the chapter concludes with a discussion on fluid and electrolyte management, including blood replacement. The management of adult patients is the focus, with only a passing reference to paediatric anaesthesia as it is beyond the scope of this text to discuss this specialty in detail.

PRE-ANAESTHETIC ASSESSMENT OF THE PATIENT

Prior to the patient undergoing an anaesthetic, a full assessment must be carried out. The preoperative assessment and preparation of the patient has been discussed in detail in Chapter 2. It is important to note the family history, especially of metabolic disease, as certain drugs and anaesthetic agents may affect patients who have a history of malignant hyperthermia. A drug history, including current medications and allergies, should be noted as the interaction of drugs can have serious consequences. A social history, including smoking, alcohol intake and use of illegal drugs, is important to note, as is the use of herbal dietary supplements that are known to produce central nervous system (CNS) stimulation or depression or interact with psychotropic drugs. All these issues can adversely affect the patient's anaesthetic outcome (Marley, 2005).

The patient assessment must take into consideration the following:

- baseline physiological state
- current and past medical and surgical history
- the planned procedure
- drug sensitivities
- past anaesthetic experience
- psychological make-up (Marley, 2005).

Assessment of the airway

As part of the pre-anaesthetic assessment, it is essential that the anaesthetist predicts airway and intubation difficulties and plans **airway management** accordingly. Assessment criteria include the following:

- length of incisors—this may impede the introduction of a laryngoscope blade into the mouth
- mobility of cervical spine, length and thickness of neck—to facilitate neck movement during intubation
- the ability to see the soft palate and uvula with the mouth open and tongue protruded, known as the Mallampati score
- the ability to sublux the mandible forward at the temporomandibular joint
- the thyromental distance (less than three fingers)—this is measured from the thyroid notch to the inner border of the mandible when the patient's head is extended.

Mallampati assessment

The Mallampati test is used to examine the patient's oral cavity and soft palate visually to predict any possible difficulties with tracheal intubation. It can be conducted during the pre-anaesthetic assessment. Figure 6-1 shows the four classifications. Classes III and VI, which indicate that viewing of the soft palate is difficult or impossible, suggest a higher degree of difficultly with intubation in these patients (Fell & Kirkbride, 2007).

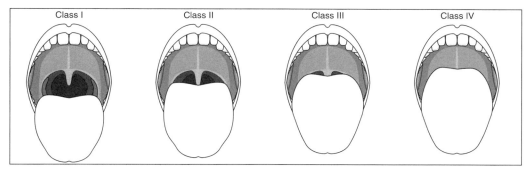

Figure 6-1 Classification of the pharyngeal view when performing the Mallampati test (Aitkenhead et al., 2007, p 285).

Further preoperative considerations

The grading system of the American Society of Anesthesiologists (ASA) was introduced in the 1960s as a description of the physical state of the patient, along with an indication of whether surgery is elective or emergency (Fell & Kirkbride, 2007). The ASA physical status classification system is presented in Table 2-2. The ASA classification of the patient will influence the anaesthetist's decisions about anaesthetic care and postoperative management. These decisions include whether the patient requires postoperative care in the day surgery unit, inpatient bed, high-dependency unit or adult intensive care unit.

After the patient's history, examination and relevant investigations have been collated, the anaesthetist is able to plan the patient's care more accurately. The decisions being considered regarding anaesthetic care, pain management and possible blood transfusions should be discussed with the patient and opportunities to ask questions should be made available. Patients should also be given relevant information regarding fasting times and whether to take their regular medications with a sip of water on the day of surgery.

It is important that anaesthetic nurses make themselves familiar with their patient's history and assessment as soon as patients are admitted into the perioperative environment in order to plan nursing care and to prepare equipment to ensure safe patient outcomes. This will be carried out in conjunction with the anaesthetist to ascertain any special requirements.

Identification and preparation of the patient

The patient is accompanied to the operating suite by a nurse from the ward, who will hand over care of the patient to a member of the perioperative team, usually a nurse in the arrival/waiting area of the operating suite, often termed the 'holding bay'. Both nurses and the patient will participate in completing a preoperative patient checklist (see Figs 2-2 and 2-3) as part of the admission procedure, which will vary according to hospital policy but will include the following:

- identification of the patient, confirming name and medical record number using the patient's medical history and identification bands
- fasting times
- allergies
- confirmation of consent—the patient confirms procedure, the site and side of surgery; in most hospitals the site of surgery should already be marked by the surgeon, although this may be carried out following admission to the operating suite
- any preoperative medications given.

In addition, it is imperative that an anaesthetic consult is present and complete. Any discrepancies should be noted, reported to the surgical team and rectified before commencement of anaesthesia (ACORN, 2006). The verification of patient details continues throughout each stage of the patient's care according to local policy.

Prior to the induction of anaesthesia, base line observations of pulse and blood pressure will be taken, electrocardiograph (ECG) monitoring devices and warming devices will be attached, and intravenous (IV) access will be secured. This can be a highly anxious time for the patient and, throughout this time, good communication skills are necessary to explain the procedures to the patient and provide quiet reassurance. Therapeutic touch and other anxiety-reduction measures (e.g. music) may be used.

TYPES OF ANAESTHETICS

Anaesthesia is defined as the 'loss of the sensations of pain, pressure, temperature and touch in a part of the whole of the body' (Bryant & Knight, 2007). The main categories of anaesthesia are:

- general
- local infiltration
- regional—spinal and epidural—these can be combined to provide the patient with pain relief in the postoperative period.
- sedation/analgesia.

General anaesthesia

General anaesthesia is a reversible, unconscious state characterised by amnesia, analgesia and suppression of reflexes (DeLamar, 2007). The drugs and gaseous agents used to induce and maintain anaesthesia have a profound physiological effect on body systems, notably the CNS. The area in the CNS that is most affected is the sensory pathways from the thalamus to the cortex, thus depressing conscious thought, motor control, perceptions, memory and sensations. The medullary centres are the final cerebral area to be affected by anaesthesia and unconsciousness occurs, with both respiratory and cardiovascular centres temporarily depressed. These stages of anaesthesia were first described by the American anaesthetist, Arthur Guedel, and are outlined in Table 6-1 (Fell & Kirkbride, 2007).

Pharmacological agents used in general anaesthesia

Intravenous induction agents

IV induction agents are commonly used to induce general anaesthesia because they provide a smoother and more rapid induction than most inhalational agents. Short-acting IV induction agents (e.g. thiopentone, propofol) induce a pleasant sleep, and anaesthesia is maintained for the duration of the surgical procedure by using a combination of oxygen, nitrous oxide and volatile inhalational agents (e.g. sevoflurane). Some anaesthetists may use an IV induction agent as a continuous infusion to maintain anaesthesia, eliminating the need for inhalational agents (Brown & Edwards, 2007).

Table 6-1 Stages of anaesthesia (modified from Guedel)

Stage	Respiration	Pupils	Eye reflexes	Upper respiratory tract and respiratory reflexes
1. Analgesia	Regular, small volume			
2. Excitement	Irregular		Eyelash absent	
3. Anaesthesia				
Plane I	Regular, large volume		Eyelid absent, conjunctival reflex depressed	Pharyngeal and vomiting reflexes depressed
Plane II	Regular, large volume		Corneal reflex depressed	
Plane III	Regular, becoming diaphragmatic, small volume			Laryngeal reflex depressed
Plane IV	Irregular, diaphragmatic, small volume			Carinal reflex depressed
4. Overdose	Apnoea			

Aitkenhead et al. (2007)

Inhalational agents

Volatile and gaseous inhalational anaesthetic agents remain popular for the maintenance of anaesthesia, and may be used to induce anaesthesia in paediatrics to avoid the need to insert IV cannulae, which can be traumatic for a child.

Inhalational agents include nitrous oxide, which is colourless, essentially odourless and the only inorganic anaesthetic gas in clinical use. Although it possesses some analgesic properties, it will not maintain narcosis. The addition of a volatile inhalational agent will maintain the patient in an unconscious state.

Volatile agents are liquid at room temperature and administered through a specialised vaporiser that is attached to the anaesthetic machine. Oxygen, which is another gas that must be used in all general anaesthesia, passes through the vaporiser and mixes with the liquid agent, changing the volatile agent into a gas. The mixture is delivered to the patient via the variety of airway and delivery equipment attached to the anaesthetic machine. The percentage of inhalational agents delivered to the patient can be adjusted by the anaesthetist depending on the depth of anaesthesia required. Table 6-2 provides a summary of the IV and inhalational agents used in general anaesthesia.

Table 6-2 Intravenous and inhalational anaesthetic agents

Drugs	Advantages	Disadvantages	Nursing interventions
Intravenous agents			
Barbiturates			
Thiopentone Methohexitone	Rapid induction, duration of action less than 5 min	Adverse cardiac effects, hypotension, tachycardia, respiratory depression	Usually have minimal postoperative effects due to extremely short duration Repeated doses may lead to 'hangover effect'
Non-barbiturate hypnotics			
Etomidate	Produces little change in cardiovascular dynamics; useful for haemodynamically unstable patients	Associated with adverse effects of myoclonia, nausea and vomiting, hiccups and adrenocortical inhibition	Observe for transient skeletal muscle movements (myoclonia), nausea and vomiting, hiccups, hypotension and hypoglycaemia
Propofol	Ideal for short outpatient procedures because of rapid onset of action, rapid distribution and high metabolic clearance; may be used for maintenance of anaesthesia as well as induction	May cause bradycardia and other dysrhythmias, hypotension, apnoea, phlebitis, nausea and vomiting, hiccups May cause hypertriglyceridaemia	Short action leads to minimal postoperative effects; monitor injection site for phlebitis; cardiac monitoring if unstable Monitor serum triglycerides every 24 h for sedation greater than 24 h
Inhalational agents			
Volatile liquids			
Halothane Enflurane Isoflurane Desflurane Sevoflurane	All volatile liquids: muscle relaxation, low incidence of nausea and vomiting Halothane: bronchodilation Isoflurane: less cardiac depression, devoid of toxicity to body organs Desflurane: rapid induction and emergence, widely used volatile agent Sevoflurane: predictable effects on cardiovascular and respiratory systems, rapid acting, non-irritating to respiratory system	All volatile liquids: myocardial depression, early onset of pain because of rapid elimination Halothane: hypotension and possible hepatotoxicity Enflurane: increased intracranial pressure, seizures, unpredictable duration of action Sevoflurane: may be associated with emergence delirium	Assess and treat pain during early anaesthesia recovery; assess for adverse reactions such as cardiopulmonary depression with hypotension and prolonged respiratory depression; monitor for nausea and vomiting

(contd)

Drugs	Advantages	Disadvantages	Nursing interventions
Gaseous agents			
Nitrous oxide	Potentiates volatile agents, allowing a reduction in their dosage and their negative side-effects and increases the rate of induction; has high analgesic potency	Weak anaesthetic, rarely used alone; must be administered with oxygen to prevent hypoxaemia; nausea and vomiting more common than with other inhaled anaesthetics	Produces little or no toxicity at therapeutic concentrations; monitor for effects of volatile liquids when nitrous oxide used as an adjunct
Dissociative anaesthetics			
Ketamine	Can be administered intravenously or intramuscularly; potent analgesic and amnesic	May cause hallucinations and nightmares, increased intracranial and intraocular pressure, increased heart rate, hypertension	Anticipate administration of a benzodiazepine if agitation and hallucinations occur, calm quiet environment is essential in postoperative care

(Lewis et al., 2007)

Adjuncts to general anaesthesia

Table 6-3 provides a summary of the most commonly used adjunct drugs to general anaesthesia. As can be seen from Tables 6-2 and 6-3, many of the agents used to induce anaesthesia and as adjuncts have a powerful effect on the patient's cardiovascular and respiratory systems. This requires the anaesthetist and anaesthetic nurse to monitor the patient closely using a variety of invasive and non-invasive haemodynamic monitoring devices (see p 151), as well as observational skills.

Table 6-3 Adjuncts to general anaesthesia			
Agents	**Uses during anaesthesia**	**Adverse effects**	**Nursing interventions**
Opioids			
Fentanyl Sufentanil Morphine sulfate Pethidine Alfentanil Remifentanil Methadone	Induce and maintain anaesthesia, reduce stimuli from sensory nerve endings, provide analgesia during surgery and anaesthetic recovery	Respiratory depression, stimulation of vomiting centre, possible bradycardia and peripheral vasodilation (when combined with anaesthetics), high incidence of pruritus with both regional and intravenous administration	Assess respiratory status, monitor pulse oximetry (for a late sign of hypoxaemia), protect airway in anticipation of vomiting, use standing orders for antipruritics, such as diphenhydramine
Benzodiazepines			
Midazolam Diazepam Lorazepam	Induce and maintain anaesthesia	Potentiation of the effects of opioids, increasing the potential for respiratory depression, hypotension and tachycardia	Monitor cardiopulmonary status, level of consciousness

(contd)

Table 6-3 Adjuncts to general anaesthesia *(contd)*

Agents	Uses during anaesthesia	Adverse effects	Nursing interventions
Neuromuscular blocking agents			

Depolarising agents:
  Suxamethonium
Non-depolarising agents:
  Vecuronium
  Atracurium
  Pancuronium
  Tubocurarine
  Pipecuronium
  Doxacurium
  Rocuronium
  Mivacurium
	Facilitate endotracheal intubation, promote skeletal muscle relaxation (paralysis) to enhance access to surgical sites; effects of non-depolarising agents are usually reversed towards the end of surgery by the administration of anticholinesterase agents (e.g. neostigmine, pyridostigmine, edrophonium)	Apnoea related to paralysis of respiratory muscles, prolonged muscle relaxation due to longer action of non-depolarising agents than reversal agents, cardiac alterations. Recurrence of muscle weakness with correction of hypothermia	Monitor respiratory rate and pattern until patient able to cough and return to previous levels of muscle strength; maintain patent airway; ensure availability of non-depolarising reversal agents and respiratory support equipment, monitor temperature and levels of muscle strength with temperature changes

Antiemetics			
Droperidol Ondansetron Dolasetron Metoclopramide Prochlorperazine Promethazine	Prevention of vomiting with aspiration during surgery, counteract the emetic effects of inhalation agents and opioids; droperidol often used during surgery; others more often used postoperatively	Droperidol: dysrhythmias, laryngospasm, bronchospasm, tachycardia, hypotension, central nervous system alterations, extrapyramidal reactions, contraindicated in patients with Parkinson's disease or hypomagnesaemia Other antiemetics: headache, dizziness, sedation, malaise, fatigue, musculoskeletal pain, shivers, diarrhoea, acute dystonic reactions, cardiovascular alterations, contraindicated in patients with hypomagnesaemia	Monitor cardiopulmonary status, level of consciousness, and ability to move limbs Droperidol: administer with caution in patients with heart disease

(Lewis et al., 2007)

Analgesics

In addition to the drugs designed to keep the patient under general anaesthesia, opioid analgesic drugs will be given to provide pain relief. Opioid is a term used to refer to a group of drugs, both naturally occurring and synthetically produced, that possess opium or morphine properties. One of the most commonly used opioids is fentanyl (Faut-Callahan & Hand, 2005).

Muscle relaxants

The discovery of curare, a naturally occurring muscle relaxant, by Harold Griffith and Enid Johnson in 1942, was a milestone in anaesthesia. Curare greatly facilitated endotracheal intubation and provided excellent relaxation for abdominal surgery. For the first time, surgery could be performed on patients without having to administer large doses of anaesthetic agents to produce the required muscle relaxation. A wide range of muscle relaxant agents have been developed since, giving today's anaesthetist a variety of drugs for use in clinical practice (Hunter, 2007).

Muscle relaxation is achieved by blocking neuromuscular activity at the motor end plate of skeletal muscles where the receptors for acetylcholine are located. Acetylcholine, a naturally occurring neurotransmitter, plays an important role in facilitating the transmission of nerve impulses. Interference with the transmission of nerve impulses results in paralysis of skeletal muscle, which includes the muscles of respiration. There are two types of neuromuscular blocking agents: depolarising and non-depolarising agents (Bryant & Knight, 2007).

Suxamethonium is a short-acting *depolarising* muscle relaxant that acts in 30–60 seconds and lasts 3–5 minutes before it is metabolised by plasma cholinesterase, a naturally occurring enzyme. It is the only agent that creates good conditions for tracheal intubation in emergency airway management or rapid sequence induction. Its onset of action is characterised by facial twitching or fasciculations. However, the effect wears off due to the build-up of plasma cholinesterase (Bryant & Knight, 2007).

To maintain muscle paralysis for the duration of the surgical procedure, a longer acting muscle relaxant is required. These agents are known as *non-depolarising* muscle relaxants (e.g. rocuronium) and they have a different mode of action to the depolarising agents. Non-depolarising muscle relaxants compete with naturally occurring acetylcholine for receptors at the motor end plate of skeletal muscles, thus causing paralysis. To terminate the action of non-depolarising muscle relaxants, a reversal drug, such as neostigmine, has to be administered towards the end of the procedure. This allows acetylcholine to build up to normal levels and enables normal muscle contraction to return. This results in the patient commencing unassisted respiration once all other anaesthetic agents have been stopped. A side-effect of neostigmine is bradycardia, which is counteracted by the simultaneous administration of an antimuscarinic drug (e.g. atropine, glycopyrrolate), which has a parasympathetic effect and increases pulse rate (Simpson & Popat, 2001).

Antiemetics

In order to minimise nausea, vomiting and possible aspiration of stomach contents into the lungs, the anaesthetist may administer an antiemetic drug. The effects of antiemetic drugs will continue into the immediate postoperative period, providing the patient with a more comfortable recovery period.

PROCEDURE FOR GENERAL ANAESTHESIA

Anaesthetic preparation and equipment checking

Prior to the commencement of the operating list, it is important that the anaesthetic machine is checked in accordance with the Australian and New Zealand College of Anaesthetists (ANZCA) guidelines by both the anaesthetist and anaesthetic nurse (ANZCA, 2003b). Anaesthetic machines deliver gases and volatile agents to the patient via delivery tubing that attaches to the patient's airway management equipment (e.g. endotracheal tube). Oxygen, nitrous oxide and air are piped into the operating room via a network of pipes from a central bulk store of gases within the hospital. A pendant attached to the ceiling delivers the gases to the anaesthetic machine through colour-coded tubes (white for oxygen, blue for nitrous oxide). The fixtures for each gas outlet are gas-specific, which is an important safety feature to ensure that the oxygen tubing cannot physically be attached to the nitrous oxide outlet and vice versa. The same feature exists for the back-up gas cylinders attached to the anaesthetic machine. The anaesthetic machine is more than a gas delivery unit. It also contains a range of sophisticated equipment necessary to monitor the patient's condition throughout the perianaesthesia period (e.g. ECG, oximetry and capnography).

Other preoperative equipment checks include suction, airway equipment, drugs, additional equipment such as infusion pumps, warming devices and all monitoring equipment. These must be available and in working order prior to the patient's arrival in order to ensure a smooth and safe anaesthesia process for the patient. Figure 6-2 shows an anaesthetic machine complete with monitoring equipment.

Induction of anaesthesia

Induction is defined as the administration of a drug or combination of drugs that results in a state of general anaesthesia (Bryant & Knight, 2007). Preoxygenation of the patient may be carried out to avoid transient hypoxaemia, which can occur before the establishment of an effective airway and ventilation.

During induction it is important that the environment is as quiet as possible to facilitate a smooth induction. Extraneous noise from people talking or the instrument and circulating nurses setting up equipment should be minimised during induction (Fell & Kirkbride, 2007).

Establishment of the airway

Once anaesthesia is induced, the patient will proceed through the stages of anaesthesia shown in Table 6-1. The establishment of an airway now becomes a priority. Depending on the type of procedure being undertaken, and the patient's history and condition, suitable airways will be selected. To understand how artificial airways are used, it is important to review the anatomy of the airway.

The airway is divided into two sections, upper and lower, which are separated at the level of the cricoid cartilage (Chipas et al., 2005). Figure 6-3 shows the anatomy of the upper airway.

Artificial airways

Artificial airways include oropharyngeal airways, or Guedel airways, which are used in patients whose tongue is obstructing the airway. This can occur when the patient loses upper airway muscle tone, causing the tongue and epiglottis to fall back against the posterior wall of the pharynx. Guedel airways may be used in conjunction with other manoeuvres, such as chin lift and jaw thrust. Nasopharyngeal airways are also available and these require lubrication before insertion via the patient's nose (Smith et al., 2007).

Face masks

Face masks used in anaesthesia are made of silicone or polyvinyl chloride (PVC) and are designed to fit firmly over the nose and mouth, following the contours of the face as this will assist in providing effective ventilation of an unconscious patient. Several types of face masks are available, including transparent masks, which allow observation of exhaled gas and immediate recognition of vomiting, and cushioned masks, which allow for contouring to facial bone structures (Smith et al., 2007).

Holding face masks requires correct technique to maintain a patent airway. It involves holding the mask with a downward pressure using the thumb and index finger, while the middle and ring fingers grasp the mandible to extend the atlantomaxillary joint. The

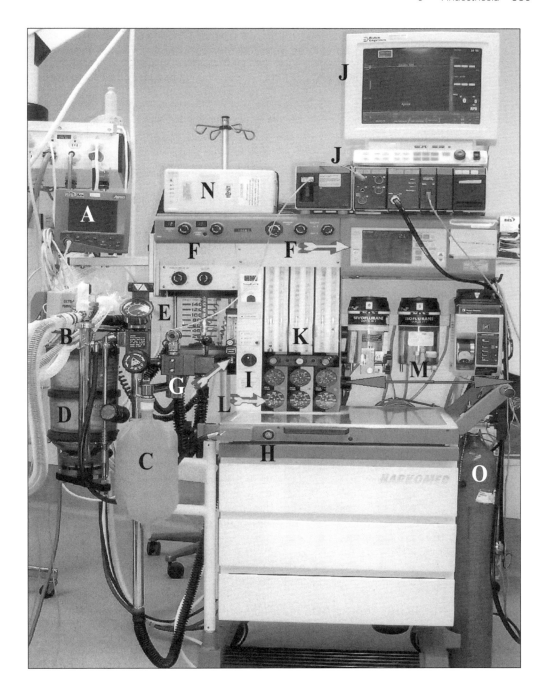

Figure 6-2 Anaesthetic machine and monitoring equipment (Rothrock, 2007, p 108). **A**, BIS monitor display. **B**, Patient breathing circuit. **C**, Reservoir ('breathing') bag. **D**, Carbon dioxide absorber. **E**, Ventilator. **F**, Integrated ventilator controls, monitor and displays. **G**, Oxygen auxiliary outlet. **H**, Oxygen flush valve. **I**, On/off switch. **J**, Monitor display and controls for ECG, temperature, blood pressure, pulse oximetry and end-tidal carbon dioxide. **K**, Flow meters for air. **L**, Gauges for pipeline and E-tank pressures (air, nitrous oxide, oxygen). **M**, Flow-through vaporisers (e.g. desflurane, isoflurane, sevoflurane). **N**, Power surge protector for anaesthesia machine. **O**, E-cylinder with oxygen.

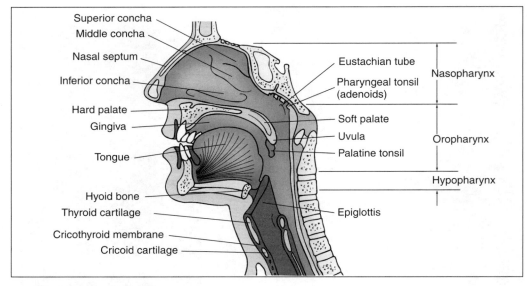

Superior concha
Middle concha
Nasal septum
Inferior concha
Hard palate
Gingiva
Tongue
Hyoid bone
Thyroid cartilage
Cricothyroid membrane
Cricoid cartilage

Eustachian tube
Pharyngeal tonsil (adenoids)
Nasopharynx
Soft palate
Uvula
Palatine tonsil
Oropharynx
Hypopharynx
Epiglottis

Figure 6-3 Anatomy of the upper airway (Elliott et al., 2007, p 264).

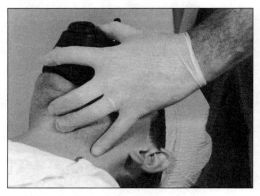

Figure 6-4 Technique for holding a face mask with one hand (Drain, 2003, p 410).

little finger slides under the angle of the jaw and pulls it anteriorly.

Poor technique when applying a face mask can result in pressure on the soft tissues of the face and neck, which can result in obstruction and excessive bag pressure, resulting in inflation of the stomach.

Difficulties in obtaining an effective seal with face masks may be experienced in denture-less patients, and those patients with congenital abnormalities, facial and eye trauma, tumours, infections or those who have limited neck extension.

Laryngeal mask airway

A laryngeal mask airway (LMA) provides an alternative to face masks or endotracheal tubes (ETTs). It consists of a silicone or PVC tube that is slightly shorter than an ETT, with an inflatable elliptical cuff at the distal end, which resembles a miniature face mask. LMAs are designed, when the cuff is inflated, to provide a relatively airtight seal around the perimeter of the larynx, but do not pass through the vocal cords. LMAs are inserted by hand without the aid of a laryngoscope.

LMAs are available in sizes for both paediatric and adult patients. Their indications for use include:

- patients who do not require tracheal intubation to facilitate their surgical procedure and are breathing spontaneously
- providing a clear airway without the need for the anaesthetist's hands to support a mask
- facilitating tracheal intubation in patients when difficulties in intubation are experienced, thus allowing the passage of an ETT.

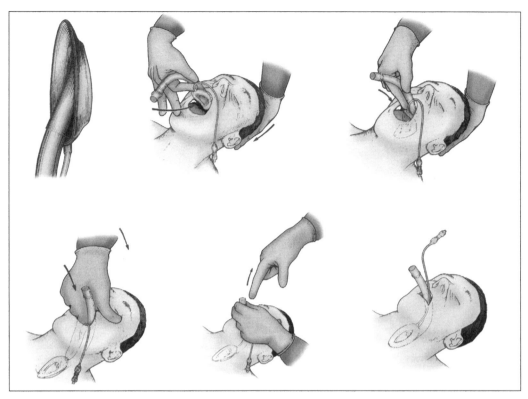

Figure 6-5 Insertion of laryngeal mask airway (Rothrock, 2007, p 118).

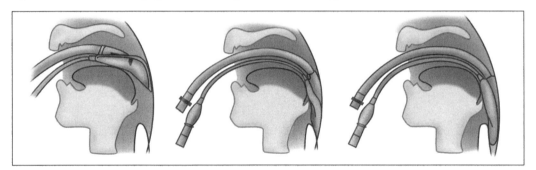

Figure 6-6 Laryngeal mask airway in situ (Rothrock, 2007, p 119).

Contraindications include patients who are at risk of aspiration due to:

- a full stomach
- pregnancy
- hiatus hernia
- high airway resistance
- pharyngeal abscess
- low pulmonary compliance, such as obesity.

Intubation

A secure airway for the purposes of delivering anaesthesia and emergency airway management can be achieved by the insertion of an ETT. This involves the anaesthetist

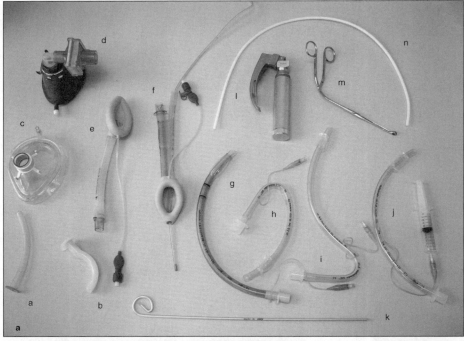

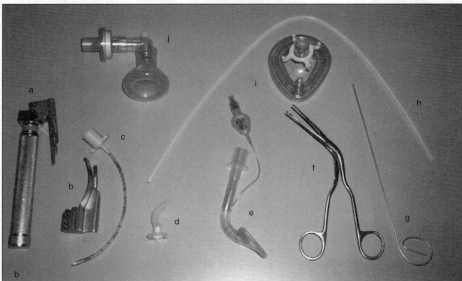

Figure 6-7 Equipment used for intubation. (a) Adults. **A**, Nasopharyngeal airway. **B**, Oral airway (Guedal). **C**, Face mask (disposable). **D**, Face mask with filter. **E**, Laryngeal mask (LMA). **F**, Proseal LMA. **G**, Reinforced endotracheal tube (ETT). **H**, Oral RAE ETT. **I**, Nasal RAE. **J**, ETT with inflating syringe. **K**, Introducer (malleable). **L**, Laryngoscope. **M**, Magill forceps. **N**, Teflon bougie (introducer). (b) Paediatrics. **A**, Laryngoscope with Miller blade. **B**, Laryngoscope blade (Mackintosh). **C**, Uncuffed endotracheal tube (ETT). **D**, Oral airway (Guedal). **E**, Laryngeal mask airway (LMA). **F**, Magill forceps. **G**, Introducer (malleable). **H**, Teflon bougie (introducer). **I**, Face mask (disposable). **J**, Neonate's face mask with elbow.

passing a tube, under direct vision using a laryngoscope, through the vocal cords into the trachea. This tube is connected to the anaesthetic delivery system. A cuff (balloon) located at the distal end of the ETT is inflated to facilitate positive pressure ventilation and to prevent the stomach contents from being aspirated into the patient's lungs, a condition which can lead to serious pulmonary consequences.

Indications for intubation include:

- patients who are at risk of aspiration and require the airway to be protected (e.g. unknown fasting time, trauma, obesity, bowel obstruction, Caesarean section)
- position of patient for surgery where a secure airway is vital—sitting, prone position
- specific surgical procedures—ear, nose and throat, facial, plastics or dental surgery— where the airway must be protected from blood loss at the operative site and also to facilitate access to the surgical site
- abdominal surgery requiring muscle relaxation and mechanical ventilation
- thoracic surgery that requires specific control of ventilation and sometimes one lung ventilation
- patients with a Mallampati score of class III or IV, where a difficult airway is anticipated (Fell & Kirkbride, 2007).

Endotracheal tubes

ETTs are designed to deliver gases directly into the trachea. They are disposable and made of PVC or silicone, with the distal end bevelled to aid visualisation and insertion through the vocal cords. The Murphy eye is an additional hole at the distal end and is designed to lessen the risk of obstruction by secretions, blood or other matter. Resistance to air flow depends primarily on the tube diameter but is also affected by tube length and curvature. Cuffed tubes permit positive pressure ventilation and decrease the risk of aspiration.

ETTs have been modified for a variety of specialised applications. Reinforced ETTs have been designed to reduce obstruction in the prone position. Ring-Adair-Elwyn (RAE) tubes are used in orofacial surgery. They are angled for use in ear, nose and throat surgery, plastic surgery and ophthalmology to avoid encroachment into the surgical site. Nasal RAE tubes are also used for oral surgery and faciomaxillary surgery.

Complications of intubation

Complications may include:

- oesophageal intubation or endobronchial intubation, which will not provide effective ventilation and could be fatal
- airway trauma, such as damage to the teeth, lip and mucosal laceration, sore throat, dislocation of the mandible, tube malfunction, cuff perforation and laryngospasm
- complications when in situ, which may include malposition due to changes in patient position, unintentional extubation or ignition during use of lasers
- obstruction of the Murphy eye with secretions, which could compromise the ability to ventilate the patient.

Intubation equipment

The anaesthetic nurse must be aware of the requirements for intubation in order to provide effective assistance to the anaesthetist and a safe outcome for the patient. The equipment required includes:

- laryngoscope handle and blades in working order
- appropriately sized tube
- syringe for cuff inflation
- tape to secure tube in place
- suction equipment, including Yankauer and Y-suction catheters.

Additional requirements that should be available include:

- a malleable introducer
- Magill forceps
- intubating bougie (for difficult or awkward airways).

Technique for direct laryngoscopy and intubation

Prior to intubation the patient will have received induction agents and muscle relaxant drugs. This is a crucial time in the patient's anaesthetic procedure and all the required equipment must be ready and the anaesthetic team prepared to proceed with intubation as soon as muscle relaxation has been achieved.

Successful intubation depends on:

- correct patient positioning, head extension and flexion (the patient appears to be 'sniffing the morning air')
- the height of the patient trolley or the operating table, which should be adjusted to facilitate access by the anaesthetist.

Direct laryngoscopy and intubation

The procedure for intubation is outlined below.

1. The laryngoscope is an instrument designed to be used in the left hand. The blade is inserted into the right side of the patient's mouth and the tongue is swept to the left, locating the epiglottis.
2. The blade is inserted into the vallecula (posterior oropharynx) and the patient's head is lifted perpendicular to the patient's mandible to expose the vocal cords.
3. The anaesthetic nurse holds the ETT so that it can be taken by the anaesthetist's right hand. The tube is inserted so that the cuff is just below the vocal cords, noting the level on the tube and at the lips.
4. The ETT is then connected to the anaesthetic delivery tubing.
5. The anaesthetic nurse, on instruction from the anaesthetist, will inflate the cuff to seal any air leak around the tube and permit positive pressure ventilation (Fell & Kirkbride, 2007).

Correct placement of the ETT (Fig 6-10) is confirmed by the anaesthetist using a stethoscope, visualisation and end-tidal carbon dioxide displayed waveform. To avoid accidental extubation during this process, the nurse assists by holding the tube until it is secured by the anaesthetist's preferred method.

Rapid sequence induction

On occasions it is necessary to undertake a rapid sequence induction, which is a technique used to secure the airway rapidly to reduce the risk of pulmonary aspiration of the stomach

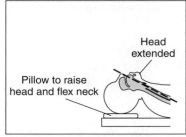

Figure 6-8 Head position for laryngoscopy (Aitkenhead et al., 2007, p 305).

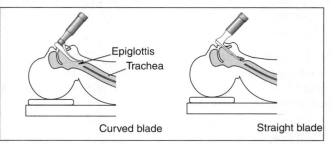

Figure 6-9 Using a laryngoscope (Aitkenhead et al., 2007, p 304).

contents. Aspiration could result in severe pneumonitis, which is known as Mendelson's syndrome and is often fatal (Hardman, 2007). The technique involves using the fingers of the anaesthetic assistant to apply pressure on the cricoid cartilage, pressing it firmly backwards onto the cervical vertebral bodies behind it and occluding the upper end of the oesophagus, thus preventing the aspiration of gastric contents. This is known as a Sellick's manoeuvre and was first described in 1961 (DeLamar, 2007).

The indications for rapid sequence induction include patients who are at risk of aspiration due to:

- unknown fasting time
- pregnancy
- hiatus hernia
- bowel obstruction
- gastrointestinal bleeding
- gastric reflux
- trauma sustained after eating.

The sequence of the technique is as follows.

- Appropriate equipment (e.g. ETT, laryngoscope and suction) are prepared.
- IV access is secured.
- Haemodynamic monitoring is applied.
- Preoxygenation using face mask.
- Location of cricoid cartilage and application of cricoid pressure.
- Administration of IV induction agent and short-acting muscle relaxant (e.g. suxamethonium).
- Intubation and cuff inflation.
- Confirmation of correct position of ETT (i.e. equal chest inflation and end-tidal carbon dioxide displayed waveform).
- Release of cricoid pressure only on the advice of the anaesthetist once the position of the ETT has been confirmed (Turner, 2007).

It is important that patients are warned that they will feel pressure on their neck as their anaesthetic is being induced. Once the airway is established, the patient will be positioned and additional equipment, such as warming devices and monitoring equipment, may be applied.

Note that Sellicks's manoeuvre is different from external laryngeal pressure or BURP—backwards, upwards rightwards

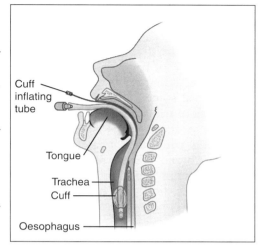

Figure 6-10 Endotracheal tube in correct position (Rothrock, 2007, p 116).

Cuff inflating tube

Tongue

Trachea

Cuff

Oesophagus

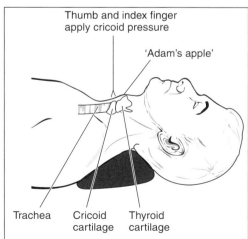

Thumb and index finger apply cricoid pressure

'Adam's apple'

Trachea   Cricoid cartilage   Thyroid cartilage

Figure 6-11 Applying cricoid pressure — Sellick's manoeuvre (Aitkenhead et al., 2007, p 28).

pressure—which the anaesthetist may request the nurse to apply to facilitate a view of the larynx for routine intubation.

Management of patients with difficult airways

In about 10% of patients, some difficulty is experienced with tracheal intubation due to congenital abnormalities or acquired conditions, such as trauma to the head, neck and cervical spine or tumours in the mouth. Of these patients, 10% (or 1% overall) present significant difficulty in intubation (Hardman, 2007). A range of options are available for the anaesthetist to achieve control of the airway depending on the patient's presenting condition. These include different sizes and designs of laryngoscopes, fibreoptic bronchoscopes and crycothyroidotomy needles. Local and regional anaesthetic modalities may be an option and negate the need for a general anaesthetic and airway management. Thorough preoperative assessment is essential to prepare a care plan for such patients and ensure that all necessary equipment is available.

Maintenance of anaesthesia

Once the patient is anaesthetised and the airway is secure, anaesthesia must be maintained for the duration of the operative procedure using a combination of oxygen, nitrous oxide gas and volatile agents (e.g. sevoflurane). Narcotics and antiemetics are adjunct drugs that may also be administered. Haemodynamic monitoring equipment is discussed on page 151.

Awareness under anaesthesia

The possibility of awareness during anaesthesia is a concern for both anaesthetists and patients. Dramatic accounts in the media of patients experiencing awareness during anaesthesia have heightened patient fears. Awareness occurs when the patient is paralysed with muscle relaxants but has been given insufficient anaesthetic agents to maintain the unconscious state. Paralysed patients have no way of indicating their awareness to the anaesthetic team. Fortunately it is a rare occurrence (about 0.2% of patients; DeLamar, 2007), but nonetheless it a distressing event for those who experience it.

The possibility of awareness can be reduced by constant observation in the form of monitoring, such as using the bispectral index (BIS) or entropy. This monitors the patient's brain waves relative to the depth of anaesthesia and can alert the anaesthetist to the patient becoming aware. An electrode attached externally to the patient's forehead provides a numerical reading on a monitor between 0 and 99. A BIS value of 0 equals electroencephalograph (EEG) silence, whereas near 100 is the expected value in a fully awake adult, and between 40 and 60 indicates a recommended level for general anaesthesia (Hardman, 2007).

Emergence from general anaesthesia

At the conclusion of the surgical procedure or anaesthetic, the patient is awoken from the general anaesthesia. This is termed *emergence*. As the procedure nears completion, inhalational agents are ceased, and reversal agents administered if muscle relaxants have been used. This is a crucial time in the care of the patient and the anaesthetic team must be prepared with the extubation equipment, including suction and oxygen delivery equipment, ready for post intubation.

When all anaesthetic agents have been ceased and the patient is breathing spontaneously, is haemodynamically stable and responding to commands, extubation occurs. The anaesthetist will suction the pharynx and give 100% oxygen to replace the gas mixture to avoid the potential effects of diffusion hypoxia. A syringe is available for ETT cuff deflation and extubation is performed during inspiration when the larynx dilates. The tube is withdrawn along its curved axis. Further suctioning may be necessary before an oxygen mask or nasal prongs are placed on the patient. The patient will then be transferred from the operating table onto a trolley/bed. The lateral position may be adopted unless the anaesthetist is satisfied that this is unnecessary. The patient is turned on one side, with the upper leg flexed and lower leg extended; the head is on one side so that the tongue falls forward under gravity, thus avoiding airway obstruction (Fell & Kirkbride, 2007). This position is known as the *recovery position*.

OTHER TYPES OF ANAESTHESIA

Sedation/analgesia

Sedation/analgesia refers to the administration of sedatives (e.g. midazolam) and analgesia (e.g. fentanyl) to produce a depressed level of consciousness, but where patients retain the ability to maintain their own airway. Patients may also be able to respond to commands or physical stimuli (DeLamar, 2007). This method is often used for colonoscopy and facilitates a rapid recovery and return to normal activities, although patients must be warned not to drive or operate machinery for 24 hours post sedation (Bryant & Knight, 2007).

Local anaesthetic techniques

Local anaesthesia refers to a group of procedures that involve using local anaesthetic drugs (e.g. lignocaine, bupivacaine) to block sensory nerve pathways, thus allowing surgery to proceed without pain and without loss of consciousness. These techniques include **epidural** and **spinal anaesthesia**, peripheral nerve blocks, local infiltration at the site of surgery, local anaesthetic sprays to the vocal cords prior to intubation and topical anaesthetic gels, which are often used prior to cannulation in paediatric patients.

These techniques are particularly useful for patients who may have comorbidities that may contraindicate the use of general anaesthesia. In many cases, they may be used in combination with general anaesthesia, providing a degree of postoperative pain relief for the patient. Other advantages for the patient include:

- minimal respiratory impairment
- less nausea and vomiting
- being able to eat and drink sooner
- more rapid mobilisation and discharge
- simplicity of administration
- sympathetic blockade (Coventry, 2007).

Central nerve blocks

Central nerve blocks refer to the administration of local anaesthetic drugs into the subarachnoid or epidural space, thus blocking nerves as they exit the spinal cord and causing large areas of the lower body to lose sensation (hence, the term 'block'). These techniques are particularly useful for surgery of the abdomen and lower limbs.

Spinal (subarachnoid) anaesthesia refers to a single administration of local anaesthetic directly into the subarachnoid space at the level of lumbar vertebrae L3–4 or L5–6, thus blocking the spinal nerve roots and producing a loss of sensation to the areas supplied by the nerves from this level of the spinal cord. The anaesthetist advances a hollow spinal needle through the intervertebral space into the subarachnoid space until drops of cerebrospinal fluid (CSF) appear. The local anaesthetic, which can be combined with opioids such as fentanyl, can be injected into the subarachnoid space and the needle is then removed (DeLamar, 2007).

Local anaesthesia injected into the CSF can cause complications such as hypotension as a result of blocking the sympathetic nerves that control vasomotor tone, thus resulting in vasodilation. This effect can be managed by rapid infusion of IV fluids and the administration of adrenaline. If the local anaesthetic agent inadvertently reaches the nerves controlling respiration, the patient may require ventilator support. The patient must, therefore, be closely observed in the immediate post-injection period.

Postoperatively, some patients may complain of a severe headache caused by the hole in the dura and the leakage of CSF. The patient may have to remain supine for 24 hours and receive additional IV fluids until the headache subsides. Occasionally, the anaesthetist may perform a 'blood patch', which involves injecting 5–20 mL of blood into the epidural space at the puncture site to seal up the hole in the dura (DeLamar, 2007).

Epidural anaesthesia involves the intermittent or continuous injection of local anaesthesia through a catheter that is inserted between the vertebrae at the L3–4 or L5–6 level into the epidural space. The epidural space is not really a space but an area of loose adipose tissue, lymphatic and blood vessels that lies between the dura mater and the ligamentum flavum (Bryant & Knight, 2007).

The anaesthetist uses a hollow Tuohy needle attached to an empty syringe, which is marked at 1 cm intervals and has a Huber point that allows the fine catheter to be directed along the axis of the epidural space. When the needle penetrates the ligamentum flavum, there is a sudden loss of resistance to pressure on the plunger of the syringe, indicating to the anaesthetist that the correct location has been reached. Advancing the needle further would result in the dura being penetrated. A fine catheter is then inserted via the needle into the epidural space and local anaesthetic is injected (Aitkenhead et al., 2007). The catheter is secured to the patient and is available to provide 'top-up' doses of local anaesthetic drugs at intervals to maintain effectiveness of the block. This may continue during the postoperative period as part of the patient's pain management.

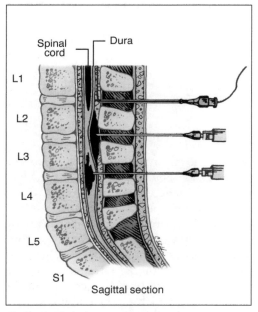

Figure 6-12 Location of needle points (Rothrock, 2007, p 120).

Figure 6-12 shows the location of epidural and spinal needles. Table 6-4 outlines the differences between subarachnoid and epidural block.

As with spinal anaesthesia, epidural blocks can also cause hypotension, although onset is usually slower. However, if a blood vessel in the epidural space is inadvertently punctured and the local anaesthetic agent is released into the bloodstream, sudden and profound hypotension, convulsions and respiratory compromise can occur. Also postoperative backache and urinary retention have been reported (Bryant & Knight, 2007; DeLamar, 2007).

It may not be possible for some patients to receive either spinal or epidural anaesthesia. Patients for whom these are contraindicated include patients with:

• no consent given
• hypovolaemia—increased risk of hypotension

Table 6-4 Differences in the effect of subarachnoid and epidural anaesthetics

	Subarachnoid	Epidural
Dose of drug used	Small: minimal risk of systemic toxicity	Large: possibility of systemic toxicity after intravascular injection or total spinal blockade after subarachnoid injection
Rate of onset	Fast: 2–5 min for initial effect; 20 min for maximum effect	Slow: 5–15 min for initial effect; 30–45 min for maximum effect
Intensity of block	Usually complete anaesthesia	Often not complete anaesthesia for all segments
Pattern of block	May be dermatomal for first few minutes but rapidly develops appearance of cord transection	Dermatomal
Addition of vasoconstrictor	Reliably prolongs block with tetracaine but not with other drugs	Reliably prolongs block with lignocaine; may prolong block with bupivacaine but not in all patients

Aitkenhead et al. (2007)

- local sepsis—danger of septicaemia and meningitis
- raised intracranial pressure—can dangerously alter intracranial pressure
- previous spinal surgery—anatomy may be altered
- coagulopathies—if a blood vessel is accidentally punctured there is a risk of haemorrhage (Bryant & Knight, 2007).

Management of the patient undergoing spinal or epidural anaesthesia

With both spinal and epidural anaesthesia, patients are positioned with their back arched into the shape of a C in order to maximise the space between the spinous processes and to facilitate access for positioning the spinal/epidural needles. The position is similar to that used for a lumbar puncture (Williams, 2005). For those patients with physical disabilities this position is difficult and they can be sat upright, a position that some anaesthetists also favour.

Prior to administration of either block, the routine checks of the anaesthetic machine and equipment must be carried out. This is because if the regional block should fail or resuscitation is required, all resuscitation equipment must be available and in working order. Monitoring, IV access and baseline observations are obtained to determine variations during the administration of the regional block. In many instances, patients will receive a combination of regional and general anaesthesia, particularly for complex abdominal surgery where the regional route can provide postoperative pain relief.

The procedure to insert both spinal and epidural anaesthesia must be undertaken using aseptic technique. The anaesthetic nurse assists by assembling the necessary equipment and by providing physical and emotional support to the patient, who is likely to be awake during the administration of regional anaesthesia.

Once the block has been administered, the patient must be closely monitored for any of the complications listed above. The effectiveness of the block must also be assessed

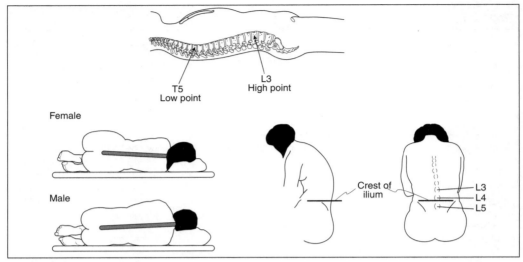

Figure 6-13 Spinal curvature for the insertion of central nerve blocks (Aitkenhead et al., 2007, p 324).

prior to surgery taking place. This may be accomplished by using ice to test the numbness in the required area and by asking the patient for feedback as to any sensations.

The patient should receive explanations and reassurance at all times. Patients must understand that although regional anaesthesia will block painful stimuli, they may still be aware of pressure in the area of the surgical procedure. They will also receive drugs (e.g. midazolam) to make them drowsy and unaware of the activity around them. Oxygen may be applied by a Hudson mask or nasal prongs. The surgical and anaesthetic team must be aware of not making unnecessary noise, especially conversations, as the patient may still be semi-conscious and able to hear. During the procedure the anaesthetic nurse may sit at the head of the patient and use verbal and non-verbal communication to reduce the patient's anxiety. Close haemodynamic monitoring by the anaesthetic team is important to detect any complications or unwanted effects of the regional anaesthesia.

Local infiltration

To facilitate minor surgery or the insertion of invasive monitoring devices, an infiltration of local anaesthetic agent will be used. This involves direct injection into tissues to block sensory nerve pathways, thus resulting in an absence of pain, which may continue post procedure to provide the patient with pain relief for a period of time. Patients must remains conscious and aware of their surroundings, although mild sedation may also be given depending on the patient's condition (Bryant & Knight, 2007). Examples of drugs used in local infiltration are lignocaine and bupivacaine.

Regional anaesthesia

Techniques of **regional anaesthesia** (often termed 'blocks') involve injecting drugs anywhere along a pathway of a nerve, thus resulting in anaesthesia to a region of the body without a loss of consciousness (DeLamar, 2007). Regional anaesthesia may be administered by:

- a single dose
- intermittent bolus—repeated injections or indwelling catheter for repeat administration
- continuous infusion via a catheter.

Regional blocks, which are available using local anaesthetics (e.g. bupivacaine, lignocaine), include:

- upper limb—axillary nerve blocks for elbow, forearm and hand surgery
- lower limb—femoral nerve blocks for femoral fractures and knee surgery (Coventry, 2007).

HAEMODYNAMIC MONITORING DURING ANAESTHESIA

Regardless of the type of anaesthesia or sedation the patient receives, **haemodynamic monitoring** is a vital component of the patient's management and safety. Advances in haemodynamic monitoring have greatly decreased the mortality and morbidity of patients, and minimum standards for monitoring are provided by ANZCA (2000) and the Australian College of Operating Room Nurses (ACORN) (2006). These minimum requirements are shown in Box 6-1.

Box 6-1 Minimum requirements of haemodynamic monitoring

1. Circulation
   (a) Arterial pulse
   (b) Blood pressure—direct or indirect
   (c) ECG—not required for local anaesthesia

2. Ventilation—direct and indirect

3. Oxygenation—oximetric values in conjunction with clinical observation of the patient, including provision of adequate lighting

ANZCA (2000)

Figure 6-2 shows the haemodynamic monitoring equipment that is used. To comply with the minimum monitoring requirements, the following monitoring equipment must be available (ANZCA, 2000):

- oxygen supply failure alarm
- oxygen analyser
- pulse oximeter
- breathing system disconnection or ventilator failure alarm
- electrocardiograph
- temperature monitor
- carbon dioxide monitor
- neuromuscular monitor
- volatile anaesthetic agent monitor
- other equipment, when clinically indicated—cardiac output, spirometry.

Circulation

Electrocardiograph

Monitoring of the patient's cardiovascular system involves observation of the patient's blood pressure and continuous ECG analysis. The ECG will detect arrhythmias, myocardial ischaemia, electrolyte imbalance and pacemaker dysfunction. Electrode placement requires the minimum of two sensing electrodes and a third reference (grounding) lead. The lead that displays the most prominent P waves on the ECG monitor is the preferred option because it follows the direction of the normal electrical impulse (Lee, 2000).

When using a three-lead ECG, the electrodes can be placed on each shoulder and one on the left side of the rib cage. The anaesthetic nurse must ensure correct placement of ECG monitoring electrodes and be alert to the proposed surgical site. Five-lead ECG monitoring provides a more accurate view, with more accurate detection of myocardial ischaemia, and is used if the patient has a history of cardiac disease (Skubas et al., 2006; Wolfgang & Rossaint, 2003).

Blood pressure

Indirect blood pressure monitoring is a minimum requirement for all patients. Changes in systolic blood pressure correlate with changes in myocardial oxygen requirements and changes in diastolic blood pressure reflect coronary perfusion pressure (Murphy & Vender, 2006).

Care must be taken to ensure that the blood pressure cuff is the correct size, being 40% of the circumference of the extremity upon which it is being placed. The cuff must also not be too tight or too loose as it will affect the readings, giving false results.

Direct blood pressure monitoring involves direct cannulation of an artery to provide continuous measurement of arterial blood pressure. This invasive method is required when the surgery could cause the patient to become haemodynamically unstable or the patient has comorbidities that require close observation (Wolfgang & Rossaint, 2003). Indicators for invasive blood pressure monitoring are listed in Box 6-2.

Box 6-2 Indicators for invasive blood pressure monitoring

1. Patient-dependent factors
   (a) Haemodynamic instability (shock)
   (b) Cardiac disease
   (c) Respiratory insufficiency
   (d) Increased intracranial pressure
   (e) Polytrauma

2. Type of surgery

   (a) Cardiac surgery
   (b) Craniotomy
   (c) Major thoracic surgery
   (d) Major abdominal surgery

Wolfgang & Rossaint (2003, p 1804)

Central venous pressure

A central venous pressure (CVP) catheter is often inserted prior to commencement of anaesthesia to:

*   measure right heart filling as a guide to intravascular volume
*   administer drugs
*   provide access in patients with poor peripheral veins.

    Additional reasons for CVP insertion include to:

*   provide a route for long-term parenteral nutrition
*   inject dye
*   remove air emboli.

Sites used for CVP catheter insertion include the internal jugular, subclavian, external jugular, cephalic, axillary and femoral veins. The CVP catheter is inserted using the Seldinger technique, which involves insertion of a needle and use of a guidewire to thread the CVP catheter over the guidewire. Chest X-ray is carried out post insertion to check the position and to exclude pneumothorax.

Complications of CVP catheter placement include:

- arrhythmias (atrial and ventricular)
- carotid or subclavian artery puncture (subclavian cannulation is contraindicated in patients on anticoagulants due to the inability to compress the vessel)
- pneumothorax, hydrothorax, infection or air embolism.

Additional invasive monitoring can include the insertion of a pulmonary artery catheter, sometimes known as a Swan-Ganz catheter, which is inserted into a neck vein and is manoeuvred through the superior vena cava, the right atrium and ventricle into the pulmonary artery. A balloon at the distal tip is inflated and pressures are measured via a transducer and displayed on a monitor. The ability to measure the filling pressure of the left ventricle provides valuable information about the cardiac condition of the patient and will assist with the management of unstable patients and those undergoing complex surgical procedures (Byrne, 2007; Murphy & Vender, 2006).

Respiration

Monitoring the patient's respiratory function during anaesthesia involves the use of pulse oximetry and capnography, and both should be available for all patients.

Pulse oximetry

Pulse oximetry is a non-invasive measurement of haemoglobin oxygen saturation (Sao_2) at the arteriole level by measuring changes in the light absorbed by an extremity (Al-Shaikh & Stacey, 2001). It works by detecting the differences in absorption of oxygenated and deoxygenated blood (Wolfgang & Rossaint, 2003). Normal values are 95% or above. If the patient's saturation levels drops below 95%, the anaesthetist should consider a higher oxygen concentration in the patient's anaesthesia. The pulse oximeter probe is usually placed on the fingers or toes and the reading is displayed on a monitor as a percentage. Cold or poorly perfused extremities can affect the accuracy of the pulse oximeter, and newer technologies using forehead oximetry may be more effective, providing more accurate readings (Schallom et al., 2007).

Capnography

Capnography is the graphical representation of expired carbon dioxide (CO_2) and maybe termed end-tidal CO_2 (Drain, 2003). Monitoring end-tidal CO_2 assists in the early detection of either technical catastrophes (e.g. inadvertent oesophageal intubation, breathing circuit leaks) or changes in the patient's respiratory, circulatory or metabolic condition, particularly indicating malignant hyperthermia, which can be an anaesthetic emergency. The normal value of end-tidal CO_2 is 35–45 mmHg. CO_2 is collected by an adapter that is placed in the breathing circuit close to the airway so that the CO_2 collected will approximate the alveolar concentration. The expired CO_2 is then analysed using an infrared ray, which converts it to a wave form displayed on a monitor.

Temperature

Normothermia is described as a temperature between 36°C and 38°C and hypothermia as a temperature below 36°C (Bitner et al., 2007). Planned hypothermia is common for neurosurgery and cardiac surgery to reduce oxygen requirements deliberately so as to create the necessary operating conditions. Unplanned hypothermia can occur for a variety of reasons (e.g. exposed areas of the body, open body cavities, cold dry gases, low ambient temperatures within the operating room). Neonates are more prone to hypothermia due immature temperature regulation centres, as are elderly patients, owing to lower metabolic rates. Patients undergoing lengthy surgery, surgery in which there is a large blood loss or burns patients are also at risk of hypothermia.

Unplanned hypothermia can lead to a variety of complications, including increased recovery times by increased demand for oxygen consumption, increased wound infections due to suppression of the immune system, impaired cardiac function, coagulopathy and increased morbidity and mortality (Bitner et al., 2007; Byrne, 2007). For major surgery, a temperature probe, which can be placed orally, nasally or in the bladder (incorporated as part of a urinary catheter), is used to measure core temperature.

Forced air warming devices are commonly used to maintain normothermia during the perioperative period. Various commercial devices exist but they generally consist of a disposable warming blanket connected to a hose and warming unit. The warm air inflates the blanket and the temperature can be regulated as required. The blankets are available in various configurations (e.g. full length or half length) to facilitate warming while allowing access to the surgical site for the surgeon.

Other methods of maintaining normothermia are:

- controlling the operating room temperature
- warming IV fluids
- humidifying the anaesthetic gases (especially for neonates)
- overhead heating lamps for paediatric patients
- use of cotton or 'space' blankets
- avoiding unnecessary exposure of the body.

FLUID AND ELECTROLYTE BALANCE

The average adult requires water to replace gastrointestinal losses (100–200 mL/day), loss through respiration and perspiration (500–1000 mL/day) and excretion of urine at a rate of 1000 mL/day (Prough et al., 2006). Adults needs to consume about 2500 mL/day of fluids to ensure their renal function is adequate (Yates, 2005).

Electrolyte balance

When electrolyte values are abnormal, this affects the **fluid and electrolyte balance** and acid–base balance, resulting in renal, neuromuscular, endocrine or skeletal dysfunction (Elgart, 2004).

The levels of serum electrolytes affect the movement of fluid between the body compartments (Elgart, 2004). The major extracellular electrolytes are sodium, calcium, chloride and bicarbonate (Table 6-5). Sodium is the most common cation and chloride the most common anion (Elgart, 2004). Potassium, magnesium and phosphate are the major intracellular electrolytes, potassium being the most common cation and phosphate the most common anion. An imbalance in the serum electrolyte levels has ramifications for metabolic activity.

Table 6-5 Normal electrolyte values	
Sodium	137–145 mmol/L
Potassium	3.2–5.0 mmol/L
Chloride	98–111 mmol/L
Bicarbonate	22–31 mmol/L
Magnesium	0.75–1 mmol/L

Hsiao & Matten (2007)

Fluid and blood loss

When patients arrive in the operating room, they have usually been fasting for some hours. They may also endure some losses of blood and other fluids during the surgical procedure. This can put the patient at risk of hypovolaemia, which can lead to other complications, such as tachycardia, hypotension and reduced urine output (Yates, 2005). Signs and symptoms of hypovolaemia include:

- pallor
- weak, thready pulse
- increased heart rate
- falling blood pressure
- peripheral vasoconstriction
- oliguria
- thirst (Yates, 2005).

The fluid requirements of a patient undergoing surgery for trauma where considerable blood loss may occur can be difficult to estimate, and patients may experience losses of up to 20 mL/kg/h (Forman & Yang, 2007). The circulating nurse may be asked to weigh used sponges to provide the anaesthetist with an estimate of blood loss. In addition, the anaesthetist will monitor the suction canisters for blood that has been suctioned from the surgical site.

A patient who is adequately hydrated before, during and after surgery will have a better outcome (Jacob et al., 2007). Therefore, all patients undergoing surgery or any procedure requiring an anaesthetic or sedation must have some form of venous access to facilitate induction and maintenance of anaesthesia, and provision of fluids during and after the procedure (Yates, 2005). Fluid overload can be determined by the following signs and symptoms:

- vasodilation
- breathlessness
- tachycardia
- increasing blood pressure
- bounding pulse (Yates, 2005).

A wide range of cannulae must be available, as well as a variety of IV fluids. The usual practice for most general anaesthetic procedures is to have a litre of IV fluid on an administration set ready for the beginning of the case. The ability to warm the IV fluid is also required, as well as a rapid infuser if there is a risk of severe haemorrhage. The anaesthetist determines the site of placement of the IV cannulae after considering the type of surgery, the IV fluid requirements, and the surgeon's and patient's preferences.

The range of IV solutions available include the following:

1. *Crystalloid solutions*. These fluids (e.g. normal saline, 5% dextrose, Ringer's lactate solution) are isotonic and are equivalent to plasma in osmolarity. They are used to replace maintenance fluid requirements, evaporative losses and third space losses (Forman & Yang, 2007).
2. *Colloid solutions*. These fluids (e.g. albumin) are hypotonic and are greater in osmolarity than plasma . This causes the solutes to move from the blood stream into the cell, causing the cell to swell. They can be used to replace blood loss or restore intravascular volume.
3. *Blood transfusions*. These are used to replace lost blood volume or a specific component (e.g. red cells, platelets or coagulation factors) (Forman & Yang, 2007).

Blood transfusions

If the patient's hypovolaemia is moderate and due to loss of blood, the anaesthetist may decide to give a blood transfusion, which, in the moderately hypovolaemic patient, will improve oxygen-carrying capacity. There are numerous potential complications with massive blood transfusion, including transfusion reactions, coagulopathies, hypothermia and sepsis (Elliott et al., 2007).

One of the most common causes of a transfusion reaction is the administration of the wrong blood type. Therefore, local protocols for the checking of blood must be followed (Greenwood & Murgo, 2007). Signs and symptoms of an acute transfusion reaction include:

- mild allergic—localised urticaria, pruritus and rash
- severe allergic—flushing, wheezing, hypotension, anaphylaxis
- febrile—unexpected fever (e.g. a temperature rise >1°C may have accompanying chills and rigors).

A guide to the management of a suspected transfusion reaction includes the following:

- Stop the transfusion immediately.
- Check vital signs.
- Maintain IV access.
- Check the right pack has been given to the right patient.
- Notify the medical officer and transfusion service provider.
- Send freshly collected blood and urine samples along with the blood pack and IV line as required by the transfusion service provider (SA Department of Health, 2006).

ANAESTHETIC EMERGENCIES

Despite the patient being closely monitored while under anaesthesia, emergencies can still occur that require prompt and effective action.

Anaphylaxis

Anaphylaxis is an antibody-mediated reaction to an antigen that can cause a sudden life-threatening response involving the skin, respiratory and cardiovascular systems. Anaphylaxis is a rare occurrence of anaesthesia (one in every 5000–10,000 anaesthetics) and is caused by the administration of muscle relaxants, opioids, antibiotics, dextrans, haemaccel, mannitol, blood and blood products, or contrast media (Currie et al., 2005). More than 90% of these reactions usually occur within 3 minutes of administration of the agent and it is vital for the anaesthetic nurse to remain with the anaesthetist at the beginning of the anaesthetic to assist in resuscitating the patient (Levy, 2006).

Treatment of anaphylaxis

Treatment of anaphylaxis includes:

- if the causative agent is known, stopping administration immediately
- administering 100% oxygen while maintaining the airway
- ceasing all anaesthetic drugs
- commencing fluid replacement with colloid or crystalloid
- treating bronchospasm with salbutamol
- administering adrenaline—bolus IV 0.001 mg/kg (adult dose 1:10,000).

Adrenaline is the drug of choice for anaphylactic reactions. It is a direct-acting sympathomimetic agent that exerts its effect on alpha and beta adrenoreceptors. It is a powerful cardiac stimulant with vasopressor and antihistamine actions. It also is an excellent bronchodilator and has a rapid onset. Once the patient is stabilised, an adrenaline infusion may be commenced and other drugs, such as hydrocortisone, administered. It is recommended that the patient is followed-up once this episode is resolved to determine the cause (Hepner & Castells, 2003).

Laryngospasm

Laryngospasm is irritation of the vocal cords that results in a complete or partial obstruction of the cords. This can occur during a light plane (e.g. Stage 3, Plane I) of anaesthesia and can be caused by secretions, vomitus, blood inhalation agents, oropharyngeal or nasopharyngeal airway placement, the laryngoscope blade or painful stimuli.

The larynx can become completely closed by a reflex closure of the cords and the anaesthetist will not be able to ventilate the patient. A less severe reaction is characterised by a 'crowing' sound or stridor and by a 'rocking' obstructed pattern of breathing. If left untreated, hypoxia, hypercarbia and acidosis will result, leading to hypertension and tachycardia and, finally, to cardiac arrest (Yates, 2005).

Management

Initially, deepening the anaesthetic and removing the stimulus (e.g. suctioning any blood or mucus from the airway) will remove the irritant and relieve the laryngospasm. Positive end-expiratory pressure (PEEP) is used to force 100% oxygen into the lungs. If this is ineffective, suxamethonium (1–2 mg/kg in an adult) may be given, which will relax the vocal cords and intubation can take place.

Bronchospasm

General anaesthesia can alter airway resistance and cause reactions within the bronchial tree, which may result in bronchospasm. This is characterised by an expiratory wheeze, which, if the patient is intubated, may make ventilation difficult. Bronchospasm can be caused by local airway irritation due to secretions, airway equipment, pulmonary aspiration or drug hypersensitivity. Bronchospasm can be precipitated by the rapid introduction of volatile anaesthetic agents. Patients who smoke, have a history of asthma or have suffered a recent respiratory tract infection are more susceptible to suffering bronchospasm.

Management

If the patient is intubated, repositioning the ETT may reduce the physical irritation to the bronchial tree. Deepening the anaesthetic by increasing the level of inhalational agent will frequently overcome the bronchospasm. Bronchodilators such as salbutamol can be administered intravenously and other drugs, such as steroids, ketamine and adrenaline, can also be used.

Aspiration

A patient's airway reflexes are depressed by general anaesthesia, which increases the risk of aspiration of gastric contents into the lungs. Vomiting and regurgitation with an unprotected airway can lead to bronchospasm, hypoxaemia, atelectasis, tachypnoea, tachycardia and hypotension. Aspiration is responsible for 10–30% of anaesthetic deaths (DeLamar, 2007). The severity of the symptoms can depend on the volume and pH of the gastric contents. Patients who have aspirated may require ventilatory support in the intensive care unit for a period of time depending on the severity of the condition.

As discussed on page 144, patients who are at risk of aspiration are most likely to undergo a rapid sequence induction.

Malignant hyperthermia

Malignant hyperthermia (MH) is a rare, autosomal-dominant muscle disorder. It is a life-threatening disease that is regarded as one of the true emergencies within the perioperative environment (Hommertzheim & Steinke, 2006). The condition can be triggered by any of the commonly used inhalational anaesthetic agents or muscle relaxants, particularly suxamethonium. If left untreated, MH can result in death.

Clinical features

MH has very clear, discernable clinical manifestations. These include:

- a sudden unexplained increase in end-tidal CO_2 levels
- unexplained tachycardia, tachypnoea, labile blood pressure and arrhythmias
- hypercarbia in the spontaneously breathing patient
- acidosis, hypoxaemia, hyperkalaemia
- muscle rigidity, in particular of the masseter (jaw) muscle
- fever, which is described as a late sign and occurs in only 30% of MH cases
- myoglobinuria, with dark coloured urine
- mottled cyanotic skin (Hommertzheim & Steinke, 2006).

Treatment

Dantrolene sodium for injection is the only effective treatment for MH and functions by inhibiting calcium uptake. It is administered at 2.5 mg/kg IV initial push and repeated as necessary to a maximum dose of 10 mg/kg. The dose is the same for paediatric patients. Each ampoule contains 20 mg of dantrolene sodium and 3 mg of mannitol in powder form and requires reconstitution with 60 mL of sterile water for injection. A well-stocked MH kit with at least 36 ampoules of dantrolene sodium for injection and drawing-up equipment is important to assist with the management of MH, together with as many people as possible to mix and draw up the drug.

Management of an acute episode

The following is recommended practice for a case of unexpected MH:

- Call an emergency using local protocols.
- Discontinue all anaesthetic agents and hyperventilate with 100% oxygen.
- Change the anaesthetic machine as soon as possible or change the breathing circuit, CO_2 absorber.
- Administer dantrolene sodium 2.5 mg/kg IV up to 10 mg/kg.
- Administer sodium bicarbonate (guided by arterial blood gas results).
- Correct hyperkalaemia with insulin and glucose.
- Treat hyperthermia by:
  - turning off warming blanket if one is being used
  - use of refrigerated IV fluids
  - gastric, rectal and bladder lavage with cold saline
  - extracorporeal cooling in extreme hyperthermia
- Cease hyperthermia treatment once the temperature is reduced to 38°C.
- Maintain urine output at 2 mL/kg/h.

Arrhythmias usually subside with resolution of the hypermetabolic state. Dantrolene sodium therapy should be continued and the patient transferred to the intensive care unit for observation and further treatment as required (Rosenberg et al., 2006).

Prompt diagnosis and treatment of MH can reduce mortality and morbidity. The patient can, however, be left with some serious problems following an episode of MH (e.g. disseminated intravascular coagulation, acute tubular necrosis). The anaesthetic nurse plays an important role in the management of an acute episode of MH and, even though the condition is rare, knowledge of the condition and the treatment is vital.

For patients who are known to have had MH or have a known family history, a number of alternative anaesthetic modalities are available to enable them to undergo safe anaesthesia and surgery (e.g. central nerve blocks, local or regional anaesthesia, total IV anaesthesia (TIVA) using a continuous propofol infusion) (McNeil, 2005; Rosenberg et al., 2006).

PAEDIATRIC CONSIDERATIONS IN ANAESTHESIA

Even though this is an anaesthetic specialty in its own right, a brief summary of paediatric anaesthetic considerations follows. The equipment (e.g. face masks, ETT, laryngoscopes and anaesthetic delivery systems) used for paediatric patients is scaled down to match the size and differing anatomy of the paediatric patient and modified to manage the different ventilator pressures required. Uncuffed ETTs are often used in children under 8 years of age to reduce the risk of trauma to the trachea, as the narrowest part of the airway is the cricoid ring (Stow, 2007). Anaesthetic induction is usually carried out using inhalational agents and with a parent present to provide comfort to the child. IV access is usually secured following induction to reduce distress. Maintaining normothermia is extremely important in babies and neonates as their capacity to regulate temperature is not well developed and this is accomplished by the use of the devices described on page 154. Drugs and IV fluids are titrated according to the child's weight and delivered through micro IV burettes to prevent fluid overload (Stow, 2007).

CONCLUSION

The focus of this chapter has been some of the main features of anaesthesia, and the modalities and agents commonly used. Pre-anaesthetic assessment of the patient was followed by a discussion of the different types of anaesthesia and the procedures involved in anaesthetising patients. The importance of haemodynamic monitoring and maintenance of fluid and electrolyte balance were also addressed. It is important that perianaesthetic nurses work in collaboration with the anaesthetist and other members of the surgical team to ensure patient safety throughout surgical procedures.

CRITICAL THINKING EXERCISES

1. Case study

Mr Rudi, a 74-year-old, is booked as an emergency admission with a suspected bowel obstruction. He has been vomiting for the past 2 days and is in severe abdominal pain. He is a poorly controlled, insulin-dependent diabetic. He is also very overweight (106 kg) and has smoked a packet of cigarettes a day since he was a teenager.

In the emergency department his vital signs were as follows:
1. temperature: 37°C
2. pulse: 118 beats/min
3. blood pressure: 160/70 mmHg

- What other information will you, as the anaesthetic nurse assigned to care for Mr Rudi, wish to know prior to his arrival in the operating suite?
- How will you prepare for his arrival?
- Identify the equipment, drugs and anaesthetic agents you will require for the induction and maintenance of Mr Rudi's anaesthetic.
- Describe the sequence of events when assisting in intubating Mr Rudi.
- Describe the monitoring you will undertake for Mr Rudi during his surgical procedure.

RESOURCES

Australian and New Zealand College of Anaesthetists
www.anzca.edu.au
Malignant Hyperthermia Association of the United States
www.mhaus.org

REFERENCES

ACORN. (2006). *ACORN standards for perioperative nursing including nursing roles, guidelines, position statements and competency standards.* Adelaide: Australian College of Operating Room Nurses.

Aitkenhead, A., Smith, G., Rowbotham, D. (Eds.). (2007). *Textbook of anaesthesia* (5th ed.). Edinburgh: Churchill Livingstone.

Al-Shaikh, B., & Stacey, S. (2001). *Essentials of anaesthetic equipment* (2nd ed.). Edinburgh: Churchill Livingstone.

ANZCA. (2000). *Professional documents of the Australian and New Zealand College of Anaesthetists. Recommendations on monitoring during anaesthesia.* Melbourne: Australian and New Zealand College of Anaesthetists.

ANZCA. (2003a). *Professional documents of the Australian and New Zealand College of Anaesthetists. Guidelines on the assistant for the anaesthetist.* Melbourne: Australian and New Zealand College of Anaesthetists.

ANZCA. (2003b). *Professional documents of the Australian and New Zealand College of Anaesthetists. Recommendations on checking anaesthesia delivery systems.* Melbourne: Australian and New Zealand College of Anaesthetists.

Bitner, J., Hilde, L., Hall, K., Duvendack, T. (2007). A team approach to the prevention of unplanned postoperative hypothermia. *AORN Journal, 85(5),* 921–929.

Brown, D., & Edwards, H. (2007). *Lewis's medical-surgical nursing* (2nd ed.). Sydney: Elsevier.

Byrne, A. J. (2007). Monitoring. In A. R. Aitkenhead, G. Smith, D. J. Rowbotham (Eds.). *Textbook of anaesthesia* (5th ed.). (pp. 345–366). Edinburgh: Churchill Livingstone.

Bryant, B., & Knight, K. (2007). *Pharmacology for health professionals* (2nd ed.). Sydney: Elsevier.

Chipas, A., Ellis, W., Zaglaniczny, K. (2005). Airway management. In J. Nagelhout, & K. L. Zaglaniczny (Eds.). *Nurse anesthesia* (3rd ed.) (pp. 408–424). St Louis: Elsevier.

Coventry, D. M. (2007). Local anaesthetic techniques. In A. R. Aitkenhead, G. Smith, D. J. Rowbotham (Eds.). *Textbook of anaesthesia* (5th ed.). (pp. 315–344). Edinburgh: Churchill Livingstone.

Currie, M., Kerridge, R. K., Bacon, A. K., Williamson, J. A. (2005). Crisis management during anaesthesia: anaphylaxis and allergy. *Quality & Safety in Health Care, 14(3),* e19.

DeLamar, L. (2007). Anesthesia. In J. C. Rothrock (Ed.), *Alexander's care of the patient in surgery* (13th ed.) (pp. 103–125). St Louis: Mosby.

Drain, C. B. (2003). *Perianaesthsia nursing* (4th ed.). St Louis: Saunders.

Dunn, P. F., Alston, T. A., Baker, K. H., Davison, J. K., Kwo, J., Rosow, C. E. (2007). *Clinical anesthesia procedures of the Massachusetts General Hospital.* Philadelphia: Lippincott, Williams & Wilkins.

Elgart, H. N. (2004). Assessment of fluids and electrolytes. *AACN Clinical Issues, 12(4),* 607–621.

Elliott, D., Aitken, L., Chaboyer, W. (2007). *ACCCN's critical care nursing.* Melbourne: Australian College of Critical Care Nurses.

Faut-Callahan, M., & Hand, W. R. (2005). Pain management. In J. Nagelhout, & K. L. Zaglaniczny (Eds.). *Nurse anesthesia* (3rd ed.) (pp. 1157–1182). St Louis: Elsevier.

Fell, D., & Kirkbride, D. (2007). The practical conduct of anaesthesia. In A. R. Aitkenhead, G. Smith, D. J. Rowbotham (Eds.). *Textbook of anaesthesia* (5th ed.). (pp. 297–214). Edinburgh: Churchill Livingstone.

Forman, S. A., & Yang, R. P. H. (2007). Administration of general anesthesia. In P. F. Dunn, T. A. Alston, K. H. Baker, J. K. Davison, J. Kwo, C. E. Rosow (Eds.). (2007). *Clinical anesthesia procedures of the Massachusetts General Hospital* (7th ed.) (pp. 228–237). Philadelphia: Lippincott, Williams & Wilkins.

Greenwood, M., & Murgo, M. (2007). Management of multi-organ dysfunctions. In D. Elliott, L. Aitken, W. Chaboyer (Eds.). *ACCCN's critical care nursing* (pp. 435–461). Sydney: Elsevier.

Hardman, J. G. (2007). Complications during anaesthesia. In A. R. Aitkenhead, G. Smith, D. J. Rowbotham (Eds.). *Textbook of anaesthesia* (5th ed.) (pp. 367–399). Edinburgh: Churchill Livingstone.

Hepner, D. L., & Castells, M. C. (2003). Anaphylaxis during the perioperative period. *Anaesthesia and Analgesia 97, (5),* 1381–1395.

Hommertzheim, R. & Steinke, E. E. (2006). Institution home study program. Malignant hyperthermia—the perioperative nurse's role. *AORN 83(1),* 149, 151–156, 159–160.

Hsiao, J. G., & Matten, E. C. (2007). Appendix 1: Supplemental drug information. In P. F. Dunn, T. A. Alston, K. H. Baker, J. K. Davison, J. Kwo, C. E. Rosow (Eds.). *Clinical anesthesia procedures of the Massachusetts General Hospital* (7th ed.) (pp. 725–754). Philadelphia: Lippincott, Williams & Wilkins.

Hunter, J. M. (2007). Muscle function blockade. In A. R. Aitkenhead, G. Smith, D. J. Rowbotham (Eds.). *Textbook of anaesthesia* (5th ed.) (pp. 367–399). Edinburgh: Churchill Livingstone.

Jacob, M., Chappell, D., Rehm, M. (2007). Clinical update: perioperative fluid management. *The Lancet 369,* 1984–1986.

Lee, J. (2000). ECG monitoring in theatre. *World Anaesthesia Online,* 11, 5, Retrieved January 8, 2008, from http://www.nda.ox.ac.uk/wfsa/html/u11/u1105_01.htm.

Levy, J. (2006). The allergic response. In P. G. Barash, B. F. Cullen, R. K. Stoelting (Eds.). *Handbook of clinical anesthesia* (5th ed.) (pp. 1298–1312). Philadelphia: Lippincott, William & Wilkins.

Marley, R. (2005). Preoperative evaluation and preparation of the patient. In J. Nagelhout, & K. L. Zaglaniczny (Eds.). *Nurse anesthesia* (3rd ed.) (pp. 332–372). St Louis: Elsevier.

McNeil, B. (2005). Healthcare challenges: malignant hyperthermia. *British Journal of Perioperative Nursing* 15, (9), 376–382.

Murphy, G. S., & Vender, J. S. (2006). Monitoring the anesthetised patient. In P. G. Barash, B. F. Cullen, R. K. Stoelting (Eds.). *Handbook of clinical anesthesia* (5th ed.) (pp. 668–687). Philadelphia: Lippincott, Williams & Wilkins.

Prough, D. S., Wolf, S. W., Funston, J. S., Svensen, C. H. (2006) Acid-base, fluids and electrolytes. In P. G. Barash, B. F. Cullen, R. K. Stoelting (Eds.). *Handbook of clinical anesthesia* (5th ed.) (pp. 175–207). Philadelphia: Lippincott, Williams & Wilkins.

Rosenberg, H., Bramdom, B. W., Nyamkhishig, S., Fletcher J. E. (2006). Malignant hyperthermia and other pharmacogenetic disorders. In P. G. Barash, B. F. Cullen, R. K. Stoelting (Eds.). *Handbook of clinical anesthesia.* (5th ed.) (pp. 529–556). Philadelphia: Lippincott, Williams & Wilkins.

Rothrock, J. (2007). *Alexander's care of the patient in surgery* (13th ed.). St Louis: Mosby.

SA Department of Health. (2006). BloodSafe Program. Australian Red Cross Transfusion Medicine Service: SA Department of Health.

Schallom, L., Sona, M., McSweeney, M., Mazuski, J. (2007). Comparison of forehead and digit oximetry in surgical/trauma patients at risk for decreased peripheral perfusion. *Heart & Lung: The Journal of Acute and Critical Care 36, (3),* 188–194.

Skubas, N., Lichtman, A. D. Sharma, A., Thomas, S. J. (2006). Anesthesia for cardiac surgery. In P. G. Barash, B. F. Cullen, R. K. Stoelting (Eds.). *Handbook of clinical anesthesia* (5th ed.) (pp. 886–932). Philadelphia: Lippincott, Williams & Wilkins.

Simpson, P. J., & Popat, M. (2001). *Understanding anaesthesia.* Sydney: Elsevier.

Smith, G., Aitkenhead, A. R., Mushambi, M. C. (2007). Anaesthetic apparatus. In A. R. Aitkenhead, G. Smith, D. J. Rowbotham (Eds.). *Textbook of anaesthesia* (5th ed.) (pp. 220–264). Edinburgh: Churchill Livingstone.

Stow, J. (2007). Pediatric surgery. In J. C. Rothrock (Ed.). *Alexander's care of the patient in surgery* (13th ed.) (p. 1075). St Louis: Mosby.

Turner, D. A. B. (2007). Emergency anaesthesia. In A. R. Aitkenhead, G. Smith, D. J. Rowbotham (Eds.). *Textbook of anaesthesia* (5th ed.) (pp. 545–553). Edinburgh: Churchill Livingstone.

Williams, J. (2005). Local anesthetics. In J. Nagelhout, K. L. Zaglaniczny (Eds.). *Nurse anesthesia* (3rd ed.) (pp. 126–148). St Louis: Elsevier.

Wolfgang, B., & Rossaint, R. (2003). Perioperative management and monitoring in anaesthesia. *The Lancet* 352, 1830–1846.

Yates, J. (2005). Care of postanaesthetic patient. In K. Woodhead, & P. Wicker (Eds.). *A textbook of perioperative care* (pp. 181–196). London: Elsevier.

FURTHER READING

Baxendale, B. R. (2007). Preoperative assessment and premedication. In A. R. Aitkenhead, G. Smith & D. J. Rowbotham. (Eds.). *Textbook of anaesthesia* (5th Ed.). (pp. 280–296). Edinburgh: Churchill Livingstone.

Bothamley, J., & Mardell, A. (2005). Preoperative fasting revisited. *British Journal of Perioperative Nursing* 15(9), 370–374.

Farman, J. (2004). Acid aspiration syndrome. *British Journal of Perioperative Nursing 14(6),* 266–267, 269–270, 272–274.

McDonald, C. (2005). Emergency surgery. In K. Woodhead, & P. Wicker (Eds.). *A textbook of perioperative care* (pp. 251–264). London: Elsevier.

NSW Health. (2005). Policy directive PD 2005_490: Latex allergy—policy framework and guidelines for the prevention and management. Sydney: NSW Health.

Rose, D. (2005). Latex sensitivity awareness in preoperative assessment. *British Journal of Perioperative Nursing 15(1),* 27–33.

Stanton, J. (2006). Literature review of safe use of cricoid pressure. *Journal of Perioperative Practice 16(5),* 250–251, 253–257.

Wicker, P., & Smith, B. (2006). Checking the anaesthetic machine. *Journal of Perioperative Practice 16(12),* 585–590.

CHAPTER 7

Wound healing

Ann Parkman and Marilyn Richardson-Tench

LEARNING OBJECTIVES

After reading this chapter, you should be able to:

- briefly discuss the anatomy of the skin and associated structures
- explain the physiology of wound healing and how this relates to patients with surgical wounds
- differentiate between acute and chronic wounds
- identify and use in practice a system for the classification of wounds
- discuss the mechanisms of surgical haemostasis in depth
- discuss methods for the closure, drainage and dressing of wounds.

KEY TERMS

biochemical mediators	dressings	wound
debridement	haemostasis	wound closure
drains	inflammation	wound healing

INTRODUCTION

Wound healing is a complex issue with several interrelated and simultaneous phases. Knowledge of the anatomy of the skin and the physiology of wound healing is essential in order to care competently for patients with wounds created during a surgical procedure and those that occur as a result of pathology or trauma. An understanding of normal coagulation (i.e. blood clotting or **haemostasis**) and the methods used in surgery to enhance it are critical as this informs many of the activities of the surgeon and instrument nurse. Scientific evidence has led to changes in wound management, with a preponderance of new and varied wound care products available. Wound management requires not only knowledge of the properties of dressings but also an understanding of the healing process. The perioperative nurse requires knowledge of the various dressings and drains available and their rationale for use. Knowledge and understanding of the basic concepts of wound healing and wound care provide the new practitioner with confidence in caring for patients in the perioperative setting.

SKIN ANATOMY

Knowledge of the anatomy of the skin and its associated structures is important in order to understand the physiology of wound healing. The skin consists of the dermis (a type I collagen) and the epidermis, which together compose the outermost layer (Wysocki, 2007). The epidermis is made up of many overlapping layers of epidermal cells and has no blood vessels, so this layer is avascular, receiving its nutrients from blood vessels in the underlying dermis (Wysocki, 2007). The structures associated with the skin, including the capillaries, lymph channels, hair follicles, sebaceous glands, sweat glands and nerve endings, are located in the dermis. Other individual cells, such as mast cells, melanocytes and fibroblasts, are also found in the dermis (Fig 7-1).

The next layer of tissue is the subcutaneous layer. This layer contains adipose or fatty tissue, which is yellow, and greasy or slippery to touch, with globules of fat that frequently dislodge. Blood vessels, lymphatics and nerves are found within the subcutaneous layer. The fascia, the next layer, is a thin membrane that fully encapsulates muscle. It is often glossy in appearance, transparent and separates the subcutaneous layer from muscles, tendons and bones (Wysocki, 2007).

WOUND HEALING

A **wound** is an injury that disrupts the continuity of body tissue, with or without tissue loss, and which may be intentional or unintentional. Wounds may be surgical, traumatic or chronic (McEwen, 2007; Phillips, 2007).

Intentional wounds

Surgical site incisions and/or excision constitute intentional wounds; an incision is a cut or an opening into intact tissue, whereas an excision is the removal of tissue. Other types of intentional wounds include occlusion, such as occlusion banding, which is used to treat haemorrhoids, or occlusion using clips to block the passage of the fallopian tubes. Wounds can also be created using chemicals applied to the skin or other tissue intentionally to cause inflammation and re-epithelialisation (e.g. performing a facial peel during plastic surgery).

Unintentional wounds (or traumatic injuries)

Unintentional wounds can be classified by cause—mechanical, thermal or chemical destruction. For example, wounds can occur following trauma (mechanical), as a result of being burnt (thermal) or from contact with chemicals such as acid (chemical).

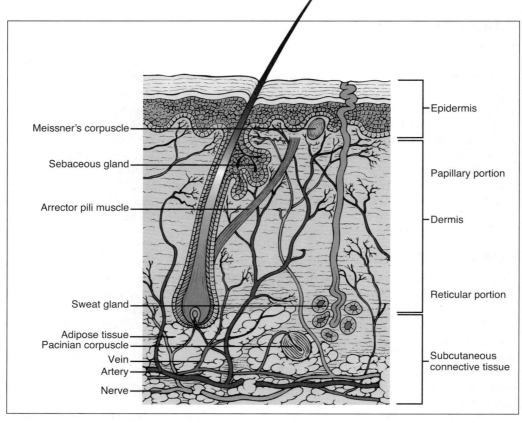

Meissner's corpuscle

Sebaceous gland

Arrector pili muscle

Sweat gland

Adipose tissue
Pacinian corpuscle

Vein

Artery

Nerve

Epidermis

Papillary portion

Dermis

Reticular portion

Subcutaneous
connective tissue

Figure 7-1 Diagram of the skin (Phillips, 2007, p 582).

Chronic wounds

A chronic wound has not completed the usual wound healing process in the expected time frame (Ramundo, 2007). These wounds are caused by an underlying pathophysiological process. For example, a decubitus ulcer, which may be caused by compromised circulation over bony prominences or venous ulcers, develops due to venous stasis or arterial insufficiency. On assessment, a wound that does not appear to be healing by approximately 14–21 days is at risk of becoming a chronic wound.

THE PHASES OF WOUND HEALING

Wound healing depends on many local and systemic factors and is a complex process that involves a series of cellular processes and biochemical events. There is disagreement among researchers about the exact number of phases of wound healing but all agree that it is complex and that there is some overlapping of these phases because they occur almost simultaneously (Benbow, 2007; Doughty & Sparks-Defries, 2007; Karukonda et al., 2000; Schultz, 2007; Schultz et al., 2003). Following haemostasis, healing progresses through three phases:

1. inflammatory phase
2. proliferative phase
3. remodelling phase.

The same basic biochemical and cellular processes are involved in the healing of all soft tissue injuries, whether they are acute or chronic.

Haemostasis and the inflammatory phase

The process of **inflammation** produces classic symptoms: redness, heat, swelling, pain and decreased function. Early and late inflammatory responses differ and each phase involves different **biochemical mediators** and cells that respond by:

- destroying injurious agents and removing them from the inflamed site
- walling off and confining these agents to limit their effect upon the host
- stimulating and enhancing the immune response
- promoting healing.

The inflammatory response is immediate, non-specific, self-limiting and lasts for 3–4 days. It is also referred to as the defensive phase of healing because it is essential to enable healing to occur (Trask et al., 2006). It is induced by:

- nutrient and oxygen deprivation
- lethal and non-lethal cellular injury due to trauma (mechanical forces)
- genetic and immune defects
- chemicals
- temperature extremes
- ionising radiation
- microorganisms
- presence of dead cells (host or foreign)
- parasites.

Haemostasis

Following injury, bleeding in large vessels must be artificially stopped or the patient will suffer from hypovolaemia and, without treatment, death will occur. Following injury, blood vessels briefly constrict. Platelets accumulate at the damaged site, adhere to one another and form a platelet plug (Benbow, 2007). When damage occurs to endothelial cells, which line the blood vessel walls, collagen fibres are exposed. When collagen fibres contact the platelets, an important release of adenosine phosphate (ADP), histamine and serotonin occurs. The coagulation cascade is also triggered (Karukonda et al., 2000; Trask et al., 2006). The mechanism of haemostasis is shown in Figure 7-2.

Biochemical mediator release

Mast cells are found in the extracellular spaces close to blood vessels. These are the most important activators of the inflammatory response. Activation occurs in two ways. Firstly, as a result of degranulation, preformed granular contents are released into the extracellular matrix (e.g. histamine release). Secondly, certain pain-producing mediators (e.g. prostaglandins) are synthesised in response to the injury

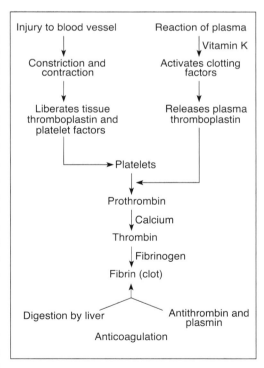

Figure 7-2 Mechanism of haemostasis (Phillips, 2007, p 548).

stimulus; leukotrines, which cause increased vascular permeability and exudation, are also produced. Mast cell degranulation also attracts leucocytes to the site of injury; these cells phagocytose damaged tissue and fight bacteria (Trask et al., 2006).

Vasodilation

Some mediators, such as serotonin and histamine, are termed vasoactive amines because they cause vasodilation and increased vessel permeability. Increased blood flow to the injured tissue causes redness. This arteriolar dilation increases pressure in the microcirculation, which causes development of an exudate made up of plasma and cells; the exudate pushes into the surrounding tissue, which causes localised oedema and swelling.

Increased capillary permeability

As blood becomes more viscous and sticky due to plasma leakage, the microcirculation slows down. Consequently, leucocytes in circulation migrate to the cell walls and adhere there. Released biochemical mediators stimulate the endothelial cells lining the capillaries and venules, causing them to retract, and a space is created at the cell junction. Consequently, leucocytes are then able to squeeze out of circulation into the surrounding tissue.

Phagocytosis

Phagocytosis is the process whereby neutrophils, monocytes and macrophages remove debris and bacteria by engulfing them. In the process, neutrophils die and pus may form. Importantly, macrophages produce growth factors by releasing angiogenesis factor, which is needed for production of capillary and lymphatic buds, and fibroblast-activating factor, which attracts fibroblasts. This process initiates wound repair.

Plasma protein systems

The inflammatory response activates three key plasma protein systems. The *complement system* activates and assists inflammation and the immune process, and directly destroys cells. The *clotting system* traps bacteria in injured tissue and interacts with platelets to prevent haemorrhage. The *kinin system* helps control vascular permeability.

Generally, most surgical wounds are sealed within hours of closure. This seal unites the wound and is a barrier, to a degree, to bacterial invasion.

Reconstructive phase (proliferative)

The reconstructive phase occurs 3–4 days after injury and lasts for about 2 weeks. During this phase the wound is filled in, sealed and then shrinks. The wound is initially sealed by a blood clot containing fibrin, which traps erythrocytes, leucocytes and platelets. Fibrin is created by the activation of the coagulation cascade, and the fibrin in the clot provides a framework for collagen molecules.

Fibroblasts

Fibroblasts synthesise collagen and other connective tissue proteins. They multiply rapidly and enter the wound, forming fibres that bridge the wound edges and restore tissue continuity (Trask et al., 2006). Collagen is the most abundant protein in the body and is the material of tissue repair. It cannot be produced without iron, vitamin C or oxygen. Collagen is produced within 6 days of fibroblasts entering a wound.

Granulation

Repair continues as granulation tissue grows inwards from the surrounding healthy tissue. Granulation tissue is filled with new capillaries, giving it a red, granular appearance. It is surrounded by fibroblasts and macrophages. Capillary buds sprout out of vascular endothelial cells and extend into the debrided areas, eventually forming capillaries. Loops form when these capillaries anastomose and leak neutrophils and erythrocytes, causing further debridement of the wound. Capillaries differentiate into arterioles and venules as repair continues; lymphatics are formed in the same way.

Epithelialisation

As a clot is being dissolved and granulation tissue formed, the healing wound must be protected. This occurs during a process by which epithelial cells grow into the wound from surrounding healthy tissue. Macrophages secrete a factor that attracts epithelial cells, which migrate under a clot or seal. Eventually these epithelial cells contact other migrating cells and seal the wound; migration/proliferation then ceases. However, the epithelial cells remain active, undergoing differentiation and giving rise to various epidermal layers (Trask et al., 2006). This process is hastened when the wound is moist.

Wound contraction

Wound contraction occurs over 6–12 days and is the final reconstructive phase necessary to close all wounds, especially those that heal by secondary intention. Granulation tissue contains specialised cells called myofibroblasts, which cause wound contraction (Trask et al., 2006). The scar will form at this point and may appear red to pink in colour (Myers, 2004). (*Note:* Wounds heal side to side and not end to end.)

Maturation phase

The maturation phase is the final phase, commencing 2–3 weeks after injury and continuing for several years. Scar tissue is remodelled as collagen type III is replaced by collagen type I, which is much stronger. Capillaries regress, leaving the wound avascular and thus pale, and localised itching subsides. Within 2–3 weeks after maturation begins, the scar has gained two-thirds of its maximal strength. However, at best, the repaired tissue will regain only 80% of its original tensile strength. Only epithelial, hepatic and bone marrow cells are capable of mitotic regeneration (i.e. they can regenerate and function as before). Other cells are replaced by fibrous tissue. The healing process is the same for all wounds, although the composition of healed tissue may differ.

TYPES OF WOUND CLOSURE

The three mechanisms by which surgical wounds may be closed and subsequently heal are: primary intention, secondary intention and delayed primary closure or tertiary intention (Fig 7-3).

Primary intention

Surgical (and other) clean wounds heal by a process of collagen synthesis, which seals

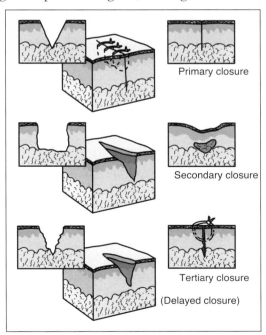

Primary closure

Secondary closure

Tertiary closure

(Delayed closure)

Figure 7-3 Mechanisms of wound healing (Phillips, 2007, p 584).

the wound. This is facilitated by minimal tissue loss and approximation of wound edges, with sutures, clips or tapes. There is no dead space on closure and contamination is held to a minimum by adherence to aseptic technique. Very little epithelialisation is required for healing and most wounds are sealed with fibrin several hours after closure (McEwen, 2007; Phillips, 2007).

Secondary intention

Secondary intention (granulation) healing occurs when there is loss of tissue and the wound cannot be closed; consequently, the wound edges are not approximated. Healing occurs by granulation, eventual re-epithelialisation and wound contraction (Harvey, 2005). The wound will heal spontaneously as long as the dermal base is preserved. Secondary intention healing takes longer than primary intention healing and produces extensive scarring. However, it is often the best option for large open wounds (e.g. decubitus ulcers), traumatic wounds or in wounds where infection is present (McEwen, 2007; Myers, 2004).

Delayed primary closure

When approximation and suturing is delayed intentionally by 3 or more days, or is secondary for the purpose of walling off an area of gross infection or where extensive tissue has been removed, then healing by tertiary intention/delayed primary closure occurs. This method may also be used for haemodynamically unstable trauma patients (McEwen, 2007). The wound edges are closed 4–6 days postoperatively/post-trauma after meticulous debridement (Benbow, 2007).

Box 7-1 Subcutaneous management of vertical incisions with 3 cm or more of subcutaneous fat

---

Surgical wound infections have been shown to be multifactorial. Obesity or an increased depth of subcutaneous fat have been regarded as a significant risk factor for developing a surgical site infection. The multifactorial nature of wound infection was explored in a study by Cardosi et al. (2006), with no definitive conclusion as to the causative factors in any given patient. The researchers found no significant correlation between the depth of subcutaneous fat and the incidence of wound complications or wound disruption.

WOUND CLASSIFICATION

Wounds are classified into the following four types (Box 7-2):
- Class I Clean wound
- Class II Clean–contaminated wound
- Class III Contaminated wound
- Class IV Dirty (infected) wound

Class I Clean wounds

Clean wounds are defined as uninfected operative wounds in which no inflammation is encountered and the respiratory, alimentary, genital or uninfected urinary tract are not entered. Additionally, clean wounds are a result of elective surgery with primary closure and, if necessary, drained with a closed drainage device. Examples include eye surgery, hernia repair, breast surgery, neurosurgery (non-traumatic), cardiac or peripheral vascular surgery (Phillips, 2007).

Box 7-2 Classification of surgical wounds from the Centers for Disease Control

Class I Clean wound

Expected infection rate: 1–5%

- Elective procedure with wound made under ideal operating room conditions
- Primary closure, wound not drained
- No break in sterile technique during surgical procedure
- No inflammation present
- Alimentary, respiratory and genitourinary tracts or oropharyngeal cavity not entered

Class II Clean–contaminated wound

Infection rate: 8–11%

- Primary closure, wound drained
- Minor break in aseptic technique occurred
- No inflammation or infection present
- Alimentary, respiratory and genitourinary tracts or oropharyngeal cavity entered under controlled conditions without significant spillage or unusual contamination

Class III Contaminated wound

Infection rate: 15–20%

- Open, fresh traumatic wound of less than 4 hours' duration
- Major break in aseptic technique occurred
- Acute, non-purulent inflammation present
- Gross spillage/contamination from gastrointestinal tract
- Entrance into genitourinary or biliary tracts with infected urine or bile present

Class IV Dirty (infected) wound

Infection rate: 27–40%

- Old traumatic wound of more than 4 hours' duration from dirty source or with retained necrotic tissue, foreign body or faecal contamination
- Organisms present in surgical field before procedure
- Existing clinical infection: acute bacterial inflammation encountered, with or without purulence; incision to drain abscess
- Perforated viscus

Phillips (2007)

Class II Clean–contaminated wounds

Clean–contaminated wounds are operative wounds in which the respiratory, alimentary, genital or uninfected urinary tract is entered under controlled conditions and without unusual contamination. Specifically, operations involving the biliary tract, appendix, vagina and oropharynx are included, providing there is no evidence of infection or no major break in aseptic technique. Examples include gastrectomy, cholecystectomy (without spillage), elective appendicectomy, cystoscopy and/or cystoscopy/transurethral resection (negative urine cultures), total abdominal hysterectomy, dilation and curettage of the uterus, Caesarean section and tonsillectomy (not infected at time of surgery) (Phillips, 2007).

Class III Contaminated wounds

Contaminated wounds are classified as those contaminated in surgery that involves open, fresh, traumatic wounds, or with major breaks in sterile technique, or with gross spillage from the gastrointestinal tract, and incisions in which acute non-purulent inflammation is encountered. Examples include rectal surgery, laparotomy (with significant spillage), traumatic wounds (e.g. gunshot, stab wounds—non-perforation of viscera) or acute inflammation of any organ without frank pus present (e.g. acute appendicitis or cholecystitis) (Phillips, 2007).

Class IV Dirty (infected) wounds

Old traumatic wounds with retained devitalised tissue and wounds that involve existing clinical infection or perforated viscera and/or delayed primary closure wounds are classified as dirty wounds. This classification suggests an infectious process was present prior to surgery. Examples include debridement, incision and drainage of, for example, an abscess, total evisceration, perforated viscera, amputation or patients with positive preoperative blood cultures.

Debridement

Debridement involves the removal of dead or necrotic tissue and the manual removal of microorganisms, often by irrigation. The aim of debridement is to provide a clean surface with a minimum of microorganisms and dead tissue that provides a focus for infection and physically obstructs contraction of the wound and closure of the wound edges. Different types of debridement materials are available (Ramundo, 2007). Sharp debridement has been described as what usually happens in the operating room (Ramundo, 2007).

SURGICAL HAEMOSTASIS

Surgical haemostasis is the deliberate halting of blood flow. It is essential to wound management and is a necessary and ongoing process during surgery. It is necessary to prevent the patient experiencing the physiological effects of excessive blood loss, which would lead to an increased length of stay in hospital. Additionally, bleeding from the operative site reduces visibility for the surgeon, and is a risk factor for developing a surgical site infection (Rubin, 2006). The mechanisms used encourage the formation of a blood clot, thereby stopping the flow of blood into the surgical site. Surgical haemostasis is achieved by several means, which are classed as mechanical, chemical or electrosurgical; several other methods are unclassified.

Methods of surgical haemostasis

Mechanical haemostasis

Mechanical haemostasis is achieved by compressing the ends of severed vessels until the normal clotting mechanisms have sealed the vessel. Various methods are used to achieve mechanical haemostasis:

- instruments
- ligatures/ties
- ligating clips
- bone wax
- packing
- pledgets
- patties
- tourniquet
- simple digital pressure (Phillips, 2007).

Instruments
Instrument clamps are used to hold a small amount of tissue or the end of a blood vessel. The haemostat or artery forceps is the most commonly used instrument for achieving haemostasis. Often, the pressure of clamping a blood vessel is sufficient to achieve haemostasis.

Ligature/ties
Ligatures are made from suture material and are available in pre-packaged standard lengths, pre-cut lengths or as ligature reels, in which the material is wound around a spool. Ties may be passed to the surgeon in several ways depending on the surgery being performed and the individual preference of the surgeon. Standard length ties may be divided and cut into halves, thirds or quarters, depending on the depth of the tissue being ligated. Ties can be grasped within the jaws of a haemostat/artery or tissue forceps, threaded through an 'eyed' needle or simply handed to the surgeon. Ties handed to the surgeon should be held taut like a guitar string.

Ligating clips
Ligating clips are small, V-shaped, staple-like devices that are designed to be pinched shut over the ends of tissue. They are made from surgical stainless steel, titanium or absorbable polymer. When placed on a blood vessel and closed shut, ligating clips occlude the lumen and stop the bleeding from the vessel (Fig 7-4). Ligating clips are available in small plastic carriers, preloaded with multiple clips, which require individual loading onto a sterile instrument. Ligating clips are also available in a purpose-designed, disposable, preloaded instrument that delivers and closes the clips.

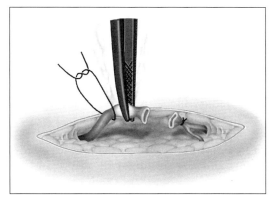

Figure 7-4 Ligating a bleeding vessel (Henry & Thompson, 2005, p 110).

Bone wax
Bone wax is small balls of processed bees wax, which is smeared along the open edge of the bone, acting as a barrier to stop oozing from the cut bone surface.

Packing
Surgical sponges or packs are used for packing a wound site, and effectively place pressure on the wound edges or in a body cavity to reduce bleeding. The surgeon may require the packs to be moistened with a warm sterile irrigating solution. Warm packs promote haemostasis by accelerating the coagulation mechanism (Phillips, 2007).

Pledgets
Pledgets are small pieces of Teflon material that are used to reinforce a suture line where bleeding may occur through the needle holes, effectively placing pressure on the site to reduce bleeding. The pledgets remain in place as part of the suture.

Patties
Compressed, absorbent, radiopaque, cottonoid patties are available in various sizes and are used to absorb blood and compress delicate areas to stop blood flow. They are commonly used in surgical procedures on the brain, spine and spinal cord. The instrument nurse counts the patties, moistens them with normal saline, presses out excess moisture and keeps them flat before use.

Tourniquets

A tourniquet compresses the underlying vessels, thus restricting the blood flow to a limb or digit, creating a bloodless field for the procedure. A pneumatic tourniquet is used when the compression of blood flow to a limb will reduce blood flow (e.g. this might be required during open reduction and internal fixation of a fractured ankle). Applying an elastic band, Penrose drain or the finger of a glove can reduce blood flow to the toes and fingers (Phillips, 2007).

Chemical haemostasis

A number of products are available to provide chemical haemostasis. The effect of these products is the formation of a blood clot. Some examples of the most commonly used products are outlined below.

Absorbable gelatin

Absorbable gelatin (Gelfoam) is an absorbable haemostatic agent made from porcine gelatin, which is compressed into a pad or powder form. As a pad, it is available in an assortment of sizes that can be cut to the desired size without crumbling. The gelatin sponge is not soluble and absorbs up to 45 times its own weight in blood. It is frequently soaked in thrombin or adrenaline solution. It is handed moist to the surgeon for use. When placed in an area of capillary bleeding, fibrin is deposited in the interstices and the sponge swells, forming a clot. Gelatin powder is mixed with sterile saline to make a paste for absorbing blood (Phillips, 2007).

Absorbable collagen sponge

Haemostatic sponges (Colostat) of bovine collagen origin are applied dry to oozing or bleeding sites. The collagen activates the coagulation mechanism, especially the aggregation of platelets, to accelerate clot formation. The material dissolves as haemostasis occurs and any residual will absorb in the wound. The sponge must be kept dry and should be applied with dry gloves or instruments. It is applied directly to the bleeding surface as supplied from the sterile package. Absorbable collagen is contraindicated in the presence of infection or where blood or other fluids have pooled (Phillips, 2007).

Oxidised cellulose

Absorbable oxidised cellulose comes in the form of a knitted fabric (Surgicel) and is applied dry to bleeding areas. It may be sutured to, wrapped around or held firmly against a bleeding site, or laid dry on an oozing surface until haemostasis is obtained. Oxidation of the cellulose acts rapidly to form a clot when it comes in contact with whole blood. As it reacts with blood, it increases in size to form a gel, and stops bleeding in areas in which bleeding is difficult to control by other means of haemostasis. If left on oozing surfaces, it will absorb 10 times its own weight with minimal tissue reaction. Oxidised cellulose is inactivated in the presence of thrombin (Phillips, 2007).

Thrombin

Thrombin (Thrombostat) is an enzyme that is extracted from dried beef blood; it is used topically. Thrombin accelerates coagulation of blood and controls capillary bleeding. It unites rapidly with fibrinogen to form a clot. It is available as a powder that is reconstituted immediately prior to use. It can be used alone or soaked into a gelatin sponge. Thrombin is used as a topical application only and is never injected (Phillips, 2007).

Oxytocin

Oxytocin is a hormone produced in the pituitary gland, which can also be prepared synthetically for therapeutic injection. It is commonly used in obstetric and gynaecological surgery. Oxytocin causes the uterine muscle to contract, thus putting pressure on the blood vessels, reducing bleeding (Phillips, 2007).

Adrenaline

Adrenaline is a naturally occurring hormone produced by the adrenal gland. It is also prepared commercially. It acts as a vasoconstrictor, reducing the flow of blood to the surgical site. Topical adrenaline can be applied to bleeding surfaces. Local anaesthesia often contains adrenaline to reduce the blood flow to the skin, promoting surgical haemostasis (Phillips, 2007).

Fibrin glue

Fibrin glue acts as a biological adhesive and haemostatic agent. It is composed of fibrinogen, cryoprecipitate from human plasma, calcium chloride and reconstituted thrombin of bovine origin (Phillips, 2007). Upon application directly to tissues, thrombin converts fibrinogen to fibrin to produce a clot. Fibrin glue may be used in deeper tissues to control bleeding and approximate tissues. A liquid gel or aerosol spray can deliver the fibrin glue.

Electrosurgical haemostasis

Electric current can be used to cut or coagulate most tissues: fat, fascia, muscle, internal organs and vessels. Electrosurgery is used to a greater or lesser extent in all surgical specialities. Electrosurgical unit (ESU), lasers and ultrasonic machines are the types most frequently seen in the operating room. These machines come with a range of disposable 'tools' that surgeons can use to achieve ongoing haemostasis.

Electrosurgical unit

The ESU provides a high-frequency electric current to cut tissue and to coagulate bleeding points. The size and flow of the current generate heat as it meets resistance in passage through tissue. The current can be passed through the tissues without causing stimulation of muscle or nerves. A grounding pad is required. Two different types of electrosurgical machines (Fig 7-5), which act to seal blood vessels using different types of energy, are available.

Laser

Laser light is used for controlling bleeding or for the ablation and excision of tissues. The laser concentrates and intensifies a light beam of a single wavelength. The thermal energy of this beam may simultaneously cut, coagulate and/or vaporise tissue. The laser wound is characterised by minimal bleeding and no postoperative oedema. Different lasers have selected uses, depending on the form of the wavelength (Phillips, 2007).

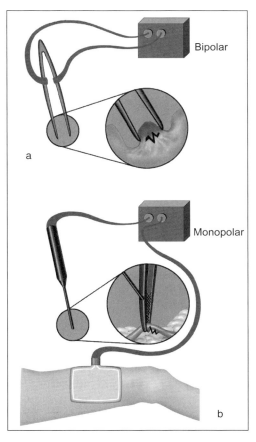

Figure 7-5 Electrosurgical haemostasis: (a) bipolar and (b) monopolar diathermy (Henry & Thompson, 2005, p 110).

Ultrasonic scalpel

The titanium blades of this scalpel move by a rapid ultrasonic motion that cuts and coagulates tissue simultaneously. It generates less heat than the ESU and, therefore, does not damage adjacent tissues. Vibrations from the tool denature protein molecules, producing a coagulum that seals bleeding vessels. The continuous vibration of the denatured protein generates heat within the tissue to cause deeper coagulation. Because electricity is not required to produce coagulative effects on tissue, a grounding pad is not required (Phillips, 2007).

Haemostatic scalpel

The sharp steel blade of the haemostatic scalpel seals blood vessels as it cuts through the tissue. When the surgeon activates the handle, the blade transfers thermal energy to tissues as the sharp edge cuts through them. The temperature can be adjusted between 110°C and 270°C. The resultant rapid haemostasis with minimal tissue damage promotes wound healing and may eliminate the need for blood replacement. Because electric current from the microcircuitry does not pass through the tissues, a grounding pad is not required (Phillips, 2007).

Additional methods of haemostasis

Embolisation

In embolisation, a haemostatic agent is placed inside a blood vessel, deliberately blocking it, in order to prevent the risk of a more serious haemorrhage. Several substances are used as embolic agents, as well as devices such as coils. This technique is often used in neurosurgery to embolise a cerebral aneurysm or the blood supply to an arteriovenous malformation, thereby negating the need for surgery, or to help the surgeon control bleeding during the surgical procedure (Phillips, 2007).

Sclerotherapy

Sclerotherapy is the injection of a coagulant to stop or reduce venous bleeding. Phenol plus alcohol is a sclerotherapy agent used to thrombose external haemorrhoids (Phillips, 2007).

WOUND CLOSURE

The goal of **wound closure** is to approximate the wound edges, eliminate dead space, distribute tension evenly along the suture line, and maintain the tensile strength across the suture line until sufficient tissue tensile strength is achieved. The closure of a surgical wound is performed after adequate haemostasis has occurred. The strength of the wound is related to the condition of the tissue and the number of stitches in the edges. Care is taken not to place more sutures than necessary to approximate the edges. The amount of tissue incorporated into each stitch directly influences the rate of healing. Wound closures often include deep and superficial sutures but may also include staples, clips, tapes and glues. There are indications for each method of closure, along with advantages, disadvantages and special considerations (Lai, 2004).

Skilful wound closure requires knowledge of good surgical technique, as well as knowledge of the properties of the suture material and needle. While the actual suturing technique is largely left to the surgeon, the perioperative nurse needs a broad knowledge of suture materials, their properties and how to handle the sutures safely in order to assist the surgeon. Chapter 8 has a detailed section on suture materials.

Wound closure methods

The traditional methods of wound closure include (Fig 7-6):

- single layer
- multiple layer
- simple continuous sutures
- simple interrupted sutures
- continuous running/locking
- subcutaneous sutures
- retention sutures
- drain suture.

Figure 7-7 demonstrates suturing techniques for wound closure.

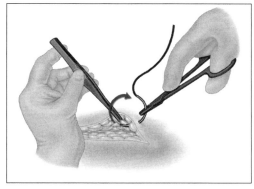

Figure 7-6 Wound closure (Rothrock, 2007, p 239).

Single layer closure

A single layer continuous suture line is commonly used in abdominal closure. It is subject to great pulling forces, and the 'bites' of the needle are deliberately large so that the force is more evenly distributed over the area.

Multiple layer closure

As the name suggests, the wound is closed in multiple layers, effectively eliminating the dead space, thus promoting wound healing.

Simple continuous sutures

In this method, the suture is anchored at one end of the wound and proceeds towards the opposite end, taking even bites of tissue. The suture is then anchored at the other end of the wound. This method is quicker than tying several knots, as for interrupted sutures (see below).

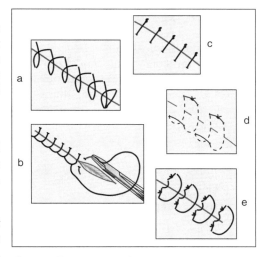

Figure 7-7 Examples of suturing techniques (Phillips, 2007, p 557): (a) simple continuous; (b) continuous locking; (c) simple interrupted; (d) horizontal mattress; (e) vertical mattress.

Simple interrupted sutures

With simple interrupted sutures, each suture is placed and tied individually. This method is generally considered to be the most secure method of suturing. Variations in the configuration of the stitch itself are designed to exert forces in different ways.

Knot placement

Interrupted stitches require individual knots and, therefore, placement of the knot can influence how well the wound heals and the cosmetic result. Principles concerning knots and knot tying include the following:

1. The knot should be tied away from:
   - (a) vital structures, such as the eye
   - (b) sources of contamination, such as the mouth
   - (c) potential irritants, such as the nares
   - (d) potential sources of increased inflammation, such as the incision line.

2. The knot should be tied towards:
    (a)   the better blood supply
    (b)   the area that provides the best security of the knot
    (c)   if possible, where the mark would be less noticeable (Phillips, 2007).

Continuous running/locking (blanket stitch)

In this method, a single suture is passed in and out of the tissue layers and looped through the free end before the needle is passed through the tissue for another stitch. Each new stitch locks the previous stitch.

Subcutaneous sutures

Subcutaneous sutures are placed under the epidermis of the skin. This method of closure provides good cosmetic results as there is no skin perforation with the suture needle. It is suitable in the absence of oedema or infection.

Retention sutures

Interrupted, non-absorbable retention or stay sutures are placed alongside the primary suture line to relieve lateral tension on the suture line, with the aim of reducing the risk of wound dehiscence. The tissue through which retention sutures are passed includes skin, subcutaneous tissue and fascia, and may include the rectus abdominis muscle and peritoneum in an abdominal incision. After abdominal surgical procedures, retention sutures are used frequently in patients in whom slow wound healing is expected because of:

*   malnutrition
*   obesity
*   carcinoma
*   infection
*   older age
*   cortisone therapy
*   respiratory problems (Phillips, 2007).

Drain suture

Drains are often anchored to the skin by a suture to prevent the drain being inadvertently pulled out or slipping into the wound. Silk sutures are the most commonly used 'drain stitch'.

Other methods of wound closure

Staples

Most operating suites have a large collection of mechanical stapling devices that are used for internal ligation, division, resection, anastomosis and closure of the skin and fascia layers. These disposable devices provide the important benefit of reducing tissue handling, thereby reducing the length of the procedure. When fired, the staples take on a 'B' shape, permitting nutrients to permeate the tissue and promote healing. Stapling devices fire a single staple, one or two straight rows or circular rows of staples. Refills are also available for some stapling devices. Some stapling devices incorporate blades; this permits the simultaneous division of tissue that has been ligated between rows of staples (Phillips, 2007).

Skin staples/clips are used to close the skin layer of an incision (Fig 7-8). The clips are made from non-corroding metal and delivered by a preloaded disposable device.

Skin staples can be used in the presence of infection as the strength of the material is not affected by the increased inflammatory response, which can weaken some suture materials (Phillips, 2007).

Tapes

Skin tapes are adhesive-backed nylon or polypropylene tapes, which can be used separately or in conjunction with subcuticular skin closure, providing extra strength (Fig 7-9). Other examples of surgical tapes include an adherent device that is laced up the centre to reduce the tension in a large wound (Phillips, 2007).

Tissue adhesives

Tissue adhesives have been available for some 20 years and have been used most commonly in the emergency room, particularly for children with minor traumatic wounds. Tissue adhesives provide good closure without causing any pain, plus there is no need to remove sutures at a later time. Patients are able to shower because the adhesive also provides a waterproof barrier. Synthetic adhesives are glue-like adhesives that polymerise to bind tissue edges together. Biological and synthetic adhesives, such as fibrin glue (Box 7-3), have great potential application in the area of haemostasis as previously presented (Phillips, 2007). Tissue adhesives may be used for microsurgical anastomoses of

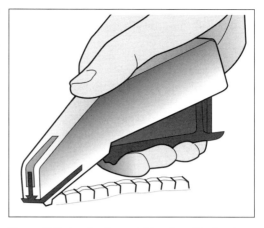

Figure 7-8 Application of skin clips (Curtis et al., 2007; p 174).

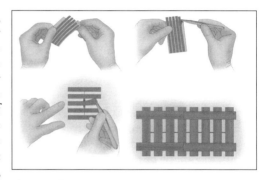

Figure 7-9 Tapes for wound closure (Copyright 3M, St Paul, MN).

blood vessels, nerves and fallopian tubes. They may also be used for reconstruction of the middle ear, to fix ocular implants, to close superficial lacerations and fistula tracts, and to secure skin grafts.

Implantable tissue repair and replacement material

Tissue deficiencies may require additional reinforcement or bridging material (Table 7-1) to obtain adequate wound healing. Sometimes, the edges of fascia, for example, cannot be brought together without excessive tension. In obese patients or older patients the fascia cannot withstand this tension because of weakness caused by the infiltration of fat. Biological or synthetic mesh materials are used to fill congenital, traumatic or acquired defects in fascia or a body wall and to reinforce fascia, as in hernia repair (Phillips, 2007). Implants must be sterile and compatible with the recipient. They should not be handled excessively to prevent damage to the surface or contamination from the field. Implants can be permanent or temporary and composed of many materials. Some implants used are mechanical.

> **Box 7-3** Sample fibrin glue compound and supplies
>
> Equipment
>
> - Sterile specimen cup
> - Two 20-mL disposable syringes
> - Two 14-gauge intravenous (IV) catheters
> - 6 units thawed cryoprecipitate
> - 1 ampoule calcium chloride (CaCl) (10%, 1 g)
> - 50,000 units thrombin
>
> Instructions
>
> Mix CaCl and thrombin in the specimen cup. Draw mixture into a 20-mL syringe and attach a 14-gauge IV catheter. Draw cryoprecipitate into the second syringe with a 14-gauge catheter on the end. Both syringes are discharged over the wound at the same time. The fibrin glue will form a clot over the wound.
>
> Phillips (2007)

WOUND CARE

Dressings

Dressings are applied to a surgical incision or wound site for the first 24–48 hours to provide the best environment for wound healing to occur. A dressing serves several purposes:

1. protection of the wound from trauma and gross contamination
2. keeping the wound free of microorganisms, both exogenous and endogenous
3. absorption of exudate and secretions
4. enhancement of patient physical comfort and aesthetic appearance
5. support and immobilisation of the incisional area and/or body part
6. provision of additional haemostasis, minimising dead space and oedema
7. maintenance of a moist environment, which supports healing
8. application of medications (McEwen, 2007).

When considering the most suitable dressing, each wound is assessed in terms of the type of wound, its location, depth and the patient's comorbidities. The type of dressing selected is also based on the surgeon's or specialty preference.

Types of dressings

Dressings are classified according to their main function: primary or secondary dressings. Primary dressings are placed directly over the wound. The function of these dressings is to absorb drainage away from the wound edge. This layer of dressing should be non-stick unless debridement is necessary. Secondary dressings are placed directly over the primary dressing. The function of secondary dressings can include haemostasis by compression, absorption of excess drainage and protection of the wound from trauma (McEwen, 2007).

One layer dressings

One layer dressings are sterile, transparent, occlusive dressings that are suitable for clean, incised wounds. Multiple studies have shown that the use of occlusive dressings promotes wound healing two to six times faster than in a wound exposed to air; surgical site infection rates are significantly lower under an occlusive dressing compared to a non-occlusive dressing (Fletcher et al., 2007).

Table 7-1 Implants: tissue repair and replacement material

Natural (biological)

Autologous	Allogeneic	Xenograft	Biomaterials
Skin	Bone	Porcine dermal collagen	Biodegradable fixation S-1 (CO_2 and H_2O)
Cartilage	Tendon and ligament	Tricalcium phosphate	Hydroxyapatite ceramic
Bone	Cornea	Porcine heart valve	Bioengineered stent endothelial
Muscle	Alloderm	Bovine xenograft screws	Bovine collagen polyester graft
Gut	Tissue matrix: periosteal, chondrium	Calcium alginate gel	
Hair follicles	Fascia	Coral	
Vessels	Saphenous veins	Bovine collagen dressing	
	Heart valve	Bovine collagen matrix	
	Ossicles	Porcine collagen matrix	

Synthetic

Chemical	Metallic	Polymer	Mechanical
Glial antibiotic disc	Plates/screws	Solid	Pacer
Bone cement	Rods	Expandable	Penile hydraulics
Drug-eluting stent	Stent	Shunts	Medication pump
Conduit graft	Joint	Stents	Cochlear components
Mesh graft	Grid	Thermoplastic polymer	Heart assist device
	Clips and staples	Liquid	Internal defibrillator
	Metallic oxide, ceramic	Polyethylene	Nerve stimulator
	Zirconium oxide	Polyurethane	
	Chromium oxide	Non-absorbable ligating clip	
	Aluminium oxide		
	Dental ceramic		

Phillips (2007)

Skin closure dressing (island dressing)

Skin closure or island dressings consist of a non-stick pad in the centre (to absorb drainage) and either an occlusive-type material or adherent woven gauze, which anchors the dressing to the skin. Fletcher et al. (2007) recommend the use of surgical island dressings on clean, incised surgical wounds.

Dry sterile dressing

Dry sterile dressings are applied to dry incised wounds where there is no drainage. Dry dressings are not used on denuded wounds or those with large amount of drainage as they adhere to the wound, causing trauma on removal.

Three layer dressings

Three layer dressings are used when moderate to heavy drainage is expected. The *contact* layer acts as a passageway for the secretion and exudates that emanate from a draining wound. It must conform to body contours regardless of the site and extent of the wound, and must stay in intimate contact with the wound surface for at least 48 hours, yet be non-adherent for painless removal. The *intermediate* layer absorbs secretions that pass through the contact layer. It should be layered but not excessively bulky, nor apply pressure that could compromise circulation. The *outer* layer holds the contact and intermediate layers in proper position. It should be conforming and stretchable to avoid constriction if oedema develops.

Non-allergenic tape is the most frequently used material to hold the dressing in place. Depending on the site of the wound, an elastic bandage may be used because it provides gentle even pressure and gives firm support. Montgomery straps (Fig 7-10) are used to hold bulky dressings in place that require frequent changes or wound inspections (Henry & Thompson, 2005).

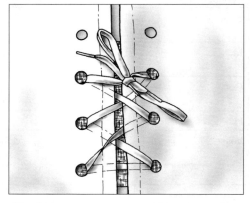

Figure 7-10 Montgomery straps (Henry & Thompson, 2005).

Pressure dressing

Bulky dressings are added to the immediate layer of a three layer dressing. This dressing acts to eliminate dead space and prevent haematoma or oedema. They also distribute pressure evenly; absorb extensive drainage; encourage wound healing and minimise scarring by influencing wound tension; and immobilise a body area or support soft tissues when muscles are being moved. A pressure dressing helps to provide comfort to the patient postoperatively. These dressings are often used in plastic, knee and breast surgery (Henry & Thompson, 2005).

Stent dressing

A stent dressing is a method of applying pressure and stabilising tissues when it is impossible to dress an area, such as on the face or neck.

Bolster/tie-over dressing

Dressing materials may be sutured in place to exert an even pressure over autografted wounds to prevent haematoma or seroma formation.

Wet-to-dry dressings

Wet-to-dry dressings are used when debridement of the wound is required; the saline-soaked gauze dries and debrides the wound on removal. This process is used to facilitate new tissue growth. These dressings are painful and their removal and/or replacement may be conducted in the operating room under anaesthetic.

Wet-to-wet dressings

Normal saline or other medicinal solutions are applied to dressings to maintain an optimal environment for wound healing. Wet-to-wet dressings are less painful than wet-to-dry dressings but may also be applied or changed in the operating room under sterile conditions.

Vacuum-assisted dressings

These dressings are a closed-system dressing used for difficult to heal wounds with large amounts of drainage. The dressing comprises an absorbent sponge to draw away fluid, an occlusive adherent dressing to seal the system, tubing to facilitate the drainage and a vacuum pump, which gently aspirates the fluid and holds it in a storage unit (Fig 7-11). The use of vacuum-assisted dressings has increased in recent years for the treatment of wounds in patients with compromised healing (Heller et al., 2006). However, some evidence suggests that the drains may contribute to the formation of fistulas (Rao et al., 2007).

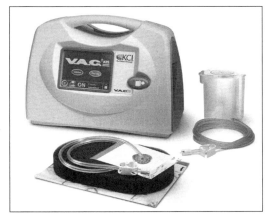

Figure 7-11 Vacuum-assisted dressings (Copyright KCI, San Antonio).

Application of dressings

The application of surgical dressings is regarded as part of the surgical procedure. The surgeon is assisted by the instrument and circulating nurse to dress the wound properly.

Drains

Drains are often inserted during surgery to provide a pathway allowing blood, lymph, intestinal secretions, bile, pus, air or urine to be transported away from the surgical site (Box 7-4). Drains can be used prophylactically or therapeutically. A drain is inserted prophylactically to remove unwanted fluid, air or secretions from around the surgical site, to promote wound healing, to provide a mechanism to observe for haemorrhage (Gurusamy & Samraj, 2007) and to reduce postoperative pain (Shen et al., 2003). The presence of a collection of fluid, air or secretions is thought to act as a medium in which microbes grow, leading to a surgical site infection.

Box 7-4 Routine abdominal drainage for uncomplicated laparoscopic cholecystectomy

In this study, the benefits and harm caused by the insertion of a closed suction drain after an uncomplicated laparoscopic cholecystectomy were assessed. The study analysed a group of six trials involving 741 patients: 361 with drain versus 380 with no drain. The study explored the reason why drains are often used, which was prevention of intra-abdominal collections, postoperative shoulder pain, nausea and vomiting. The authors concluded that the use of a drain after a laparoscopic cholecystectomy increased wound infection and delayed discharge from hospital.

Gurusamy et al. (2007)

The use of prophylactic drains in surgery continues to be controversial. Several recent studies have found insufficient evidence to support their use (McCarthy et al., 2005; Parker et al., 2007; Tjeenk et al., 2005;). The presence of a wound drainage system does not necessarily reduce the incidence of surgical site infection or haematoma (Gurusamy & Samraj, 2007; Gurusamy et al., 2007). Indeed, in some cases the presence of a drain is thought to increase the risk of surgical site infections by providing a route for the migration of bacteria around the tube into the wound (Fletcher et al., 2007).

A drain that is inserted therapeutically is used to reduce the amount of an already present collection, which may be necrotic or purulent material. Drains are usually inserted at the time of surgery primarily through a small stab incision near the operative site. Drains may or may not be sutured to the skin.

Some drains act by directing the fluid away through the lumen of the tube itself, other drains have a small fenestration at the tip, which drains into a closed system, and other drains act by 'wicking' the fluid away by capillary action into an absorbent dressing or drainage bag (Phillips, 2007).

The perioperative nurse must document clearly in the patient's medical record the type of drain, its location and whether the drain is sutured in place, and ensure that the drain is working properly before the patient leaves the operating room.

Drain types

Passive drains
Passive drains use gravity and capillary action to move unwanted fluids away from the operative site. A Penrose drain (Fig 7-12) is a soft latex tube, of varying sizes, often used for the superficial drainage of abscesses. A Yeates drain is a soft, silicone corrugated drain, which acts by capillary action and gravity into a dressing or drainage bag; it is often used to drain post-appendicectomy wounds (Phillips, 2007).

Active drains
Active drains are attached to an external source of vacuum to create a negative pressure in the wound. Active drains include closed wound suction systems, sump drains and chest drains.

Closed wound suction
Closed drainage systems, such as the Jackson-Pratt or haemovac drains (Fig 7-12), are sterile, self-contained drainage units. The closed unit minimises the pathway of pathogens to the wound site. They may be used with or without suction; that is, they can be active or passive drains. The negative pressure in the reservoir acts to draw fluid gently away from the wound site into the reservoir.

Specialised drains
The T-tube drainage system is a soft latex drain that is inserted into the common bile duct, allowing bile to be drained away.

Urinary drainage
A urinary or ureteral catheter provides continuous drainage of the bladder or kidneys during and after the surgical procedure. The balloon of a urinary catheter maintains pressure on the bladder neck, which helps control bleeding after a transurethral prostatectomy and can be used to facilitate bladder irrigation. The urinary catheter is also used to monitor the patient's haemodynamic status.

Gastric decompression
A nasogastric tube can be used as a drain to decompress the stomach of flatus or gastric fluids. It is used to drain gastric secretions, thus preventing aspiration. It can also be used to decompress the stomach to aid the surgeon's view.

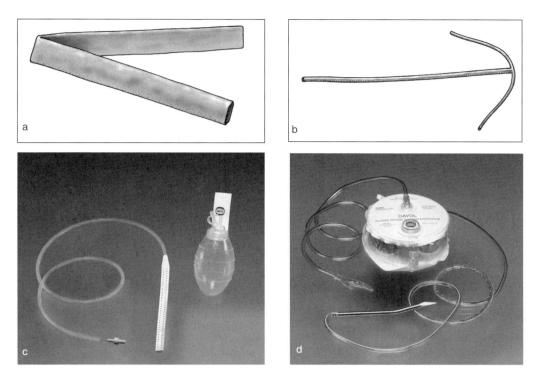

Figure 7-12 Various drain tubes: (a) Penrose drain; (b) T-tube drain by gravity; (c) Jackson-Pratt and (d) haemovac closed active drains (Copyright CR Bard, Inc, Murray Hill, NJ).

CONCLUSION

The perioperative nurse must show sound assessment, planning, implementation and evaluation of all aspects of wound management during the perioperative period. The results of a surgical site infection may be devastating to patients and their family and continue to be a costly problem for hospitals. Wound healing, assessment, haemostasis, wound closure and wound management have been explored in this chapter in more detail to empower the perioperative nurse to care for patient wounds skilfully.

CRITICAL THINKING EXERCISES

1. Potential wound problems

Mr Jones is scheduled for a liver resection on tomorrow's list. He weighs 60 kg, is 175 cm tall and has a previous history of alcohol abuse.

Identify three potential problems that Mr Jones may encounter. Address the following:

- Why has the normal mechanism of haemostasis been disrupted?
- What methods of haemostasis would you consider necessary for his procedure?
- What method of wound closure is likely to be performed?
- Discuss the most appropriate method of skin closure for Mr Jones.
- The consultant surgeon asks for a closed system drain. What does the perioperative nurse document?
- Describe the dressing that is most appropriate for Mr Jones.

2. Wound classification

Alan Bright is 12 years old and is undergoing an appendicectomy. He is febrile and quite nauseous before the procedure. The surgeon removes the appendix but finds it had ruptured before Alan's arrival in operating room.

- How would you classify Alan's wound?
- Discuss the methods and layers of wound closure?
- Would this wound require a drain? Why?

3. Drainage management

Mrs Tulip has had a left breast mastectomy and axillary clearance. She has a haemovac drain in situ. You notice that the drain reservoir is inflated.

- How would you manage this situation?

REFERENCES

Benbow, M. (2007). Healing and wound classification. *Journal of Community Nursing, 21(9)*, 26–32.

Cardosi, R., Drake, J., Holmes, S., et al. (2006). Subcutaneous management of vertical incisions with 3 or more centimetres of subcutaneous fat. *American Journal of Obstetrics & Gynecology, 195*, 607–616.

Corbett, L. Q., & Milne, C. T. (2001). Wound care in the age of PPS: tools for survival. *Home Health Care Management Practice, 13*, 93.

Curtis, K., Ramsden, C., Friendship, J. (2007). *Emergency and trauma nursing.* Sydney: Elsevier.

Doughty, D., & Sparks-Defries, B. (2007). Wound healing physiology. In R. Bryant, & D. Nix (Eds.). *Acute and chronic wounds: current management concepts* (3rd ed.) (pp. 56–81). St Louis: Mosby.

Fletcher, N., Sofianos, D., Brantling Berkes, M., Obremskey, W. T. (2007). Prevention of perioperative infection. *Journal of Bone & Joint Surgery, 89*, 1605–1618.

Gurusamy, K. S., & Samraj, K. (2007). Wound drains after incisional hernia repair. *Cochrane Database of Systematic Reviews, 1*, CD005570.

Gurusamy, K. S., Samraj, K., Mullerat, P., Davidson, B. R. (2007). Routine abdominal drainage for uncomplicated laparoscopic cholecystectomy. *Cochrane Database of Systematic Reviews, 4*, CD006004.

Harvey, C. (2005). Wound healing. *Orthopaedic Nursing, 24(2)*, 143–159.

Heller, L., Levin, S. L., Butler, C. E. (2006). Management of abdominal wound dehiscence using vacuum assisted closure in patients with compromised healing. *American Journal of Surgery, 191*, 165–172.

Henry, M., & Thompson, J. (2005). *Clinical surgery* (2nd ed.). London: Saunders.

Karukonda, S., Flynn, T., Boh, E., et al. (2000). The effects of drugs on wound healing: part 1. *International Journal of Dermatology, 39(4)*, 250–257.

Lai, S. Y. (2004). Sutures and needles. *eMedicine.* Retrieved April 29, 2007, from http://www.emedicine.com/ent/topic38.htm.

McCarthy, C. M., Disa, J. J., Pusic, A. L., et al. (2005). The effect of closed-suction drains on the incidence of local wound complications following tissue expander/implant reconstruction: a cohort study. *Plastic and Reconstructive Surgery, 119(7)*, 2018–2022.

McEwen, D. (2007). Wound healing, dressings and drains. In J. Rothrock (Ed.). *Alexander's care of the patient in surgery* (13th ed.). (pp. 263–273). St Louis: Mosby.

Myers, B. (2004). *Wound management: principles and practice.* New Jersey: Prentice Hall.

Parker, M. J., Livingstone, V., Clifton, R., McKee, A. (2007). Closed suction surgical wound drainage after orthopaedic surgery. *Cochrane Database of Systematic Reviews, 3*, CD001825.

Phillips, N. (Ed.). (2007). *Berry & Kohn's operating room technique* (11th ed.). St Louis: Mosby.

Ramundo, J. (2007). Wound debridement. In R. Bryant, & D. Nix (Ed.). *Acute and chronic wounds: current management concepts* (3rd ed.) (pp. 176–192). St Louis: Mosby.

Rao, M., Burke, D., Finan, P. J., Sagar, P. M. (2007). The use of vacuum-assisted closure of abdominal wounds: a word of caution. *Colorectal Discourse, 9*, 266–268.

Rothrock, J. (2007). *Alexander's care of the patient in surgery* (13th ed). St Louis: Mosby.

Rubin, R. (2006). Surgical wound infection: epidemiology, pathogenesis, diagnosis and management. *BMC Infectious Diseases, 6*,171.

Shen, C. C., Wu, M. P., Lu, C. H., et al. (2003). Effects of closed suction drainage in reducing pain after laparoscopic-assisted vaginal hysterectomy. *American Association of Gynaecologic Laparoscopists, 10(2)*, 210–214.

Schultz, G. (2007). Molecular regulation of wound healing. In R. Bryant, & D. Nix (Eds.). *Acute and chronic wounds: current management concepts* (3rd ed.) (pp. 82–99). St Louis: Mosby.

Schultz, G., Sibbald, G., Falanga, V., et al. (2003). Wound bed preparation: a systematic approach to wound management. *Wound Repair and Regeneration, 11,* 1–28.

Tjeenk, R. M., Peeters, M. P., van den Ende, E., et al. (2004). Wound drainage versus non-drainage for proximal femoral fractures: a prospective randomised study. *International Journal of Trauma Surgery, 36,* 100–104.

Trask, B. C., Rote, N., Huether, S. (2006). Innate immunity: inflammation. In K. McCance, & S. Huether (Eds.). *Pathophysiology the biologic basis for disease in adults and children* (5th ed.) (pp. 175–209). St Louis: Mosby.

Wysocki, A. (2007). Anatomy and physiology of skin and soft tissue. In R. Bryant, & D. Nix (Eds.). *Acute and chronic wounds: current management concepts* (3rd ed.) (pp. 39–55). St Louis: Mosby.

FURTHER READING

Carless, P. A., Henry, D. A., Anthony, D. M. (2003). Fibrin sealant use for minimising peri-operative allogenic blood transfusion. *Cochrane Database of Systematic Reviews, 2,* CD004171.

Choy, P. Y. G., Bissett, I. P., Docherty, J. G., et al. (2007). Stapled versus handsewn methods for ileocolic anastomoses. *Cochrane Database of Systematic Reviews, 3,* CD004320.

Collis, N., McGuiness, C. M., Batchelor, A. G. (2005). Drainage in breast reduction surgery: a prospective randomised intra-patient trail. *British Journal of Plastic Surgery, 58,* 286–289.

Evans, J. (2007). Massive tissue loss: burns. In R. Bryant, & D. Nix (Eds.). *Acute and chronic wounds: current management concepts* (3rd ed.) (pp. 361–390). St Louis: Mosby.

Hall, J. C., & Hall, J. L. (2004). The measurement of wound infection after breast surgery. *The Breast Journal, 10(5),* 412–415.

Hangstrom, A. (2006). Perceived barriers to implementation of a successful sharps safety program. *AORN Journal, 83(2),* 391–397.

Hess, C., & Kirsner, R. (2003). Orchestrating wound healing: assessing and preparing the wound bed. *Advances in Skin and Wound Care, 16(5),* 246–257.

Lusby, P. E., Coombes, A., Wilkinson, J. M. (2002). Honey: a potent agent for wound healing? *Journal of Wound, Ostomy and Continence Nurses, 29(6),* 295–300.

McCallum, I., King, P. M., Bruce, J. (2007). Healing by primary versus secondary intention after surgical treatment for pilonidal sinus. *Cochrane Database of Systematic Reviews, 4,* CD006213.

Nadkarni, M. S., Rangole, A. K., Sharma, R. K., et al. (2007). Influence of surgical technique on axillary seroma formation: a randomized trial. *Australian and New Zealand Journal of Surgery, 77(5),* 385–389.

Parker, M. J., Livingstone, V., Clifton, R., McKee, A. (2007). Closed suction surgical wound drainage after orthopaedic surgery. *Cochrane Database of Systematic Reviews, 3,* CD001825.

Perry, J., & Jagger, J. (2005). Slash sharps risk for surgical personnel. *AORN Journal, 36(11),* 28–29.

Sessler, D. I. (2006). Non-pharmacological prevention of surgical wound infection. *Anesthesiology Clinics of North America, 24,* 279–297.

Vilar-Compte, D., Roldan-Martin, R., Robles-Vidal, C., Volkow, P. (2006). Surgical site infection (SSI) rates among patients who underwent mastectomy after introduction of SSI prevention policies. *Infection Control and Hospital Epidemiology, 27(8),* 829–834.

Wang, N. D., Doty, D. B., Doty, J. R., et al. (2007). BioGlue: a protective barrier after pericardiotomy. *Journal of Cardiac Surgery, 22,* 295–299.

Yarboro, S. R., Baum, E. J., Dahners, L. E. (2007). Locally administered antibiotics for prophylaxis against surgical wound infection. *Journal of Bone and Joint Surgery, 89,* 929–933.

CHAPTER 8

Surgical intervention

Serena Cole and Marilyn Richardson-Tench

LEARNING OBJECTIVES

After reading this chapter, you should be able to:

- identify the stages of surgery
- discuss the rationale for having a surgical sequence
- discuss the five instrument categories, including the names of at least two instruments from each category
- identify the two main classifications of suture material
- state the two main groups of needles available and explain their differences
- discuss the two insertion techniques used in minimally invasive surgery.

KEY TERMS

atraumatic	laparoscopic surgery	surgical sequence
endoscopic surgery	minimal access surgery	suture
instrumentation	needle	telescopic surgery
keyhole surgery	surgical instruments	ties

INTRODUCTION

This chapter provides an overview of the principles of surgical intervention. A laparotomy (exploration of the abdominal cavity) is used as an example to relate the sequence of surgery. Surgical instruments, suture materials and surgical needles are presented. Some of the innovations associated with minimally invasive surgery are also examined. The perioperative nurse plays an important role in the surgical intervention of a patient. Underpinning this role is a sound knowledge of anatomy, the physiological response to surgery, aseptic technique, safety, and legal and ethical aspects.

SURGICAL–HISTORICAL PERSPECTIVE

Surgery is as old as human beings, with archaeologists finding skulls with evidence of having had a surgical procedure performed dating back to 350,000 BC. Prior to anaesthesia and anaesthetic technique, surgery was performed only if absolutely necessary. Surgery developed along with knowledge in microbiology, disinfection and anaesthetics.

Modern surgery is the branch of medicine that comprises perioperative patient care encompassing such activities as preoperative preparation, intraoperative judgement and management, and postoperative care of patients (Phillips, 2007). Surgery as a discipline combines physiological management with an interventional aspect of treatment, which may be restorative, corrective, diagnostic or palliative (Table 8-1).

Table 8-1 Common indications for surgical procedures

Indication for surgical procedure	Example
Incision	Open tissue or structure by sharp dissection
Excision	Remove tissue or structure by sharp dissection
Diagnostics	Biopsy tissue sample
Repair	Closing of a hernia
Removal	Foreign body
Reconstruction	Creation of a new breast
Palliation	Relief of obstruction
Aesthetics	Facelift
Harvest	Autologous skin graft
Procurement	Donor organ
Transplant	Placement of donor organ
Bypass/shunt	Vascular rerouting
Drainage/evacuation	Incision of abscess
Stabilisation	Repair of a fracture
Parturition	Caesarean section
Termination	Abortion of a pregnancy
Staging	Checking cancer progression
Extraction	Removal of a tooth
Exploration	Invasive examination
Diversion	Creation of a stoma for urine

Phillips (2007)

Surgical procedures are carried out in hospitals, day surgery units or surgeons' rooms. A surgical procedure may be invasive, minimally invasive, minimal access or non-invasive in nature. Any invasive or minimal access procedures involve entry into the body through an opening in the tissues or a body orifice (Phillips, 2007). Non-invasive procedures are frequently diagnostic and do not enter the body. Advances in diagnostic methodologies and drug therapies enable more individuals to be considered for surgery; however, each patient and each procedure is unique. Surgery cannot be considered always completely safe, patient outcomes are not constantly predictable and the surgical team must, at all times, be prepared for the unexpected.

Surgery and surgical techniques continue to evolve along with technology; the result is increasingly less invasive procedures and more rapid patient recovery. Improvements in technology in perioperative patient care are attributed to:

- surgical specialisation of surgeons and teams
- sophisticated diagnostic and intraoperative imaging techniques
- minimally invasive equipment and technology
- ongoing research and technological advancements (Phillips, 2007).

All surgery has clearly defined principles of the operative technique (Phillips, 2007). These principles are listed below.

1. Plan the incision.
2. Make the skin incision with one stroke of evenly applied pressure.
3. Handle tissue carefully and as little as possible.
4. Provide haemostasis.
5. Preserve blood supply.
6. Debride necrotic and devitalised tissue.
7. Keep tissue moist.
8. Carefully and accurately approximate tissues.
9. Immobilise the wound.

SEQUENCE OF SURGERY

Every surgical procedure, no matter how simple or complex, will follow a defined **surgical sequence**. This generalised sequence is then adapted to the specific surgical procedure being performed. Knowledge of the stages of surgical intervention, instrumentation and suture material assists the perioperative nurse in ensuring safe patient outcomes. A working knowledge is required of the sequential steps for a specific surgical procedure based on four concepts that should be considered for any surgical event:

1. approach
2. procedure
3. possible complications
4. closure.

Additional knowledge required by the surgical team includes:

- understanding the anatomy involved
- knowing the surgeon's approach (position and incision)
- recognising accepted techniques for a given institution (e.g. counts, usage of equipment)
- general condition of the patient
- possible complications related to the proposed surgery (intraoperative, post-operative).

Stages of the surgical procedure

Every surgical procedure, whether invasive or minimally invasive, and regardless of the procedure undertaken, will follow a set sequence that can be broken down into five stages, as shown in Table 8-2 (Richardson-Tench & Martens, 2005).

The instrument nurse must have an in-depth knowledge of each stage of the surgical sequence in order to anticipate the surgeon's requirements. The focus for the circulating nurse is the provision of support to the surgical team, and management and coordination of the operating room. A laparotomy procedure is used below to outline the five stages in the operative procedure.

Table 8-2 Five stages of the surgical procedure

Stage	Procedure
I	Open
II	Dissection and exposure
III	Exploration and isolation
IV	Repair—revise, excise or replace
V	Close

Stage I—Open

Stage I involves two steps:

1. *Incision.* The skin and subcutaneous tissue are incised with a scalpel blade.
2. *Haemostasis.* Subcutaneous bleeding vessels are clamped with a curved artery forceps (haemostat) and ligated or cauterised according to the surgeon's preference. Refer to Chapter 7 for a detailed discussion of surgical haemostasis.

Stage II—Dissection and exposure

A clean scalpel blade, curved dissecting scissors or electrosurgery/cautery is used to incise the deep fascia and peritoneum. Toothed forceps are used to elevate the peritoneum prior to incising it as this will prevent inadvertent damage to the underlying structures.

Stage III—Exploration and isolation

Before definitive surgery, the entire abdomen is explored and the pathology isolated for further action. A self-retracting abdominal retractor, such as a Balfour-Doyen retractor, may be inserted to provide maximum exposure.

Stage IV—Repair: excision, revision or replacement

Surgery frequently focuses on the removal, reconstruction or resection of any given structure. Scissors, non-toothed tissue forceps and sponges/packs are required. Specialised instruments may be required to accomplish this task (e.g. a linear stapler for reanastomosis of the bowel). Depending on the purpose of the surgery and local anatomy, each surgical procedure will require a certain amount of dissection of surrounding tissue. As the depth increases, the length of the instrument should also increase.

Haemostasis and irrigation

In preparation for closure, the surgeon will examine the operative site, controlling any bleeding with ligation and/or electrosurgery. To assist in the examination for bleeding, some surgeons will fill the abdominal cavity with a warm solution, such as normal saline. If an anastomosis has been performed, this is examined to ensure that it is secure. The surgeon carries out a final check to ensure that no items are left behind. Oozing from the operative site may require a drain to be inserted, such as a closed wound suction system.

Collection and verification of specimen
Specimens are passed off the sterile field by the instrument nurse to the circulating nurse for processing. Verification of the specimen is carried out by the instrument nurse with the surgeon and circulating nurse.

Stage V—Close
The closing stage comprises wound closure (including surgical counts) and the application of a dressing. The principles related to the division of tissue (Table 8-3) must be understood by all members of the surgical team. This knowledge is of particular importance for the instrument nurse and the nurse assisting the surgeon.

Table 8-3 Principles of division of tissue	
Procedure	**Rationale**
Providing exposure	• Adequate traction required for surgical procedure. • Overly aggressive traction may cause injury to patient.
Stabilisation of anatomical structures	• Wet or dry packs and/or Raytec gauze are used to hold back tissue/push it out of the way. • Gentle handling prevents bruising, tearing and puncturing; firm handling prevents slippage. • Tapes, ties, vessel loops, Penrose drains or sutures may be used.
Use of retractors, grasping instruments and other devices	• Hand-held or self-retaining retractors move and hold tissue/organs. • Clamps, swabs on sticks and suction cannulae push tissue and organs away or towards the surgeon. • A misplaced retractor can compress, tear or stretch blood vessels, nerves and organs. • A grasping instrument can puncture delicate tissue. • Self-retaining retractors are normally used on muscle; smooth blades prevent tearing; toothed blades hold fasciae, subcutaneous tissue, skin. • Swabs on sticks—peanuts—are used for blunt dissection/haemostasis. • Poole and Yankauer suckers are used as exposure devices.
Clamping tissue	• Artery forceps are used to grasp superficial vessels. • Vascular clamps provide haemostasis or partial occlusion until vessel is sutured. • Non-crushing clamps are used for intestinal surgery.
Grasping tissue	• Use fingers/forceps to lift tissue. • Use non-toothed forceps on tissue that may bleed/perforate. • Toothed forceps are used on skin, dense tissue, scar tissue.

Phillips (2007)

The division of tissues is explained below in relation to a laparotomy.

Wound closure
The body is made of many different tissue layers, each having individual characteristics and roles. Historically, every layer was sutured closed. However, with research and the advent of synthetic materials, this practice has been deemed unnecessary in the majority of patients (Phillips, 2007).

Abdominal and visceral peritoneum

The first layer to be closed is that of the abdominal and visceral peritoneum. This is the serous membrane that lines the abdominopelvic cavity. The abdominal peritoneum divides at the posterior midline and surrounds the abdominal organs, creating the visceral peritoneum. The closure of either the visceral or abdominal peritoneum is dependent on the surgeon and the surgery being undertaken. The majority of surgeons will close either the abdominal peritoneum or fascia using either a continuous absorbable suture or interrupted non-absorbable sutures. However, occasionally, depending on their past experience, a surgeon may choose to close both these layers.

The second surgical count commences upon closure of the peritoneal cavity. In anticipation of this closure, the instrument nurse ensures that the surgeon has all the necessary instruments and equipment to continue surgery without interrupting the second surgical count. Clamps can be used to grasp the edges of the peritoneum during closure.

Muscle

The next layer of tissue encountered is muscle. Three layers of muscles—the rectus abdominis, internal and external obliques, and the transverse abdominis—cover the abdominal cavity. The layering effect provides greater strength. The muscle may or may not be sutured upon closure (Phillips, 2007).

Fascia

The external oblique fascia lies directly below the subcutaneous layer and is considered extremely important upon closure as the suture material must hold the wound together while resisting intra-abdominal pressure. An absorbable, monofilament suture that provides long-term wound support is the suture material of choice.

Subcutaneous layer

Closure of the subcutaneous layer will be dependent on the surgeon and the patient's physical characteristics. One of the objectives of wound closure is to remove dead space and, in doing so, achieve better wound closure, as discussed in Chapter 7. The subcutaneous layer is one layer that, if left unsutured, will provide dead space, the presence of which allows tissue fluids to accumulate, which can delay wound healing. Absorbable suture material that is broken down by hydrolytic action is preferred for suturing of the subcutaneous or subcuticular tissues.

Skin

The final surgical count commences upon closure of the skin. As before, the instrument nurse ensures that the surgeon has access to all the necessary instruments, including suture scissors, tissue forceps, moistened sponges to clean the wound, dry sponges to dry the wound area and a dressing.

An absorbable monofilament suture material with a cutting needle using a subcuticular suturing technique is the preferred option for skin closure as the sutures do not require removal and there is less associated tissue reaction. The skin may also be closed by interrupted sutures using an absorbable or non-absorbable suture material. Skin staples or skin glue can also be used, despite not belonging to the absorbable, monofilament group. In conjunction with these skin closure materials, sterile adhesive strips may be added to provide extra support to the skin edges. Tension sutures may be required to provide additional support and relieve undue strain on the wound for patients in whom wound healing may be compromised; for example, in elderly or obese patients or those on chemotherapy (see Ch 7) (Dunscombe, 2007).

Application of dressing/tape

The skin around the operative site is cleansed prior to the application of the wound dressing. The choice of dressing is dependent upon the area to be dressed and the preference of the surgeon. After its application, the instrument nurse assists with the removal of the drapes from around the surgical site. Finally, tape or other fixative is applied to the dressing by the instrument nurse, the surgeon or surgeon's assistant.

INSTRUMENTS

Surgical instruments are critical to the surgical procedure. There are many elements to learn regarding **instrumentation**, such as names, handling, function, intended use, cleaning and sterilisation. All are very important; however, for many new nurses the most important element is to follow the progression of an operation and, through observation, learn which instruments are required for the various steps in the procedure, their names and function. This knowledge enhances the performance of the instrument nurse and leads to the ability to anticipate the requirements of the surgeon throughout the operative procedure. In preparing instrumentation for an operation, the instrument nurse should check sterility, working condition and completeness of the instruments being used.

Instrument categories

Some basic manoeuvres are common to all surgical procedures. The surgeon dissects, resects or alters tissue and/or organs to restore or repair body functions or body parts (Phillips, 2007). Surgical instruments are designed to act as the tools that the surgeon needs for each manoeuvre and are commonly categorised into five major groups. Although different labels may be attributed to these groups, they are generally categorised as:

1. cutting and dissecting instruments
2. grasping and holding instruments
3. clamps
4. retractors
5. miscellaneous/ancillary/accessory.

Anatomy of a ring-handled clamp

The features of a ring-handled clamp are outlined below as an example of a surgical instrument (Fig 8-1).

- Tips should mesh together evenly when the instrument is closed.
- Jaws hold tissue or perioperative materials securely and the pattern of the jaws dictates its purpose. Artery clamps/forceps have a serrated pattern, whereas needle holders have a cross-thatched pattern.
- The box lock has a pin that holds the two sides of the instrument together.
- The shank is the area between the box lock and ringed handles; the length is appropriate to the wound depth.
- Ratchets interlock to keep the jaws locked when the instrument is closed.
- Ringed handles are for ease of holding.

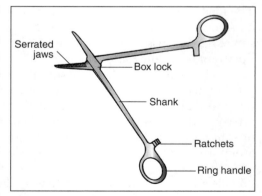

Figure 8-1 Anatomy of a ring-handled clamp (Phillips, 2007, p 334).

Cutting and dissecting instruments

Cutting and dissecting instruments have sharp edges and are used to dissect, incise, separate or excise tissues.

Scalpels

Various scalpel blades are available with configurations for different uses. The Bard Parker and Beaver scalpel handles hold disposable scalpel or knife blades. The Fischer tonsil, Smillie cartilage and Myringotome scalpel handles incorporate the blade into the handle.

Scalpel blades are a potential sharps hazard and, therefore, scalpels are passed in a receptacle (AORN, 2005a). In certain surgical specialties, such as cardiac, vascular and neurosurgery, it is not possible to pass the scalpel blade in this manner. In these circumstances, the instrument nurse should grasp the top of the handle, passing the handle towards the surgeon with the actual blade pointing downwards.

Scissors

Scissors may open and close or have a spring action. The spring action provides better control and more precision, which is important when dissecting delicate tissues, such as those within the eye. Handles can be short or long, with blades straight or angled. Four types of scissors (Fig 8-2) are available:

1. *Dissecting scissors* must have sharp edges and are available in several types. The curvature, weight and size vary according to the intended use. The two most commonly utilised are the Mayo (for dissection of heavy tissue, such as the fascia) and the much finer Metzenbaum scissors (for dissection of delicate tissue in intra-abdominal and other general surgery). Added to these scissors are sharp-tipped angled scissors with short jaws for vascular surgery, sharp-tipped scissors with short jaws for deep areas, such as the nasal cavity, and small scissors with specially shaped tips, such as tenotomy scissors.
2. *Suture scissors* have round tips to prevent trauma to the delicate surrounding structures and the blades are most commonly straight.
3. *Dressing scissors* are heavier to prevent damage to the scissors themselves.
4. *Wire cutters* are used to cut stainless steel wires; the blades are short and heavy.

When holding suture scissors, the ring finger and thumb are placed into the ringed handles, and the index finger is placed along the outside of the blade to stabilise the scissors. For added stability when cutting sutures, the fingers of the opposite hand are placed under the box joint.

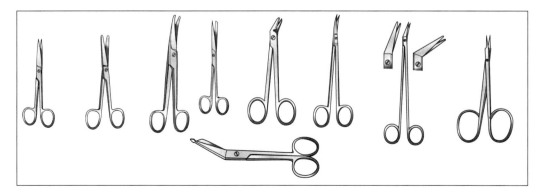

Figure 8-2 Types of surgical scissors (Phillips, 2007, p 331).

Some other instruments that also belong under this heading include bone-cutting instruments, such as chisels, gouges, rasps, osteomes, files, drills, saws, rongeurs and bone nibblers. Curettes, biopsy forceps, punches, snares and dermatomes are also included in this category.

Blunt dissection

Friable tissue or tissue planes can be separated by blunt dissection. Periosteal elevators, the scalpel handle, the blunt sides of scissors, a sponge on a stick and the surgeon's fingers may be used to achieve blunt dissection (Dunscombe, 2007).

Grasping and holding

Grasping and holding instruments are used to, as the names suggest, grasp or hold onto tissue, sutures, swabs or drapes. They include:

- dissecting/tissue forceps
- towel clips
- needle holders
- sponge-holding forceps
- bone-holding forceps
- stone/calculi forceps
- tenaculums.

Dissecting/tissue forceps

Dissecting/tissue forceps (Fig 8-3) hold tissue so that the surgeon can perform a manoeuvre, such as dissecting or suturing, without injuring the surrounding tissues. One group have a tweezer-like action; they vary in length and are available as toothed or non-toothed. Toothed dissecting forceps have opposing 'spurs' or 'teeth' on either side of the jaws, which interlock to provide extra grip. Toothed dissectors are most commonly used on thick, strong tissues, such as skin, muscle, cartilage and fascia. The size of the 'spurs' or 'teeth' indicates the type of tissue each would be used on. For example, the Gillies forceps has finer teeth and is more likely to be used on the skin, whereas the thick heavy teeth of Bonny's forceps means that it is likely to be used for the fascia, cartilage or muscle. Finer versions, such as the DeBakey forceps, have small serrated teeth and are commonly used on delicate tissues, such as blood vessels, bowel, nerves and ureters. Non-toothed forceps, as the name suggests, have no teeth and are considered atraumatic.

When preparing instrumentation, the points of forceps should be checked to ensure that they are of equal length, and that the

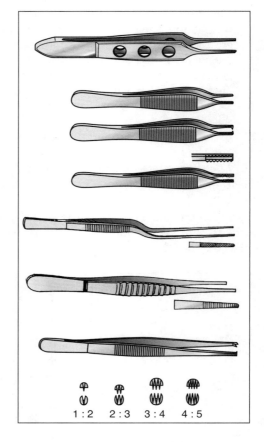

Figure 8-3 Types of tissue forceps (Phillips, 2007, p 333).

teeth or serrations mesh smoothly and evenly and remain closed, even with added pressure.

The second group of forceps are ring-handled and have a scissor action. The Allis forceps has a row of teeth at the end to hold tissue gently but securely. The Babcock forceps has a jaw with a rounded end that is designed to fit around a structure or to grasp tissue without injury. Other ring-handled forceps may be straight or curved (e.g. stone forceps), have sharp points (e.g. Lahey forceps) or have curved or angled points on the ends of the jaws (e.g. tenaculums).

Dissecting forceps should be gripped like a pencil, with the tip pointing down. When passing forceps to a surgeon, the forceps should be grasped in the middle of the handle, with the tips pointing down, and the top of the forceps should be placed into the surgeon's hand (Fig 8-4).

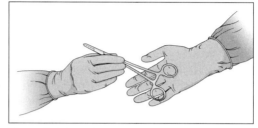

Figure 8-4 Handing an instrument (Phillips, 2007, p 347).

Towel clips

Towel clips are used to secure drapes, diathermy quivers or other items to prevent them falling off or below the level of the sterile field.

The majority of towel clips available today are blunt tipped or have a ball and socket tip; however, some sharp-tipped towel clips are still available. Care should be taken when using sharp-tipped clips. Once an item has been secured to the sterile field, it cannot be moved. The sharp tips can penetrate the sterile drapes, leaving small holes for microorganisms to enter the sterile field. Also, the sharp tips can pierce a patient's skin, or perforate gloves or other equipment, such as the diathermy lead.

Needle holders

Needle holders grasp the needle securely so that it can be passed through tissues without moving. The pattern is cross-thatched rather than grooved, like an artery clamp/forceps, and provides a smoother surface and a good grip on the needle. This pattern also prevents rotation and flattening of the needle, which prevents damage to the needle. Needle holders can be straight or curved. Most have a ratchet; however, in some surgical specialties (e.g. cardiac, ophthalmology, vascular surgery) they have spring-action handles. The spring-action handle on a needle holder provides a much smoother, gentler motion for the surgeon. The general rule of thumb is that the size of the needle indicates the size of the needle holder required.

Sponge-holding forceps

Sponge-holding forceps have several functions. Their most common use is to pick up swabs for skin preparation. Gauze squares can be wrapped around the tips to make what is referred to as a 'swab on a stick', which can be used to soak up fluid in a small space or to dissect tissues bluntly.

Clamps

Clamps occlude, manipulate, crush or hold tissues and other materials. Between the ringed handles is a ratchet that is designed to lock the jaws onto tissue or other material. Within this category are artery clamps/forceps, and crushing and non-crushing clamps.

Artery clamps

Artery clamps/forceps occlude or clamp blood vessels and other tissue with minimal trauma because of the deep transverse serrations within the jaws. They come in different sizes and styles—straight, curved, short and long. The serrations should be cleanly cut and mesh together evenly as these serrations hold the tissues within the jaws of the clamp.

Artery clamps can be damaged easily, so attention must be paid to the thickness of the tissue or blood vessel in relation to the size of the artery clamp. Artery clamps/forceps must not be used for any reason other than what they are designed for. This rule applies to all instruments.

Crushing clamps

Many variations of haemostatic forceps/clamps are used to crush tissues or clamp blood vessels. The jaws may be straight, curved or angled, and the serrations may be horizontal, diagonal or longitudinal. The tip may be pointed or rounded or have a tooth along the jaw, such as on a hysterectomy clamp. Some clamps are designed for use on specific organs, such as bowel clamps, which are used on bowel tissue that is diseased and requiring dissection.

Non-crushing clamps

Non-crushing clamps are used to occlude peripheral or major blood vessels temporarily (e.g. non-crushing vascular clamps), which minimises tissue trauma. The jaws of these clamps have opposing rows of finely serrated teeth and may be straight, curve, angled or S-shaped. Non-crushing bowel clamps are atraumatic and hold healthy bowel tissue without causing damage. This enables the bowel tissue to be reanastomosed.

Retractors

Retractors hold back wound layers and anatomical structures to allow visualisation of the operative site; they can be hand-held or self-retaining. There are two types of self-retaining retractors: those that attach to a frame, such as the Bookwalter (Fig 8-6) or Omni-Tract retractors, and those that are held in place by a ratchet, such as the Weitlaner or Gelpi retractors.

At the beginning and end of the surgical counts, any retractor with screws must be checked to ensure that the screws are present. Self-retaining retractors should be handed to the surgeon in the

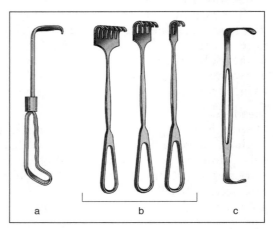

Figure 8-5 Manual retractors. (a) Solid blade appendiceal retractor. (b) Volkmann rake retractors (tips can be sharp or blunt). (c) Double-ended Army-Navy retractor (Phillips, 2007, p 335).

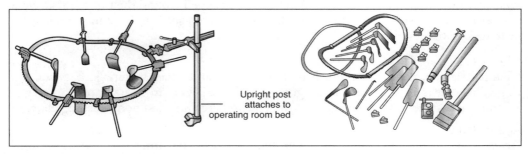

Upright post attaches to operating room bed

Figure 8-6 Bookwalter retractor (Phillips, 2007, p 338).

closed position. Hand-held retractors usually come in pairs and can be single or double ended, with a variety of shapes and sizes (e.g. Langenbeck retractors, Deaver's retractors, cats paws, skin hooks or rakes).

Care of instrumentation

Instruments are very expensive but they can last a long time if they are properly cared for and maintained. Here are some general rules for good instrument care.

1. Blood and/or tissue should be wiped off instruments intraoperatively using sterile water. Blood or tissue that dries, becoming hard on the serrations of jaws or blades of scissors, impairs the function of the instrument, makes cleaning more difficult postoperatively and causes instruments to become stiff and possibly break. Instruments with lumens or channels (e.g. Frazier suckers) should be irrigated periodically, intraoperatively, to prevent blockages.
2. Delicate or microsurgery instruments should be kept separate from other instrumentation. Never place heavy instruments on top of delicate or microsurgery instruments.
3. Instruments should be handled gently at all times and should not be thrown, bounced or dropped.
4. Keep instruments with cutting edges, pointed tips or other sharp components away from metal surfaces that could dull their edges. Ensure that their sharp edges are protected so staff members responsible for cleaning are not injured.
5. Instruments should be returned to the tray in which they were assembled.
6. Fibreoptic cables should be loosely coiled and placed on top, or separated from, other instrumentation.
7. Always use the instrument for its intended purpose! Scissors or clamps that are misused can be forced out of alignment and break. Curved tissue scissors that are used to cut sutures or dressings will soon become blunt.
8. Forceps, clamps and other hinged instruments should be inspected at the beginning and end of each procedure to ensure that the jaws or teeth align and the ratchets hold firmly but release easily. Scissors should also be checked for sharpness.
9. Damaged instruments should be set aside for repair or replacement and alternatives added.

SUTURES AND NEEDLES

Documented evidence regarding the use of sutures dates as far back as 2000 BC (Dunscombe, 2007); however, it was not until the mid 1800s, as a result of increased infection rates, pain and haemorrhage, that a wider variety of suture materials and their uses developed. Suture material and needles were not sterilised until Joseph Lister began to experiment with carbolic acid as a form of sterilisation during the 19th century (Pieknik, 2006).

Traditionally, the word **suture** referred to a strand of material used to close wounds, or ligate tissues or blood vessels. These strands were passed through the eye of a needle that resembled an ordinary household sewing needle. Today, needle and suture material are joined together as a continuous unit referred to as an **atraumatic** needle, which is eyeless and presterilised. The 'eyed' needle meant that two strands of suture material were being pulled through the tissues, causing a lot of trauma. However, the newer 'atraumatic' needles cause less tissue trauma because only one strand of suture material is pulled through the tissues.

The evolution of surgery has witnessed the use of numerous materials, ranging over the years from gold, silver, silkworm gut, cotton, silk, linen, tendon and intestinal tissue to the highly fashionable synthetic fibres of today. These include, but are not limited to, nylon, polyester, polypropylene and polymer combinations.

Properties of suture materials

The properties that are taken into consideration when choosing and evaluating the effectiveness of a suture material include:

1. physical characteristics
2. handling properties
3. tissue reaction.

Physical characteristics

There are three physical characteristics:

1. physical configuration—number of fibres comprising one strand
2. synthetic or natural fibres
3. diameter or size of the suture material.

Physical configuration

Configuration refers to the number of fibres that are contained within one strand of suture material and they way those fibres are rendered to make one strand of suture material. There are two types of configurations:

1. monofilament
2. multifilament.

Monofilament sutures are made of a single strand of suture material. This structure is less prone to harbouring microorganisms. Monofilament sutures also provide less resistance when passing through tissue. However, crushing the strand weakens monofilament sutures, which can lead to premature suture failure.

Multistranded or *multifilament sutures* are composed of multiple strands that are either braided or twisted together. These materials are more pliable than monofilament sutures and are easier to handle and tie, but generate more friction when passing through tissue.

Natural and synthetic materials

Natural suture material is derived from sources such as collagen, silk and cotton. Synthetic sutures are artificial and are made from various materials, such as nylon, polypropylene, polyethylene, polyester, polyglactin or surgical steel.

Diameter

In Australia, the diameter of a suture is determined in millimetres. The base numeral is 0, with the sizing scale ranging from 7, which is the largest, down to 11/0, which is the smallest (Fig 8-7). Sizes 0–7 have a progressively larger diameter, whereas sizes 0–11/0 are progressively smaller sizes. Once the scale falls below 0, the numbers would normally be referred to as −1, −2; however, they are referred to as 00 (2/0), 000 (3/0) and so on. Sizes 0–4/0 are the most commonly used sizes. The diameter of the suture material and the size of the atraumatic needle attached are chosen depending on the type and thickness of tissue being approximated.

Handling characteristics

The handling characteristics of a suture focus on the ease of use and include:

• pliability and coefficient friction

Smaller gauge										Zero							Larger gauge		
12–0	11–0	10–0	9–0	8–0	7–0	6–0	5–0	4–0	3–0	2–0	0	1	2	3	4	5	6	7	8	9	10

Figure 8-7 Suture material gauge (Phillips, 2007, p 560).

- elasticity and memory—ability of the suture material to retain its packet shape
- capillarity—ability to absorb fluids
- tensile and knot strength—amount of weight to break the suture material and force required to break the knot
- configuration—number of fibres comprising one strand (Dunscombe, 2007).

Pliability and coefficient friction

The pliability of the suture material is the ease in which it bends; the coefficient friction is the drag caused by the pulling of the material through the tissue and the security of the knot. Suture material may be coated to reduce tissue drag, thereby making it easier to remove; however, this, in turn, makes the knots less secure. Sutures made from nylon are not as pliable, have some elasticity, memory and a low coefficient friction, create knots that are less secure and are prone to unravelling (Dunscombe, 2007).

Elasticity and memory

Elasticity or memory is the ability of the suture strand to return to its original 'packet' shape after being stretched. Once removed from its packaging, plain gut, nylon or catgut suture material remains coiled. After the suture material has been stretched, although it appears straight, it still has small curves from where it was coiled in the original packet. To remove the elasticity of the suture material, the atraumatic needle is loaded within the jaws of a needle holder while grasping the free end of the suture material with the thumb and forefinger. Both hands are gently extended and, in doing so, the suture material is stretched, removing the elasticity. The suture material is not 'tugged' or 'snapped' as this can damage the fibres within the strand of suture material (Dunscombe, 2007).

Capillarity

The capillarity of the suture material refers to its ability to transmit fluid along its length. Multifilament sutures have more capillarity, drawing fluid into the space along and between filaments. This increased absorption of fluid along its length may act as a tract to introduce pathogens into deep tissue (Dunscombe, 2007).

Tensile strength and knot strength

The amount of force exerted on the suture material in order to make it break, is known as its tensile strength. Tensile strength also takes into consideration the time in which the suture retains its integrity before breaking down. The force necessary to cause a knot to slip or break is known as its knot strength. Sutures with a high memory and low coefficiency have poor knot strength (Dunscombe, 2007).

Tissue reaction characteristics

All suture material causes some tissue reaction. The tissue reaction begins when the suture material passes through the tissue. The inflammatory response causes the area to be infiltrated with white blood cells, macrophages and fibroblasts—the very process that initiates healing in the wound also causes the breakdown or encapsulation of the suture material. The time frame in which the suture maintains its strength is significant to the choice of suture material and is referred to as its tensile strength. Suture materials such as silk have a higher prevalence of tissue reaction compared to nylon, which is much less reactive. Other factors that influence suture material selection are tissue type, patient's nutritional status and the presence or absence of infection (Lai & Becker, 2006).

Non-absorbable suture materials

Non-absorbable suture materials are not affected by hydrolysis or enzymatic activity and can be synthetic or natural material. Non-absorbable sutures become encapsulated during the healing process and the term non-absorbable suggests that this group will remain within the body indefinitely. However, this does not equate to the suture maintaining its original strength. The strength of any suture material will slowly lessen over time. Non-absorbable sutures generally retain their suture strength for a longer period of time than do absorbable suture materials (Dunscombe, 2007). For example, Monosof, Dermalon and Surgilon (non-absorbable suture materials) lose approximately 15–20% of strength per year, with essentially no strength left after 5 years (Tyco Healthcare Australia, 2005).

Absorbable

Absorbable suture material is capable of being absorbed by living tissue, yet may be treated to modify its rate of absorption. The source may be natural or synthetic. Absorbable sutures break down by hydrolysis or are digested by the body's enzymes, initially losing strength and gradually being absorbed by the body. Accelerated absorbability of the suture may occur if the material is moistened before the suture is used or by fluid in a body cavity (Dunscombe, 2007). Table 8-4 presents the variety of suture materials available.

Ties

A **tie** is a piece of suture material without a needle attached to it. Ties are used to ligate a bleeding vessel, as discussed in Chapter 7 (Phillips, 2007).

Needles

The atraumatic **needles** of today are processed in large factories, and are prepackaged and presterilised with the suture material attached. Needles are manufactured in different shapes and sizes, and most are described in degrees of circles; however, they can also be straight.

Except for free ties, surgical needles are necessary to carry suture material through the tissue with minimal trauma. The best surgical needles are made of high-quality surgical steel that is strong enough to pass through tissue without breaking, and rigid enough to prevent excessive bending but flexible enough to prevent breaking after bending. Needles need to be approximately the same diameter as the suture material and sharp enough to pass through tissue. The needle needs to be the correct size and shape to accommodate the type of tissue, the location and accessibility of the repair (Lai & Becker, 2006).

Atraumatic needles can be single or double armed; single armed means one needle is attached and double armed means two needles are attached to both ends of the suture material. Some needles have been specially designed to release quickly and easily from the suture material without the use of scissors; these are called control release.

Anatomy of a needle

Needles vary greatly depending on the type and location of tissue being sutured. They can vary in shape, size, point design and wire diameter. Curved needles represent the majority of all atraumatic needles and are described in degrees of a circle (e.g. ½, ¾, ¼, ⅝). The size of the circle depends on how wide or large a 'bite' is required and how much room there is to insert the needle. The components of a needle are listed below.

Table 8-4 Types of suture materials

Suture name	Material	Configuration	Colour coding	Suture material colour	Use	Tissue reaction	Diameter
Caprosyn	Polyglytone 6211, synthetic	Monofilament	Pink/rose	Clear and violet	General soft tissue approximation and/or ligation but not cardiovascular, neurosurgery, microsurgery or ophthalmic surgery	Absorbable, hydrolysis	1–6/0
Monocryl	Polyglecaprone 25, synthetic	Monofilament	Coral/apricot	Coral/apricot, undyed	General soft tissue approximation and/or ligation	Absorbable	2–6/0
Biosyn	Glycomer 631, synthetic	Monofilament	Red/rose	Violet and undyed	General soft tissue approximation and/or ligation and ophthalmic surgery	Absorbable	1–6/0
Vicryl	Polyglactin 910, synthetic	Braided monofilament	Violet	Violet and undyed	General soft tissue approximation and/or ligation and ophthalmic surgery	Absorbable, hydrolysis	10/0–2/0, 0–3 and ties
Polysorb	Lactomer 9-1, synthetic	Multifilament (braided)	Violet	Violet and undyed	General soft tissue approximation and/or ligation and ophthalmic surgery	Absorbable, hydolysis	2–8/0 and ties
Dexon II, Dexon S	Polyglyclic acid, synthetic; Dexon II is coated and Dexon S is not	Multifilament (braided)	Green	Bicolour and beige	General soft tissue approximation and/or ligation and ophthalmic surgery	Absorbable, hydrolysis	Dexon II, 2–6/0 and ties; Dexon S, 2–10/0
Maxon	Polyglyconate, synthetic	Monofilament	Green	Green and clear	General soft tissue approximation and/or ligation, paediatric, cardiovascular tissue	Absorbable	1–7/0 and ties
PDS, PDS II	Polydioxanone	Monofilament	Silver	Violet and clear	Abdominal and thoracic closure, subcutaneous tissue, colon/rectal surgery, orthopaedic and plastic surgery	Absorbable	2–9/0

(contd)

Table 8-4 Types of suture materials *(contd)*

Suture name	Material	Configuration	Colour coding	Suture material colour	Use	Tissue reaction	Diameter
Coated Vicryl Rapide	Polyglactin 910, synthetic	Multifilament (braided)	Violet	Violet and undyed	Superficial soft tissue approximation of skin and mucosa	Absorbable	1–7/0
Chromic gut	Collagen from sheep mucosa or beef serosa treated with chromic salts, natural	Multifilament	Tan	Tan and blue (for ophthalmology)	Tissues that do not require extended wound support and ophthalmology	Absorbable, enzymatic	3–7/0 and ties
Surgical gut, plain gut	Collagen from sheep mucosa or beef serosa, natural	Multifilament	Yellow	Yellow	Ligation of superficial vessels and subcutaneous tissues and ophthalmology	Absorbable, enzymatic	2–7/0 (Tyco); 3–7/0 (Johnson & Johnson)
Ethilon	Polyamide polymer and nylon 6, synthetic	Monofilament	Mint green	Undyed, green, blue and black	Skin closure, retention sutures, plastic surgery, ophthalmology and microsurgery	Non-absorbable	2–11/0
Monosof, Dermalon	Long chain aliphatic polymers nylon 6 and 6.6, synthetic	Monofilament	Green	Monosof undyed or black; Dermalon blue	General soft tissue approximation and/or ligation, including cardiovascular, neurological and ophthalmic surgery	Non-absorbable	Monosof, 2–11/0; Dermalon, 2–6/0
Nurolon, Surgilon	Long chain aliphatic polymers nylon 6 and 6.6, synthetic	Multifilament (braided)	Green	Black and undyed	General soft tissue approximation and/or ligation, including cardiovascular, neurological and ophthalmic surgery	Non-absorbable	Nurolon, 1–6/0; Surgilon, 2–7/0
Mersilene	Polyester, synthetic	Multifilament	Turquoise	Green and undyed	Cardiovascular, general, plastic and ophthalmology	Non-absorbable	5–11/0

Suture name	Material	Filament	Package colour	Suture colour	Uses	Absorbable	Sizes
Ti-Cron	Polyester polyethylene terephalate, synthetic	Braided	Orange	Undyed and blue	General soft tissue approximation and/or ligation, including cardiovascular, neurological and ophthalmic surgery; particular use in cardiac valve replacement surgery	Non-absorbable	5–8/0 in both braided coated and uncoated; or 9/0–11/0 monofilament uncoated and ties
Ethibond	Polyester polyethylene terephalate, synthetic; coated with polybutylate	Braided	Orange	Undyed, green and light green	Cardiovascular, general, plastic	Non-absorbable	5–7/0
Prolene, Surgipro	Polypropylene, synthetic	Monofilament	Deep blue	Blue and undyed	General soft tissue approximation and/or ligation, including cardiovascular, neurological, plastic and ophthalmic surgery	Non-absorbable	2–10/0
Novafil	Polybutester, synthetic	Monofilament	Green	Blue and undyed	General soft tissue approximation and/or ligation, including cardiovascular and ophthalmic surgery	Non-absorbable	2–10/0 and ties
Silk, Softsilk	Natural fibre from protein of raw silk, natural	Multifilament (braided)	Light blue	Black and undyed	General soft tissue approximation and/or ligation, including cardiovascular, neurological, microsurgery and ophthalmic surgery; common use: central venous line, drains and retention sutures in cardiac surgery	Non-absorbable	5, 2–9/0 and ties
Surgical stainless steel, steel	316 stainless steel, natural	Multifilament or monofilament	Mustard	Silver/steel	Abdominal wall closure, tendon repair, skin closure, orthopaedic and neurosurgery; sternal closure in cardiothoracic surgery; hernia repair and intestinal anastomosis	Non-absorbable	7–10/0, with and without needles

Suture names are from both Tyco and Johnson & Johnson (Ethicon). Adapted from Tyco and Ethicon suture range.

1. The *point* is the extreme tip of the needle; it is the part that penetrates the tissues. Points can be either tapered, cutting or a combination of both. Tapered needle points pierce and spread the tissues without 'cutting' the tissues, which means less trauma and bleeding. Cutting needle points typically slice or cut through the tissues, causing trauma and bleeding.

2. The *body* of a needle can be rounded, triangular, rectangular or trapezoidal. The body is the part of a needle that is grasped by the needle holder and its shape determines how well it is grasped within the jaws of the needle holder. In other words, the shape of the body will depend on the type of tissues this needle is expected to penetrate, the force behind the insertion of the needle and, hence, how securely the needle needs to be grasped by the needle holder.

3. The *attachment end*, which is also known as the *swaged end*, is where the suture material and the needle are joined to become one unit (Phillips, 2007).

4. The *eye* of the needle is the segment of the needle where the suture material attaches to the needle.

Types of needle points

Both the 'body' and the 'point' of a needle determine which tissues the needle will penetrate. For simplicity, needles are classified into two main groups: cutting and taper needles. Within each classification, numerous types of each needle are available. Figure 8-8 shows the different needle points.

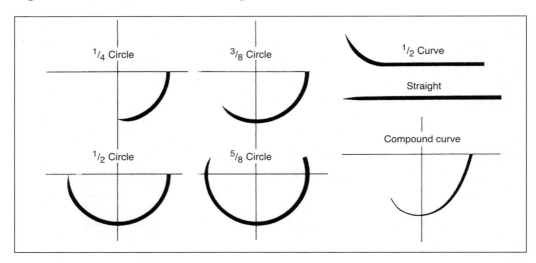

Figure 8-8 Suture needle point types (Rothrock, 2007, p 170).

Cutting point

Cutting-edge needles have two or more opposing edges, which slice through the tissues. They can be divided into two main types—conventional and reverse needles—which are determined by the location of the cutting edge. A conventional cutting-edge needle has its cutting edge on the concave (inside) side of the needle, whereas the cutting edge of the reverse cutting-edge needle lies on the convex (outside) side of the needle. Cutting-edge needles are predominantly used on skin; however, special types have been designed specifically for individual surgical specialties, such as ophthalmology and plastic surgery (Phillips, 2007).

Taper point

Typically, the body of a taper needle is flattened or rounded, which is described as either oval or rectangular. The point of a taper needle pierces the tissue while the flattened/rounded body of the needle spreads tissue without cutting. The taper point is used in softer tissue that offers less resistance to the needle as it passes through. A taper needle is considered less traumatic due to the way in which it separates the tissues and causes less bleeding. Taper needles can be used on all tissues except skin (i.e. blood vessels, muscle, viscera, peritoneum and fat) (Phillips, 2007).

Blunt point taper needles are tapered needles with a blunt point that is rounded; they are designed to pass through friable tissue, such as liver or kidney. Blunt point taper needles have also been recommended as a safety measure to prevent needlestick injuries for operating room staff and are commonly seen in hepatobiliary and gynaecological surgery (Phillips, 2007).

The taper cut needle is another type of taper needle. The taper cut needle was designed for vascular/cardiothoracic surgery, particularly for use with calcified, fibrotic blood vessels or prosthetic grafts. The cutting edges only extend a very short distance from the needle tip and blend into a rounded, tapered body. Hence, the cutting edges pass through the hard, calcified portion of the blood vessel, while the remaining rounded taper body passes through the friable section of the blood vessel.

Table 8-5 shows the different types of needles and their uses.

Table 8-5 Needle types and their uses			
Needle type	Wire type	Tissue	Surgery examples
Taper	Fine	Soft	Bowel, vascular
	Medium	Fibrous	Fascia
	Heavy	Tough	Gynaecological
Blunt	–	Fibrous	Fascia, gynaecological
Cutting	Fine	Tough	Plastic
	Medium	–	Skin closure
	Heavy	–	Orthopaedics
Taper cutting	Fine	Vessels	Vascular
	Medium	Tough	Gynaecological
Spatula	Fine	Delicate	Ophthalmic

Tyco Healthcare (2005)

Body of the needle

The gauge of the wire, length, shape and finish determine the body or shaft of the needle. Factors to consider when choosing a needle body include:

- tough tissue will require a heavier gauge needle, whereas microsurgery will require a fine-gauge needle
- the depth of bite required to penetrate the tissue determines a needle length
- the circumference of the needle body may be round, oval or triangular in shape (Phillips, 2007).

Swaged needles

The most common needle is the swaged or atraumatic needle. In this type of needle, one end of the suture material is enclosed inside the needle itself. The needle and suture material are almost the same diameter, causing less trauma to the tissues when passed through. A modified form of permanently swaged needle is the controlled-release suture, which is commonly known as a 'pop off'. The needle and suture begin as one unit; however, a light pull on the suture material will separate the two components, leaving the tie behind (Phillips, 2007).

Ordinary needles

An ordinary or eyed needle is a needle that must be threaded with the suture material. Two strands of suture material are pulled through the tissue, which is much more traumatic to tissues (Phillips, 2007).

Loading needles

Needles are loaded onto an appropriate needle holder. A needle holder has specifically designed jaws to grasp the needle securely. The gauge of the needle determines the appropriate-sized jaws. Fine, small needles are loaded onto fine-tipped needle holders. The length of the needle holder will depend on the depth of the wound closure, intra-abdominally, for example. The needle holder will be longer when working in deep cavities than that required for skin closure (Phillips, 2007).

As a general rule of thumb, load the needle one-third of the distance from the swaged/attachment end, with the needle gripped at the tip or one-third of the distance into the jaw of the needle holder and at a 90° angle. The needle should never be clamped over the swaged area as this weakens the attachment. The needle should be clamped as near to the tip of the needle holder as possible, on the first or second ratchet. The point of the needle faces in towards the body of the surgeon, unless it has been requested to load it backwards. In some specialty surgery (e.g. vascular surgery), surgeons will change the angle of the needle to suit the location/area they are suturing (Fig 8-9).

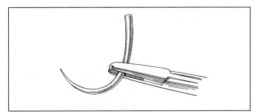

Figure 8-9 Correct position of curved needle in holder, about one-third down from swage or eye (Phillips, 2007, 171).

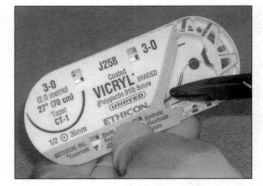

Figure 8-10 Ethicon suture (made by Johnson & Johnson Medical).

ENDOSCOPIC MINIMALLY INVASIVE SURGERY

The development of endoscopic minimally invasive surgery has been one of the most dramatic advancements in surgery over the past few decades and has evolved from a diagnostic modality to a widespread surgical technique. Minimally invasive surgery can be referred to as **endoscopic, telescopic, laparoscopic, keyhole** or **minimal access**

surgery and incorporates all fields of **endoscopic surgery**. Minimally invasive surgery, or endoscopic techniques, are prevalent in all fields of surgery, including bariatric, general, gynaecological, ear, nose and throat, urological, cardiovascular/thoracic, plastic, orthopaedic and neurosurgery on almost all anatomical areas (AORNb, 2005; Bragg et al., 2005). Minimally invasive surgery uses small incisions or no incisions, rather than the traditional open methods, and telescopes, cameras and fibreoptic light leads are used to assist with this field of surgery. The incisions are so small that they are typically closed with one or two sutures.

Box 8-1 presents an abbreviated review of the historical development of MIS. The work of a few surgeon's listed here are still recognised today (e.g. Veress needle, and Hasson cannula and trocar).

Box 8-1 History of minimally invasive surgery

1901	Dimitri Ott, German gynaecologist, performed a ventroscopy, where a speculum was introduced through an incision in the posterior vaginal fornix. Dr Ott wore a head mirror to reflect light and aid visualisation.
1901	George Kelling, also a German surgeon, reported using a cystoscope to examine the intra-abdominal viscera of a dog.
1938	Veress developed a needle with a spring-loaded obturator that allowed safe insertion and insufflation of the peritoneal cavity.
1966	Kurt Semm introduced an automatic insufflation device capable of monitoring intra-abdominal pressures. Semm also designed a high-volume irrigation/aspiration system, perfected the Endo Loop applicator, as well as intra- and extracorporeal knot-tying techniques, and developed thermocoagulation, which revolutionised laparoscopic surgery by virtually eliminating thermal injuries.
1966	Hopkins, a British optical physician, introduced the rod–lens system, which improved brightness and clarity. The fibreoptic (cold) light source was also developed, which reduced the incidence of burns to bowel and viscera.
1970s	Gynaecological surgeons had embraced laparoscopy and thoroughly incorporated the technique into their practice.
1970	Orthopaedic surgeons began utilising arthroscopy.
1977	DeKok performed the first laparoscopic appendicectomy.
1978	Hasson introduced an alternative method of trocar placement, which permitted direct visualisation of the trocar entrance into the peritoneal cavity.

Ballantyne (2000)

Minimally invasive surgery has progressed immensely over the past decade and will continue to change as more surgical procedures are performed in this manner.

The advantages of minimally invasive surgery for patients are considered to outweigh those of open surgery and include:

• smaller surgical scars
• less trauma to the body
• decreased postoperative pain and thus less requirement for pain relief
• decreased recovery period
• quicker return to normal activities (Bragg et al., 2005).

Such advantages for patients heightened surgeons' interest in minimally invasive surgery and, in consultation with medical companies, equipment and instrumentation were developed and modified. This, in turn, has allowed surgeons to perform more complex cases (e.g. hysterectomy, nephrectomy and hemi-colectomy) either completely laparoscopically or laparoscopically assisted.

However, minimally invasive surgical procedures are not without their risks to the patient. The length of operating time frequently is longer than the equivalent 'open' surgical procedure, thereby increasing anaesthesia time, which may have an impact on patient outcomes. Serious complications of endoscopy include perforation of a major vessel or organ, bleeding from a biopsy site or any area where tissue has been cut or when endoscopic sutures or clips have become dislodged, and moderate or severe hypothermia (Phillips, 2007).

There are also some important disadvantages for the surgeon, which, on occasions, can lead to the procedure becoming an open surgical procedure. These include:

- restricted vision
- difficulty handling the instruments
- restricted mobility of tissues
- no tactile perception.

All patients should be prepped and draped for conversion to an open surgical procedure when warranted because of recognised or potential complications. Instrumentation and supplies for an open surgical procedure should be precounted and readily available (Phillips, 2007).

Equipment

Although the types of endoscopic instruments available are similar to those used for open surgery and can be classified according to the five instrument categories, adaptations have been made to allow their use via a laparoscope. Figure 8-11 shows a variety of endoscopic instruments.

All instrumentation is available in reusable and disposable items. The following items are available to provide haemostasis:

1. *Endoclips.* These single metal staples are used to occlude tissue or blood vessels.
2. *Harmonic scalpel.* The tip of the scalpel rapidly vibrates, enabling precise cutting and coagulation.
3. *Laparoscopic suture.* Suturing can be performed using one of two methods—extra- or intracorporeal. Extracorporeal suturing means that the knot is tied outside the abdominal cavity. A suture is passed down one of the cannulae and the needle of the suture is passed through the desired tissue. The needle is then removed via the cannula and cut off; the knot is tied outside the abdomen and pushed back down the cannula onto the tissue. Intracorporeal suturing refers to the knot being tied within the abdominal cavity using two needle holders or a specially designed needle holder that transfers the needle from one prong of the jaw to the other.
4. *Endoloops.* These are snare-like loops of suture material that are pre-knotted within an introducer sleeve. Once the suture loop is around the designated

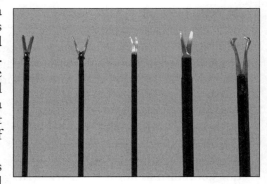

Figure 8-11 Disposable endoscopic instruments (Rothrock, 2007, p 187).

tissue, the existing suture knot is pushed down the introducer sleeve until it is tightly secured around the tissue.

5. *Endoscopic stapling devices*. These, like their open surgery counterparts, cut and staple at the same time.

Laparoscopic procedure

As with open surgery, minimally invasive surgery follows a generalised sequence of surgery. The three broad sequences involved when performing minimally invasive surgery and the instrumentation required are:

1. exposure—insufflation needle and trocar and cannula
2. visualisation—the endoscope, light source and camera
3. perform procedure, dissection, haemostasis and removal of tissue—electrocautery, ties, endoscopic suturing, stapling devices, instruments, endoscopic bags to remove tissue and wound protection devices.

Exposure

The two types of insertion techniques—open technique and closed or blind technique—indicate the type of trocar and cannula that are suitable. These two separate techniques were developed based on the experiences of both general and gynaecological surgeons.

General surgeons developed the open technique, which involves a small incision into the peritoneum under direct vision, through which a blunt trocar can be passed. The cannula can also be sutured in place to reduce gas leakage, if desired. The gas tubing is attached to the cannula and the abdominal cavity is filled with carbon dioxide before the remaining cannulas are inserted, if required. Most general surgeons utilise a Hasson-like trocar and cannula that is blunt tipped. The majority of general surgical cases will begin in the supine position; however, once the initial cannula is inserted the patient will be placed in the reverse Trendelenburg position.

The closed or blind technique, which was developed by gynaecologists, involves the insertion of an insufflation needle, filling the abdominal cavity with carbon dioxide and then the insertion of the first trocar and cannula. Sharp (self-piercing) trocars are used in this technique as they puncture the skin on the way through the peritoneum. All gynaecological cases are performed in the lithotomy position as the uterus will be manipulated during the procedure. The patient is placed into the reverse Trendelenburg position prior to the insertion of the insufflation needle.

In both techniques, the initial cannula is inserted at the inferior aspect of the umbilicus; however, alternative sites may be chosen if the patient has had previous abdominal surgery as there can be the risk that loops of bowel or adhesions have adhered to the previous incision site. The peritoneal cavity is filled with carbon dioxide to prevent damage to the abdominal structures and provide good visualisation; this is called pneumoperitoneum. Pneumoperitoneum can be achieved by the insertion of an insufflation needle (commonly referred to as a Veress needle) or via the first cannula introduced. Sterile tubing is attached to either the insufflation needle or a three-way tap on the cannula; the end of the tubing is passed off the sterile field and connected to the gas insufflator.

Trocar tips come in a range of shapes, such as triangular, conical, pyramidal or bladeless. Depending on the manufacturer, the trocar tips can also be retractable or provide a shield that covers the sharp tip once entry has been achieved. The bladeless trocar separates tissue without cutting or stretching the tissue, and provides the option of visualising the insertion of this type of trocar. Recent advancements relating to the design of cannulas have resulted in a newer version of cannula with a better grip, thus preventing accidental removal or movement of the cannula during surgery (Phillips, 2007).

Visualisation

Many types of endoscopes are available, and their size (diameter) and length depend on the access required to visualise the area. Flexible endoscopes provide a panoramic view, whereas rigid endoscopes provide either a direct (0° scope) or angled (30°, 70° or 120°) view. Table 8-6 lists the types of endoscopes that are available, and Figure 8-12 shows the set-up for a laparoscopic procedure.

Table 8-6 Types of endoscopes

Flexible scopes	Rigid scopes
Angioscope	Cystoscope
Bronchoscope	Laparoscope
Choledochoscope	Sinuscope
Colonoscope	Arthroscope
Cystonephroscope	Bronchoscope
Hysteroscope	Laryngoscope
Mediastinoscope	Hysteroscope
Ureteroscope	
Ureteropyeloscope	
Gastroscope	
Sigmoidoscope	

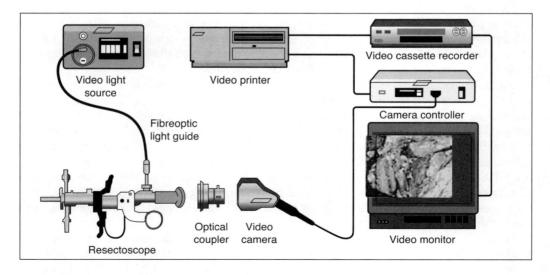

Figure 8-12 Camera with video set-up for endoscopic surgery (Phillips, 2007, p 646).

Fibreoptic light, or cold light, was developed in 1966. The heat from the light source is not transmitted down the length of the endoscope, which prevents tissue from being inadvertently damaged. However, it should be noted that the end of the fibreoptic cable is very hot. Once disconnected from the endoscope, the light source should be switched to standby or off to prevent accidental burning of the drapes and/or patient.

Performing Procedure

In order to perform an operative procedure using the minimally invasive technique, a surgeon's hands must be free to manipulate the instrumentation, and the assistant and instrument nurses must also be able to see the operative field. This has been achieved by the introduction of the video camera. The video camera enlarges the images from the endoscope and projects them onto a television screen, which means that all members of the surgical team can observe the procedure.

When tissues such as the appendix, ovary and gall bladder are removed, a specially designed endoscopic specimen bag can be used to prevent spillage of their contents. In the case of laparoscopic bowel resection, once the segment of bowel has been resected, a slightly larger incision is made through which the segment of bowel will be removed. A wound edge protector can be used to protect the wound from contamination from the diseased bowel.

Advances continue to be made in minimally invasive surgery, with different surgical specialisations developing new techniques.

CONCLUSION

The focus of this chapter has been on assisting perioperative nurses to understand the process of surgical intervention and their role in this process. Every surgical procedure, including minimally invasive surgery, follows a generalised sequence of steps. By understanding this concept and adopting the protocol of organising instrumentation, sutures and needles, and other equipment according to the sequence of surgery, the perioperative nurse can make versatile judgements based on the needs of the patient and the surgical team.

CRITICAL THINKING EXERCISES

1. Instrumentation

Identify a Frazier, Yankauer and Poole sucker, and compare the number of suction holes in the tip of each device.
- Explain the purpose of multiple suction holes in the Poole suction device.
- List the types of surgery that each suction device could be used for and the reasons why.

2. Instrument cleanliness

- Discuss the use of sterile water to clean instruments intraoperatively in preference to saline.

3. Surgical sequence

- Detail the sequence of surgery for a transurethral resection of the prostate.

4. Sutures and needles

- Discuss the advantages and disadvantages of the various suture materials and needles available.

RESOURCES

Laparoscopic procedures and research
www.obesitysurgery.com

REFERENCES

AORN. (2005a). *Recommended practices for perioperative nursing. Standard and transmission-based precautions.* Denver, CO: Association of Perioperative Registered Nurses.

AORN. (2005b). Recommended practices for endoscopic minimally invasive surgery. *AORN Journal, 81(3),* 643–660.

Ballantyne, G. H. (2000). Minimally invasive surgery for diseases of colon and rectum: the legacy of an ancient tradition. Retrieved January 11, 2008, from http://www.lapsurgery.com/history.htm.

Bragg, K., VanBalen, N., Cook, N. (2005). Future tends in minimally invasive surgery. *AORN Journal, 82(6),* 1006–1020.

Dunscombe (2007). Sutures, needles and instruments. In J. C. Rothrock, & D. R. McEwen (Eds.). *Alexander's care of the patient in surgery* (13th ed.) (pp. 170–178). St Louis: Mosby.

Lai, S. Y., & Becker, D. G. (2006). Sutures and needles. *eMedicine.* Retrieved April 29, 2007, from http://www.emedicine.com/ent/topic38.htm.

Phillips, N. (2007). *Berry & Kohn's operating room technique* (11th ed.). St Louis: Mosby.

Pieknik, (2006). *Sutures and hemostasis. A pocket book guide.* St Louis: Saunders.

Richardson-Tench, M., & Martens, E. (2005). From systems to tissues: a revolution in learning in perioperative education. *Education for Health: Change in Learning and Practice, 18(1),* 22–31.

Rothrock, J. C. (Ed.). (2007). *Alexander's care of the patient in surgery* (13th ed.). St Louis: Mosby.

Tyco Healthcare. (2005). *Suture and needle guide.* Sydney: Tyco Healthcare.

FURTHER READING

Al-Abdullah, T., Plint, A. C., Fergusson, D. (2007). Absorbable versus non-absorbable sutures in the management of traumatic lacerations and surgical wounds: a meta-analysis. *Pediatric Emergency Care, 23(5),* 339–344.

Anderson, E. R., & Gates, S. (2004). Techniques and materials for closure of the abdominal wall in caesarean section. *Cochrane Database of Systematic Reviews, 4,* CD004663.

AORN. (2005). AORN guidance statement. Sharps injury prevention in the perioperative setting. *AORN Journal, 81(3),* 662–671.

Heniford, B. T., Park, A., Ramshaw, B. J., Voeller, G. (2003). Laparoscopic repair of ventral hernias: nine years' experience with 850 consecutive hernias. *Annals of Surgery, 238(3),* 391–399.

McLeod, R. S., & Stern, H. (2004). Canadian Association of General Surgeons Evidence Based Reviews in Surgery. 10. Laparoscopy-assisted colectomy versus open colectomy for treatment of non-metastatic colon cancer: a randomized trial. *Canadian Journal of Surgery, 47(3),* 209–211.

Nelson, H., Sargent, D. J., Wieand, H. S., et al. (2004). A comparison of laparoscopically assisted and open colectomy for colon cancer. The Clinical Outcomes of Surgical Therapy Study Group. *New England Journal of Medicine, 350,* 2050–2059.

Senagore, A. J., Madbouly, K. M., Fazio, V. W., et al. (2003). Advantages of laparoscopic colectomy in older patients. *Archives of Surgery, 138(3),* 252–256.

Schindler, O. (2007). Minimally invasive surgery of the knee. *Journal of Perioperative Practice, 17(11),* 535–542.

Upton, A., Roberts, C., Ryan, M., et al. (2002). A randomised trial, conducted by midwives, of perineal repairs comparing a polylycolic suture material and chromic catgut. *Midwifery, 18,* 223–229.

Postanaesthesia recovery unit

Emma Robbins, Lyell Brougham and Beth Hooper

LEARNING OBJECTIVES

After reading this chapter, you should be able to:

- understand the purpose and function of the postanaesthesia recovery unit (PARU)
- explore the design features of the PARU
- discuss the initial management of the postoperative/postanaesthesia patient
- examine the common postoperative and postanaesthesia complications and their management
- discuss the discharge criteria for postoperative/postanaesthesia patients.

KEY TERMS

airway management
discharge criteria
handover

hypotension
laryngospasm
pain management

postanaesthesia
complications

INTRODUCTION

This chapter describes the role and function of the postanaesthesia recovery unit (PARU), the assessment and ongoing observations of the patient during the immediate postoperative period, and discharge criteria. Commonly experienced post-surgical, post-procedural and postanaesthesia complications (hereafter referred to collectively as postoperative) and their management are examined, as well as the management of pain and postoperative nausea and vomiting.

ROLE AND FUNCTION OF PARU

The PARU is a specialised area designed to care for patients in the immediate postoperative period. As discussed in Chapter 6, most anaesthetic agents have properties that have depressant effects on a number of body systems; the respiratory and cardiovascular systems are particularly vulnerable. Therefore, all patients who have received general or regional anaesthesia, or sedation, must be closely observed during the immediate postoperative period, and their condition evaluated and stabilised, with emphasis on anticipating and preventing complications resulting from anaesthesia and surgery (ACORN, 2006a).

The area is staffed by nurses and medical practitioners who are specially trained to manage and stabilise patients prior to their return to the ward or discharge home via the day surgery department. Many patients have a history of comorbidities which, when combined with the stress of anaesthesia and surgery, can affect their immediate postoperative management. The postoperative patient in the PARU is vulnerable because of altered physiological function, along with psychological and cognitive impairment. This places patients in a state of ultimate reliance on the nursing and medical staff to ensure their safety, privacy, dignity and comfort during a phase when they are unable (or inadequately able) to advocate or care for themselves (ACORN, 2006b; 2006c).

PARUs are mainly located within operating suites. However, patients may also undergo procedures that require sedation or anaesthesia in other departments, such as endoscopy, radiology, cardiac investigation laboratories and free-standing day surgery settings. These departments also require an area in which patients can be monitored post-procedure.

In some hospitals, particularly day surgery facilities, PARUs are often divided into stage 1 and stage 2 areas. The stage 1 area is where patients are admitted directly from the operating or procedural room and closely observed until they are haemodynamically stable and meet appropriate discharge criteria. Patients are then transferred to the stage 2 area, which consists of reclining lounge chairs, rather than beds or trolleys, and which has a more home-like environment to encourage a sense of wellness and normalcy, but where the patients can still be observed until they are ready to be discharged home (Burden, 2008). The history of the development of PARUs, which were originally called recovery rooms, is outlined in Box 9-1.

PARU DESIGN FEATURES

The majority of PARUs, particularly in larger, tertiary (or referral) hospitals, function as independent areas with their own staff within the operating suite environment, providing care for patients who have undergone a range of surgical procedures under various anaesthesia techniques. In smaller hospitals, with only one or two operating rooms, and which generally cater for less complex operative procedures, staff may be multiskilled in all the perioperative roles. Regardless of the size, such areas are still required to have monitoring and resuscitation equipment to manage postoperative patients (ACORN,

2006b; Australian and New Zealand College of Anaesthetists [ANZCA], 2006a). Figure 9-1 shows a typical PARU that could be found in Australia or New Zealand.

The location and design of the operating suite should provide for quick and easy access between each operating room and the PARU to enable an immediate response by surgeons, anaesthetists and others to assist in the management of postoperative patients who develop complications, should they arise. It should be an area that promotes

---

Box 9-1 History of PARUs

Florence Nightingale developed the first known PARU for soldiers following battlefield surgery during the Crimean War. However, PARUs did not become formally established until the 1940s. 'Recovery' wards evolved in Australia in response to their development in America and from recommendations arising out of studies into preventable postoperative deaths. The first known PARU in Australia, which was specifically designed to care for patients in the period immediately after surgery, was built in 1901 at Royal Adelaide Hospital. Prior to this, patients were returned to their ward immediately following surgery, most often to be cared for by a student nurse with limited experience. The nurses and medical staff in these PARU areas were seen to have advanced skills, which eventually led to larger areas being built and the admission of other longer stay, critically ill patients, such as polio victims requiring iron lung management.

During the 1950s and 1960s, intensive care units were established to provide specialised care of these critical patients and recovery wards began to be purpose-built to assist in the recovery of the increasing numbers of postoperative and postanaesthesia patients. Then, as now, these areas assisted in reducing preventable deaths and morbidity, particularly from airway complications (Hughes, 1982).

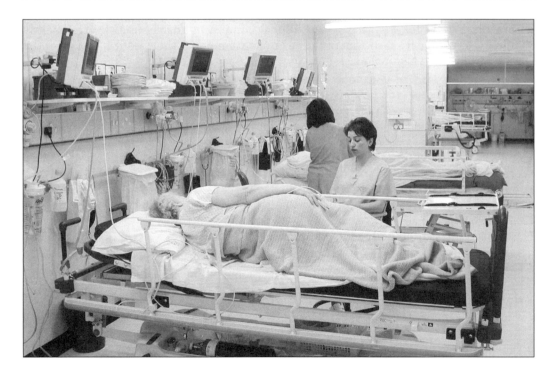

Figure 9-1 Typical PARU (Aitkenhead et al., 2007, p 485).

comfort and reduces anxiety for the postoperative patient; therefore, design features, such as indirect lighting, soft colours, good ventilation and soundproofing to reduce noise, should be considered (Hamlin, 2005). The three most critical design features of the PARU are:

1. close proximity to the procedure or operating rooms
2. an open area that enables unobstructed patient observation
3. essential monitoring and resuscitation equipment available to meet the needs of the surgical population served (ANZCA, 2006a).

The PARU is a semi-restricted area within the operating suite, although it is important that health care workers in street clothes can access the PARU directly to consult on or provide patient care if required. However, external access into the PARU should be limited as much as practical to reduce the transfer of microorganisms into this semi-restricted area. Hospital policy will dictate whether PARU staff should wear operating suite attire (ACORN, 2006b).

The space allocated to a patient bay, which will accommodate a patient's bed/trolley, should be at least 9 square metres, with easy access to the patient's head (ANZCA, 2006a), at least 1.2 metres between each patient's bed/trolley, and a specially designated area for the isolation of infectious patients when the need arises (Centre for Health Assets Australasia [CHAA], 2006). To accommodate PARU patients during peak periods, the number of allocated beds/trolley spaces within the unit should be at least 1.5 spaces per operating room; in other words, a four-room operating suite should have six PARU bays available (ANZCA, 2006a).

Equipment requirements

The set-up of each PARU bay should be standardised, with devices that are used regularly available in each bay, and emergency and other essential equipment centrally located within the PARU for easy access. Additional equipment that is used less frequently should be accessible from the operating suite environment at short notice. The essential equipment for each bay includes:

* two suction outlets with one suction container, tubing and a range of suction catheters
* two oxygen outlets with flow meters and oxygen delivery systems
* two power outlets with at least two additional outlets connected to emergency power
* pulse oximeter with finger and ear probes available
* oral airways and Y-suction catheters
* blood pressure monitoring apparatus, including cuffs suitable for all patients
* personal protective equipment
* vomit bowls or bags
* means of measuring body temperature (ACORN, 2006b; ANZCA, 2006a).

The essential equipment for the whole PARU includes:

* equipment and drugs for airway management and endotracheal intubation
* emergency equipment and drugs for resuscitation (e.g. resuscitation bag and face mask, naloxone, succinylcholine)
* call system for emergency assistance
* electrocardiograph (ECG) monitor(s)
* haemodynamic monitor(s)
* core temperature measuring devices
* forced air warming devices

- blood glucose measuring devices
- oxygen and air outlet for provision of manual ventilation (a minimum of two devices)
- personal protective equipment (ACORN, 2006b; ANZCA, 2006a).

Additionally, there must be easy access to the following:

- defibrillator
- 12-lead ECG machine
- patient ventilator
- anaesthetic machine
- equipment for difficult intubation
- devices for measuring expired carbon dioxide
- neuromuscular function monitor
- chest drains
- blood and electrolyte monitoring
- warming cupboard
- refrigerator for drugs/blood
- diagnostic imaging services (ANZCA, 2006a).

PATIENT TRANSFER FROM OPERATING ROOM TO PARU

Patients transported to the PARU from the operating room or procedure area should always be accompanied by an anaesthetist, a member of the nursing team and an orderly. This ensures the safe monitoring and transfer of the patient and minimises the manual handling risks to the staff. The patient must be continuously observed during transfer as complications, including apnoea, respiratory obstruction, hypoxia and/or vomiting, can often occur during this critical period. The patient will be receiving oxygen therapy during transfer, either by Hudson mask or nasal prongs. The transferred patient's conscious state will vary from fully anaesthetised, to semi-conscious (with the possibility of an unprotected airway), to awake and alert.

Although the anaesthetist will determine the patient's position for transfer, the supine position with the head slightly raised is a favoured position for the transportation of unconscious patients as this allows maximum observation of the patient's airway and conscious state. If there is a risk of vomiting, the patient may be transported in a lateral position with the trolley/bed in a head-down tilt. Portable emergency equipment (e.g. oxygen, suction and ventilation devices such as ventilating bag and mask) is essential and must be present/available during transfer to the PARU, regardless of the procedure or anaesthetic (Ball, 2008).

Handover of care

Members of the team transporting the patient from the operating room to the PARU must have knowledge of the patient's condition, history and interventions occurring during anaesthesia and surgery in order to provide a comprehensive **handover** of care to the PARU nurse, who will commence the patient's postoperative care. The handover will be carried out by the anaesthetist and a member of the nursing team.

The nursing handover should include, but not be limited to:

- patient's name
- surgery or procedure
- details of dressings, drains and catheters
- specific patient care details (e.g. compromised pressure areas).

Additional specific patient care details, which are extremely useful to the PARU nurses, may include:

- preferred name by which to address the patient
- physical impairments, such hearing, eyesight or movement difficulties
- whereabouts of patient's belongings, such as teeth, spectacles or hearing aids
- whereabouts of relatives who may be waiting; this is particularly important for paediatric patients because most PARUs allow parents to visit and remain with their child in the immediate postoperative period.

The anaesthetist handover should include, but not be limited to:

- patient's name
- operative procedure
- type of anaesthesia and any other drugs administered (e.g. antibiotics, narcotics)
- patient's medical history, including allergies
- significant intraoperative events/actions (e.g. significant blood loss, injection of local anaesthetic at the operative site—referred to as local infiltration)
- intravenous (IV) access and fluid orders
- postoperative orders for the administration of analgesia, antiemetics and any other medications
- any specific, relevant postoperative issues, such as airway, throat packs, intra-arterial devices, epidural catheters in situ or drug infusions (ANZCA, 2006b).

All documentation and follow-up information related to the patient's anaesthetic, surgical intervention and ongoing management must be present at handover and clarification sought by the PARU nurse when required. Postoperative surgical requirements are usually documented by the surgeon as part of the operation record and should be examined to ascertain any special orders pertaining to drains, dressings or catheters, and any special observations or other postoperative actions required (Ball, 2008).

PATIENT MANAGEMENT IN PARU

Initial PARU patient management

A member of the anaesthetic team is required to remain with the patient until the PARU nurse assigned to the patient is available to receive handover, take over care of the patient and is satisfied that the patient's condition is stable (Hegedus, 2003).

On taking over a patient's care, PARU nurses will immediately position themselves at the head of the patient's bed, preferably behind it and the patient, to allow quick and easy access to the patient's airway and also to emergency equipment, such as oxygen and ventilating equipment, which is usually wall mounted. An initial assessment is made of the patient's airway, breathing and colour (ABC) and if it is apparent that the patient is unable to maintain her or his own airway, then the nurse must remain with the patient and provide airway support. A second nurse may assist by assessing and documenting blood pressure, pulse, oxygen saturation level and the patient's level of consciousness and pain status, all of which are priorities at this time (ACORN, 2006a; Ball, 2008).

Patient observations and monitoring

Once these initial patient care priorities are met and the patient is able to maintain his or her own airway, a more thorough patient assessment can be undertaken following a 'head to toe' approach, which includes wound status and type of dressing, location of drains and nature of any drainage, presence of catheters, any IV fluids being given and temperature measurement. If necessary, comfort measures, such as the use of warm blankets, can be initiated. Assessment of pain status and the presence of postoperative nausea and vomiting can be made and interventions commenced where necessary (see pp 226 and 233).

Regular patient observations will be carried out throughout the patient's stay and accurate documentation is vital. Haemodynamic status is determined via assessment and documentation of vital signs, including:

- respiratory rate
- oxygen saturation level
- pulse rate
- blood pressure
- temperature
- urine output.

Other observations include the patient's consciousness level and, where indicated, the ECG rhythm is monitored and displayed continuously. Assessment of ABC and vital signs continue at appropriate intervals in a stable patient according to standard requirements and individual hospital policy. Unstable patients will require more frequent and prolonged assessment and documentation according to individual patient condition (ACORN, 2006a; ANZCA, 2006a, 2006b).

Assessment of airway and breathing

Airway and breathing **management** are a priority in the initial patient assessment and continue to be monitored throughout the patient's stay in the PARU. Oxygen therapy is continued on arrival into the PARU via a Hudson face mask or nasal prongs at a rate of 4 litres per minute, unless otherwise ordered.

A systematic approach to assessing the patient's airway follows a look, listen and feel approach; any untoward findings require immediate action.

Look
Assessment of the patient's airway includes looking at the following:

- Is there misting and demisting of the oxygen mask (or laryngeal mask airway tube if still in situ), indicating that effective respiration is taking place?
- Is the patient's colour pink, indicating that the patient is receiving adequate oxygen?
- Is there symmetrical chest movement, indicating that effective respiration is taking place, or is the patient using the accessory muscles of respiration, indicating ineffective respiratory effort or upper airway obstruction?
- Is the respiratory rate normal, shallow or laboured?
- Is the patient conscious and able to respond to commands to take a deep breath?
- Is the pulse oximeter showing good oxygen saturation levels? A level of 95–98% is considered the normal range (O'Brien, 2008).

Listen
Assessment of the patient's airway includes listening to the following:

- What are the breath sounds like? Are they noisy (e.g. gurgling, snoring)? These signs may indicate an upper airway obstruction, which could be caused by the tongue falling backwards or by laryngospasm.
- Is the patient wheezing, indicating a lower airway obstruction (e.g. bronchospasm)?

Feel
Assessment of the patient's airway includes doing the following:

- Placing a hand on the patient's chest, is there symmetrical chest movements, indicating effective respiration?

Monitoring airway and respiratory function

Apart from visual observation of the patient, non-invasive monitoring of the arterial oxygen saturation level is carried out using a pulse oximeter. A detailed description of pulse oximetry is given in Chapter 6. Determination of oxygen saturation via the use of pulse oximetry is a mandatory observation carried out in the PARU and a reading of 98% is normally anticipated in the postanaesthetic patient (O'Brien, 2008).

Circulation

The effects of surgery and the side-effects of anaesthetic agents are both powerful stimulators of the stress response, which can have dramatic effects on a patient's circulation (Desborough, 2000). Circulatory assessment includes:

- heart rate
- blood pressure
- skin and peripheral tissues (e.g. hands and feet)
- level of consciousness.

Heart rate

Heart rate can be monitored using pulse oximetry or ECG, although it is preferable to palpate the patient's pulse as this provides an assessment of the strength of the pulse, and determination of any irregularities. Touching the patient to palpate the pulse also allows the opportunity to assess skin temperature and determine peripheral perfusion, and provides reassurance to the patient.

Blood pressure

Blood pressure is usually measured using non-invasive blood pressure equipment, either manually or using an automated device. The patient's preoperative blood pressure readings should be noted to provide a baseline and assess whether postoperative readings are within normal limits. A blood pressure reading 20% above or below the patient's normal reading may be considered abnormal and can be attributed to a number of factors (e.g. haemorrhage and resultant hypovolaemic shock) (O'Brien, 2008).

Level of consciousness

Assessing a patient's emergence from general anaesthesia and awareness of self and surroundings requires close monitoring; it is also an excellent indicator of ABC sufficiency and neurological function. Consciousness is usually assessed concurrently with ABC using verbal or gentle tactile stimulation and includes determining a patient's:

- orientation and alertness
- ability to follow commands (e.g. 'take a deep breath')
- ability to move all limbs as per preoperative status (O'Brien, 2008).

Temperature control

While it is common practice to monitor vital signs such as blood pressure and pulse, monitoring the patient's temperature is often overlooked. It is important to take active measures to assess the patient's temperature and maintain normothermia. The issues related to the importance of monitoring for hypothermia and hyperthermia during the anaesthetic phase were discussed in Chapters 4 and 6. This must continue while the patient is in the PARU.

Assessment of temperature

Assessment of the patient's temperature can be made using tympanic, axillary or oral thermometers, although the latter may be impractical due to airway equipment and may render a lower reading than other routes (Drain & Odom-Forren, 2008). In many PARUs the tympanic route is the route of choice to monitor temperature as it is easy to use, non-invasive, non-traumatic and provides an accurate assessment of core temperature. The aim is to maintain the patient's temperature within the range 36.5–37.5°C and to provide comfort warming measures for a patient with a normal temperature but who feels cold. Patients who have a temperature below 36.5°C may require active warming measures, which include forced air warming devices, warm cotton body blankets and head caps or foil thermal blankets (Good et al., 2006).

It is also important to assess the patient with a temperature above 37.5°C for the possibility of malignant hyperthermia, and seek advice and assistance immediately if this condition develops (O'Brien, 2008).

General comfort measures

Although assessing and monitoring the patient's physiological status is paramount in the immediate postoperative period, providing comfort and reassurance is also important during this time. As part of the 'head to toe' assessment, any soiled sheets or gown should be removed and the patient made clean and as comfortable as possible. Psychological care is important as the patient may be anxious about the outcome of surgery, and the presence of a nurse speaking gently, reassuring and reorientating the patient to time and place can be very comforting. Mouth care and providing ice chips to suck will be appreciated by the patient. Some PARUs allow family members to visit, particularly for paediatric patients, where the presence of a family member may reduce patient anxiety and make the child feel more secure (Hamlin, 2005; O'Brien, 2008).

POSTANAESTHESIA COMPLICATIONS

Airway and breathing complications

The effect of anaesthetic agents and relaxant drugs is to depress the central nervous system, resulting in potentially life-threatening **postanaesthesia complications**. These drugs are the main cause of airway obstruction in the PARU (Younker, 2008). Therefore, the initial patient assessment on admission to the PARU is to determine airway patency. If obstruction has occurred, immediate action is required to identify the cause, remove it if possible and maintain the patient's airway (Hegedus, 2003). The most common causes of airway obstruction are the tongue falling backwards into the oropharynx and the presence of secretions, such as mucus, blood or vomitus (Hamlin, 2005).

Table 9-1 summarises the common postoperative respiratory complications seen in the PARU.

Obstruction by the tongue

Muscle relaxant drugs, if they have not been fully reversed, can affect the muscles of the pharynx and the tongue, causing the latter to fall back into the oropharynx and obstruct the upper airway, especially in patients who are lying supine.

The signs and symptoms of tongue obstruction are noisy, gurgling, choking sounds, irregular respirations, decreased arterial oxygen saturation readings and rapid onset of cyanosis.

Management is chin support and/or the instigation of the jaw thrust manoeuvre (Fig 9-2); the jaw thrust manoeuvre lifts the soft palate away from the pharyngeal wall, opening the airway (Younker, 2008). Additionally, the insertion of an artificial airway (oropharyngeal or nasopharyngeal) can be used to maintain an open airway. The patient must not be left unattended during this period until the PARU nurse is confident that the patient is able to maintain his or her own airway. Patients can also be repositioned on

Table 9-1 Common immediate postoperative respiratory complications

Complications and causes	Mechanisms	Manifestations	Interventions
Airway obstruction			
Tongue falling back	Muscular flaccidity associated with decreased consciousness and muscle relaxants	Use of accessory muscles Snoring respirations Decreased air movement	Patient stimulation Jaw thrust Chin lift Artificial airway
Retained thick secretions	Secretion stimulation by anaesthetic agents Dehydration of secretions	Noisy respirations Rhonchi	Humidified O_2 Suctioning Deep breathing and coughing IV hydration IPPV with mucolytic agent Chest physiotherapy
Laryngospasm	Irritation from secretions, endotracheal tube or anaesthetic gases Most likely to occur after removal of endotracheal tube	Inspiratory stridor (crowing respiration) Sternal retraction Acute respiratory distress	O_2 therapy—high flow Positive pressure ventilation IV muscle relaxant
Laryngeal oedema	Allergic drug reaction Mechanical irritation from intubation Fluid overload	Similar to laryngospasm	O_2 therapy Antihistamines Corticosteroids Sedatives Possible intubation
Hypoxaemia			
Atelectasis	Bronchial obstruction caused by secretions or decreased lung volumes	↓ Breath sounds ↓O_2 saturation	CPAP Humidified O_2 Deep breathing Incentive spirometry Early mobilisation
Aspiration	Inhalation of gastric contents	Bronchospasm Atelectasis Crackles Respiratory distress ↓O_2 saturation	O_2 therapy Cardiac support Antibiotics
Bronchospasm	Increased smooth muscle tone with closure of small airways	Wheezing Dyspnoea Tachypnoea ↓ O_2 saturation	O_2 therapy Bronchodilators

Hypoventilation			
Depression of central respiratory drive	Medullary depression from anaesthetics/ opioids/sedatives	Shallow respirations Respiratory rate/apnoea $\downarrow Pa_{O_2}$ $\uparrow Pa_{CO_2}$	Stimulation Reversal of opioids/ benzodiazepines Mechanical ventilation
Poor respiratory muscle tone	Neuromuscular blockade Neuromuscular disease	As above	Reversal of paralysis Mechanical ventilation
Mechanical restriction	Tight casts, dressings, positioning or obesity prevent lung expansion	As above	Elevate head of bed Repositioning Loosen dressings
Pain	Shallow breathing to prevent incisional pain	As above Complaints of pain Guarding behaviour	Opioid analgesic therapy in reduced dose

CPAP, continuous positive airway pressure; IPPV, intermittent positive pressure ventilation; IV, intravenous.

Brown & Edwards (2008)

their side in the recovery position as this action will assist in moving the tongue forward and relieving the obstruction (Drain & Odom-Forren, 2008).

Obstruction by secretions

The upper airway can also be obstructed by the presence of secretions such as mucus, blood or vomitus. The signs and symptoms include noisy, gurgling, choking sounds, coughing, irregular respirations, decreased oxygen saturation readings and rapid onset of cyanosis.

Management includes:

* gentle suctioning of the mouth and oropharynx using a Yankauer sucker or suction catheter
* repositioning patients on their side to assist in the drainage of secretions from the mouth
* taking care when suctioning patients following surgery on the throat as this may cause bleeding to occur (Hamlin, 2005)
* remaining with patients until they are able to swallow.

Laryngospasm

Laryngospasm is one of the most serious life-threatening airway complications. It is the partial or complete closure of the vocal cords in response to stimulation by secretions such as mucus, vomitus or blood, vigorous suctioning of the airway or inappropriate placement of an artificial airway, which touches the vocal cords (Mahajan, 2007).

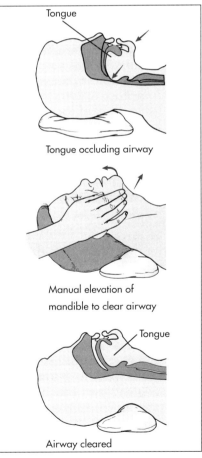

Tongue

Tongue occluding airway

Manual elevation of mandible to clear airway

Tongue

Airway cleared

Figure 9-2 Demonstration of jaw thrust manoeuvre and chin lift (Lewis et al., 2007, p 380).

The closure of the cords in response to these stimuli is a protective reflex but can become a life-threatening event as little or no air enters the lungs. Immediate action is required to restore a patent airway.

Partial closure of the vocal cords results in a 'crowing'-like noise on inspiration. This is known as stridor and is caused by air passing through partially closed vocal cords. The patient may be awake when this occurs and will show signs of panic and distress as this is a very frightening experience.

Management includes:

- if patients are awake, sitting them up, giving reassurance and asking them to take deep breaths (Odom-Forren, 2007)
- removing the cause of the irritation (e.g. gentle suctioning of secretions, or the withdrawal of an artificial airway) (Hegedus, 2003)
- providing oxygen with a Hudson mask or resuscitator bag and mask; if patients are awake they may not tolerate the latter as it may increase their distress
- assistance from nursing colleagues and an anaesthetist if required—do not hesitate to seek it.

The above actions may be sufficient to overcome the partial spasm and the patient's airway will be restored. Patients will require close monitoring to prevent a recurrence of the laryngospasm.

The patient may also suffer a total laryngospasm when the vocal cords close completely. In this situation, there is no sound and no air entry into the lungs, although the patient will still be making efforts to breath characterised by exaggerated chest movements. These patients will rapidly become hypoxic and then unconscious (Drain & Odom-Forren, 2008).

Management of total laryngospasm includes:

- calling for immediate assistance from the anaesthetist as this is an emergency situation
- asking nursing colleagues to obtain intubation equipment as this may be required
- applying positive pressure ventilation using a bag and mask in the hope that the cords will relax momentarily, allowing oxygen into the lungs (Hegedus, 2003).

If a patent airway is not restored using the above manoeuvre, then sedation and reintubation may be carried out by the anaesthetist. This will occur following administration of a sedative drug, such as midazolam and the short-acting muscle relaxant succinylcholine (Hegedus, 2003). The use of a sedative may also prevent laryngospasm from recurring following subsequent extubation as the endotracheal tube touches the vocal cords.

Bronchospasm

Bronchospasm is a lower airway obstruction caused by the bronchial tubes constricting in response to aspiration of stomach contents or secretions, pharyngeal suctioning, or a histamine release secondary to an allergic response to the drugs used during or post anaesthesia (Odom-Forren, 2007). Bronchospasm is characterised by an expiratory wheezing and use of the accessory respiratory muscles.

Management includes:

- oxygen therapy
- administration of inhalational bronchodilators (e.g. salbutamol) and/or IV salbutamol
- reassurance and explanation to the patient, who may be distressed by the inability to breath effectively.

Inadequate reversal of muscle relaxants

The initial assessment of some postanaesthesia patients reveals that they are breathing weakly and have very shallow respirations. This can be an indication that the muscle relaxants used during anaesthesia have not been adequately reversed or have not been totally eliminated from the body. As well as shallow respirations, these patients may display restlessness, and their limbs may lack tone and appear 'floppy'. The shallow respirations are not effective for adequate gas exchange and the patient can become hypoxic; this can quickly progress to respiratory arrest.

Management includes:

- providing oxygen therapy or manual ventilation via a bag and mask if required
- reassurance and asking the patient to take deep breaths
- further administration of reversal drugs.

Cardiovascular complications

Hypotension

Hypotension in the immediate postoperative period is a common occurrence and may be due to a number of factors:

1. blood loss
2. hypoventilation
3. changes in position
4. pooling of blood in the extremities
5. anaesthetic agents
6. narcotics.

Most commonly, hypotension is due to hypovolaemic shock, which is caused by blood and fluid loss either intraoperatively or in the immediate postoperative period. It is characterised by a fall in venous pressure, peripheral vasoconstriction and tachycardia (Hamlin, 2005). Other signs of shock include:

- moist, clammy skin
- rapid, often gasping respirations (sometimes termed 'air hunger')
- patient restless and apprehensive (Hamlin, 2005).

The primary goal in managing hypovolaemic shock is increasing the fluid volume to a level that is able to generate adequate cardiac output and perfusion to the tissues (Drain & Odom-Forren, 2008). The fluid is usually given as a bolus and may be a crystalloid or colloid solution, or a blood product. The hypotensive patient should always receive oxygen via a face mask to aid cellular oxygenation at a tissue level (Drain & Odom-Forren, 2008). Positioning the patient flat or slightly head down will assist in raising the blood pressure in a patient who is compromised. Close observation of the patient's vital signs must be made until his or her condition stabilises, and the cause found and treated. Accurate documentation of fluid balance must also be kept to ensure appropriate management of fluid replacement and assessment for adequate urine output.

Haemorrhage

One cause of hypotension is haemorrhage, which can occur at any time during the perioperative period and can be life-threatening if not managed quickly and effectively. As the patient recovers from the effects of the anaesthetic and surgery, the patient's blood pressure returns to normal limits; this rise may cause blood to ooze from vessels that have been tied or resected during surgery. Often the patient's natural haemostatic mechanisms will control the bleeding, but occasionally the haemorrhage will be profuse.

Active bleeding may be seen through a wound dressing or in drains, or it may occur insidiously, resulting in the patient exhibiting the range of signs and symptoms of hypovolaemic shock. Careful assessment of the patient's wound, drains and catheters for excessive bleeding should be made during the immediate postoperative period. The surgeon and anaesthetist should be informed and the cause of haemorrhage investigated at the same time as resuscitation of the patient is commenced using the measures described above. Unresolved haemorrhage may require that the patient is returned to the operating room to find the cause of the bleeding and initiation of surgical haemostasis (Hamlin, 2005).

MANAGEMENT OF PAIN IN THE POSTOPERATIVE PERIOD

Management of pain is a vital component of a successful outcome for the surgical patient. Achieving absolute and complete pain relief postoperatively is usually unattainable and the term 'optimal' pain relief best describes the PARU goals when providing analgesia to patients (Macintyre & Ready, 2001). Most patients will be anxious about the pain that they are likely to experience and will seek reassurance about the pain management techniques available.

Pain assessment and management

Pain assessment should occur early and often in the PARU and is considered one of the primary functions of the PARU nurse (ANZCA, 2007; Australian and New Zealand College of Anaesthetists & Faculty of Pain Medicine [ANZCA & FPM], 2005; Iacono, 2004). It is well documented that assessing pain intensity is considered the fifth vital sign and pain should be assessed when routine observations are undertaken (ANZCA & FPM, 2005). Importantly, pain is what the person experiencing it says it is, and patient self-report is the most reliable guide about the type and nature of pain being experienced (Bryant & Knights, 2007).

The accurate assessment of pain is of utmost importance and consistent use of a validated pain assessment tool should be used across the facility to promote awareness and correct use (Mitchell et al., 2007). Pain assessment tools that are quick and easy to use are the most suited to pain assessment in the PARU (Macintyre & Ready, 2001). Figure 9-3 shows the commonly used pain assessment scales.

Pain assessment and management in the emergence phase of anaesthesia can be difficult because the patient may be unconscious or semi-conscious, and unable to verbalise their pain adequately. In addition, normal haemodynamic responses to pain, such as tachycardia and hypertension, may be depressed in the immediate postoperative period due to the ongoing effect of anaesthetic agents (Pasero, 2003b). Observing for agitation and restlessness or changes in facial expressions, such as grimacing, evidence of clenched teeth or grinding of teeth, are all highly reliable indicators of pain (Rodriguez et al., 2004).

As well as scoring pain intensity using a validated tool, pain location should also be assessed (ANZCA & FPM, 2005). The surgical incision site is the most obvious source of discomfort or pain for the postoperative patient. However, less obvious sources of pain and discomfort, which can be equally distressing, include a sore throat from intubation, pressure points from prolonged positioning in the operating room or a distended bladder (or kinked urinary drainage tubing). Patients may also experience referred pain (e.g. following a limb amputation).

Pharmacological interventions

Drugs that may be used for **pain management** in the immediate postoperative period include opioids, non-steroidal anti-inflammatory drugs (NSAIDS) and local

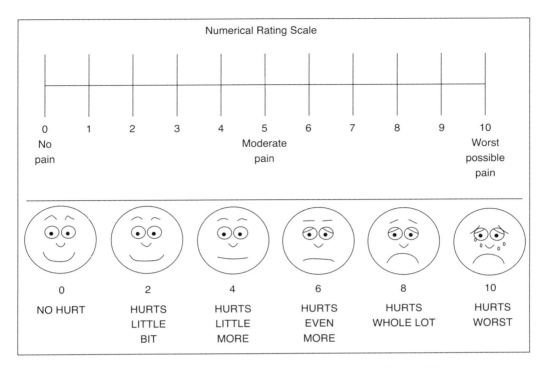

Figure 9-3 Tools commonly used for pain assessment (Hockenberry & Wilson, 2007).

anaesthetics, as well as a range of adjuvant therapies (e.g. antidepressants) and other drugs to treat analgesia-related side-effects (ANZCA, 2007; Bryant & Knights, 2007; Windle, 2004). Drugs can be administered by oral, subcutaneous, intramuscular, IV, epidural, intrathecal, rectal, transdermal, inhaled/intranasal or transmucosal routes (ANZCA, 2007; Power & Atcheson, 2007). The methods and routes commonly used in the PARU include IV, epidural and spinal analgesia (central nerve blocks), regional blocks (e.g. of limbs) or local anaesthesia, and finally, the oral route.

Opioid drugs

IV opioids are the 'gold standard' for the relief of severe acute pain in the immediate postoperative period due to their rapid onset and efficacy (ANZCA & FPM, 2005). IV opioids can be given in the form of a continuous infusion or as intermittent bolus doses, which may be nurse-initiated or patient managed. To maximise the effect of the opioid and limit the side-effects, vital signs, pain and sedation scores must be assessed prior to the commencement and throughout the administration of any IV analgesia, whether given continuously or intermittently (Macintyre & Ready, 2001).

The dose administered is titrated to the individual patient (ANZCA, 2007) and is dependent on the patient's age, pain and sedation scores and response to previous doses (Macintyre & Ready, 2001). However, titrating IV opioids in the immediate postoperative phase is a delicate balance between relieving acute pain promptly and avoiding over-sedation (Pasero, 2003b). Many PARUs use pain protocols in the form of algorithms (flow charts) to allow the nurse to play an autonomous role in assessing pain and administering prescribed analgesics by means of intermittent IV bolus doses of opioids (e.g. morphine) (Macintyre & Ready, 2001). Standard pain protocols in adult patients require the elderly to receive smaller opioid doses due to their reduced tolerance and increased susceptibility to the side-effects, particularly respiratory depression and sedation (ANZCA & FPM, 2005).

Pain protocols are for use by PARU staff who are experienced and knowledgeable in administering IV opioids, including giving loading doses, and they are only implemented where nursing goals are focused on providing rapid relief of acute pain in a monitored environment. They are not recommended for use in a general ward environment with reduced nurse-to-patient ratios (Macintyre & Ready, 2001).

Contraindications to the commencement or continuation of a pain protocol are patients who are over-sedated, hypotensive or who have poor respiratory effort (Macintyre & Ready, 2001). These patients will require review by an anaesthetist prior to the opioid loading dose being administered/continued to avoid exacerbating these conditions.

Patient-controlled analgesia

Patient-controlled analgesia (PCA) is an analgesic delivery system that allows patients to administer their own IV analgesia (usually opioids) intermittently and on demand (ANZCA & FPM, 2005). The PCA device is pre-programmed to deliver a prescribed amount of opioid or 'bolus dose' to patients when they press a hand-held button (Macintyre & Ready, 2001). After a bolus dose is received, a 'lockout system', which is incorporated into a programmable device, disables the system for a prescribed amount of time, commonly 5–8 minutes (Macintyre & Ready, 2001). This prevents over-sedation and results in the patient continuing to experience the effect of the previous dose before being able to successfully initiate another dose (ANZCA & FPM, 2005). Postoperative patients in the PARU may initially require IV loading to bring pain scores to acceptable levels before commencing this analgesia maintenance therapy (Macintyre & Ready, 2001).

The use of PCA should be discussed with patients preoperatively and education provided in the operation of the device, including reassurance that they will not be able to overdose on the drugs used.

Nursing assessment and monitoring includes regular assessment and documentation of respiratory rate, amount of opioid used, sedation and pain scores, vital signs and treatment of any side-effects (Macintyre & Ready, 2001).

The advantages of PCA include the following:

- Patients have more control, and therefore more satisfaction, when able to self-administer opioids in accordance with their current experience of pain and activity levels (ANZCA & FPM, 2005).
- Nursing time is reduced when compared to time spent in preparation of intermittent opioid analgesia (ANZCA & FPM, 2005).
- If patients become too drowsy, they are unable to administer further opioid (Macintyre & Ready, 2001).
- Patients can prescribe their dosage in accordance with individual analgesic requirements (Macintyre & Ready, 2001).
- Peaks and troughs of analgesia, sedation and pain can be avoided when compared to intermittent opioid analgesia (Macintyre & Ready, 2001).

The disadvantages of PCA include the following:

- Decreased effectiveness of device if patients are not appropriately educated in its use (Macintyre & Ready, 2001).
- Requires trained medical and nursing staff to load and program PCA device.
- More expensive method when compared to intermittent opioid doses (ANZCA & FPM, 2005).

- Not appropriate for patients who are cognitively impaired or very young children.
- Side-effects related to ongoing opioid administration, such as sedation, respiratory depression, nausea and vomiting, urinary retention, pruritus, confusion, reduced bowel motility and hypotension (Macintyre & Ready, 2001; Power & Atcheson, 2007).

Continuous opioid infusions

Continuous opioid infusions describe a system where a prescribed amount of opioid is delivered continuously to the patient via an automated delivery system. This modality is beneficial for patients who are unable to use PCA. The goal of the continuous infusion is directed at keeping consistent blood levels of analgesia, thus avoiding peaks and troughs (ANZCA & FPM, 2005). In addition to the continuous infusion, the prescription usually includes a loading dose, which allows the nurse to give a bolus dose of opioid if the analgesic effect is unsatisfactory or prior to performing potentially painful activities, such as repositioning for pressure area care (Macintyre & Ready, 2001). As a result of patients receiving continuous delivery of opioid regardless of the pain intensity or sedation levels, this modality is associated with a higher incidence of respiratory depression; therefore, patients must be closely monitored. Table 6-3 provides a summary of the commonly used agents for opioid analgesia.

Patient management following local anaesthesia infiltration

A common technique used by surgeons when a short-duration local anaesthetic is required to facilitate minor surgery is infiltration of a local anaesthetic (e.g. bupivacaine) in and around the surgical site, targeting the nerve endings (Pasero, 2003b). The same technique may also used following major surgery to provide localised postoperative pain relief, often in conjunction with other drugs. Local anaesthetics act on nerve endings to block the transmission of pain and are used to reduce the overall opioid requirements (and thus the undesired side-effects of continuously administered opioids) (Pasero, 2003b). Local anaesthetics can be given as a single dose, often on completion of the surgery and prior to the patient leaving the operating room. Alternatively, they may be continuously infused directly into and around the operative area via a catheter placed directly in the wound site, which is attached to a disposable pump device (Liu & Wu, 2007). Patients may also require oral or IV analgesia concurrently and/or prior to the locally infiltrated anaesthetic wearing off to provide ongoing multimodal pain relief (Macintyre & Ready, 2001).

Patient management following regional anaesthesia

Regional anaesthetic techniques involve injecting local anaesthetic drugs anywhere along a nerve pathway, resulting in anaesthesia to a region of the body served by that nerve without a loss of consciousness. They are usually administered by the anaesthetist pre- or intraoperatively (DeLamar, 2007). They are often termed 'peripheral nerve blocks' as they are used to facilitate surgery on peripheral areas of the body (i.e. arms or legs). They have the advantage of providing better analgesia with fewer associated side-effects compared to parentally administered opioids (Liu & Wu, 2007). The local anaesthetic is usually administered as a single bolus, which not only provides pain-free surgery, but can also provide pain relief for several hours postoperatively. It is important that other analgesic drugs are prescribed to provide ongoing pain relief when the effect of the local anaesthetic drug wears off (Macintyre & Ready, 2001).

The anaesthetist may inject local anaesthetic into the brachial plexus, which will anaesthetise the arm, or inject the sciatic nerve block, which will affect the leg (see Ch 6) (Klein et al., 2005). In the PARU, care of patients following regional anaesthesia involves prevention of injury to the affected limb that has reduced or no motor or sensory function, and monitoring the neurovascular status of the anaesthetised limb (Banks, 2007). The affected limb also requires supporting on a pillow.

Complications associated with peripheral nerve blocks include damage as a result of malpositioned needles or the side-effects of the drugs administered. Potential insertion complications detected in the PARU include, for example, pneumothorax following incorrect placement of the needle during a brachial plexus block procedure (Klein et al., 2005).

Excessive doses of local anaesthetic can cause toxicity, with signs and symptoms including dizziness, ear ringing, tingling or numbness around the lips, mouth and tongue area, which, if left untreated, can progress to seizures and cardiac instability (Pasero, 2003b).

Peripheral nerve block infusion

A method devised for prolonging the benefits of regional (peripheral) nerve block is to use a continuous peripheral nerve block infusion. This involves a fine catheter being inserted against the nerve sheath and left in situ; it is subsequently attached to a drug delivery system (Banks, 2007). Patients undergoing knee replacement or shoulder stabilisation surgery can benefit from continuous peripheral nerve block infusions. Postoperatively, the patient receives an hourly rate of local anaesthetic, with a prescription of bolus doses available in the event of unsatisfactory pain management. Peripheral nerve block infusions are commonly used in combination with other pain management strategies, such as PCA, with the benefit of reducing opioid requirements and the associated side-effects of continuous opioid administration (Pasero, 2003b).

Nursing care of patients with continuous peripheral nerve block infusions involves:

- securing the catheter insertion site with a transparent occlusive dressing for easy visualisation (Banks, 2007).
- securing the line against accidental removal
- regular observation of the insertion site for early signs of swelling or inflammation (Banks, 2007).
- regular assessment of the pain score
- monitoring the effects on motor function of the affected limb.

Patient management following central nerve blocks

Central nerve blocks refer to the administration of local anaesthetic and other drugs into the subarachnoid or epidural space, blocking the transmission of impulses along the nerves as they exit the spinal cord, and causing large areas of the lower body to lose sensation (hence the commonly used term 'block'). These techniques are particularly useful during and following surgery of the abdomen and lower limbs (DeLamar, 2007). See Chapter 6 for further details.

Epidural analgesia

The use of epidural anaesthesia to facilitate surgery has been described in Chapter 6. As well as facilitating surgery, the epidural route is well recognised as one of the most effective methods for providing postoperative analgesia as part of a multimodal approach. It is particularly effective following orthopaedic, abdominal and obstetric surgery (Pasero, 2003a), and thoracic surgery (Faber & Klein, 2008). The most common selection of drugs are low concentrations of local anaesthetics (e.g. bupivacaine) and opioids (e.g. morphine or fentanyl) (ANZCA & FPM, 2005). Used together, these drugs have a synergistic effect, with a requirement for lower doses (Power & Atcheson, 2007). Opioids administered into the epidural space work via two different pathways:

- a percentage is diffused across the dura into the cerebrospinal fluid, gaining direct access to the opioid receptors in the spinal cord
- a percentage is absorbed systemically, having similar effects to parentally administered opioids (Macintyre & Ready, 2001).

The use of epidural analgesia has a number of advantages when compared to parentally administered opioids:

- improved postoperative pain management
- decrease in pulmonary complications
- quicker return of bowel function (ANZCA & FPM, 2005)
- less patient fatigue and earlier mobilisation (Pasero, 2003a)
- a catheter technique (for continuous infusion) can be used (Power & Atcheson, 2007).

However, a number of side-effects and complications can occur, for which the patient must be closely monitored. Those associated with the opioids include:

- respiratory depression
- nausea and vomiting
- sedation
- urinary retention
- pruritus (Macintyre & Ready, 2001).

Those associated with the use of local anaesthetics include:

- hypotension
- motor and sensory nerve blockade
- urinary retention (Macintyre & Ready, 2001).

Those associated with placement of the epidural catheter include:

- headache due to puncture of the dura
- nerve or spinal cord injury
- epidural abscess or haematoma
- epidural catheter migration (Macintyre & Ready, 2001).

    Nursing care involves:

- regular monitoring and documentation of the respiratory rate, sedation and pain scores, heart rate, blood pressure and urinary output
- regular assessment and documentation of motor and sensory function
- regular assessment of the epidural site to check that the dressing is intact and for ooze or early signs of infection (Macintyre & Ready, 2001).

Spinal block

The use of spinal anaesthesia (block) to facilitate surgery has been described in Chapter 6. The direct injection of a single dose of local anaesthetic (e.g. bupivacaine) into the subarachnoid space causes a complete loss of motor function to the lower limbs and loss of sensation to those areas below the site of the injection and the lower abdomen, thus facilitating surgery (Lee et al., 2007). The effects of the spinal anaesthesia may last well into the immediate postoperative period and the patient is unlikely to require additional postoperative analgesia while in the PARU. The possible side-effects associated with local anaesthetics are:

- hypotension
- bradycardia
- nausea and vomiting
- motor and sensory block

- urinary retention
- headache due to cerebrospinal fluid leak (Lee et al., 2007; Macintyre & Ready, 2001).

Nursing care for patients with spinal anaesthesia involves:

- regular monitoring and documentation of blood pressure, pulse and urine output
- regular assessment and documentation of return of motor and sensory function—if the patient does not experience any return of function, the anaesthetist should be consulted and the patient further examined to ensure no permanent spinal damage has been sustained
- administration of antiemetics for nausea and vomiting
- if patient is complaining of a headache, placing the patient in the supine position and seeking management advice from the anaesthetist (Davis, 2008)
- support for the affected lower limbs.

Other forms of pain management

Oral analgesia

Oral analgesics are generally impractical for use in the immediate postoperative period when patients are recovering from general anaesthesia because they are unable to take oral medications. However, oral analgesia is useful in day surgery settings or if patients have had surgery using local anaesthesia infiltration (Boss et al., 2003). Examples of oral medications include paracetamol, tramadol and NSAIDs (e.g. ibuprofen) (Power & Atcheson, 2007).

Multimodal analgesia

Multimodal analgesia refers to the concurrent use of different classes of analgesics, each working at different sites and in different ways to relieve pain (Windle, 2004). Combining different drugs results in superior pain management and the requirement for smaller doses of each of them, thus reducing the incidence of side-effects (ANZCA, 2007; Pasero, 2003a; Power & Atcheson, 2007). The combined use of local anaesthetics, NSAIDs and opioids are the main components of multimodal analgesia and their administration should commence prior to surgery to optimise the effect (Pasero, 2003b). It is well documented that as increased amounts of opioids are given, the incidence of undesirable side-effects (e.g. respiratory depression) also increases, and thus to decrease these and the subsequent additional time spent in the PARU and hospital, a multimodal analgesic approach is recommended (Pasero, 2003b).

Non-pharmacological and comfort measures

In addition to the pharmacological measures, non-pharmacological and comfort measures can be initiated by the PARU nurse. Measures that can aid in relieving pain include:

- repositioning
- pressure area care
- breathing exercises
- elevation of affected limbs
- application of hot or cold packs (Mitchell et al., 2007).

Additional measures that can be considered in conjunction with the anaesthetist and other members of the surgical team include:

- psychological interventions
- physiotherapy
- acupuncture

- transcutaneous electrical nerve stimulation (TENS) (ANZCA, 2007; Bryant & Knights, 2007).

These measures generally complement rather than supplant pharmacological interventions in the PARU (ANZCA, 2007). However, they can be useful adjuncts, given that patients' attitude and beliefs about pain modify their perceptions of it and can alter their requirements for relief. Box 9-2 discusses some non-pharmacological methods of pain management.

Box 9-2 Non-pharmacological methods of pain management

A pilot study to determine the effects of guided imagery and music therapy on postoperative pain, postoperative nausea and vomiting (PONV), and length of stay for patients undergoing gynaecological laparoscopy was carried out by Laurion and Fetzer in 2003. Guided imagery audiotapes, music audiotapes or standard care were used on patients, who were randomly assigned to one of these interventions, and the outcomes evaluated. Patients who received guided imagery and music therapy reported significantly less pain on discharge from PARU to home than patients who received standard care in the control group. No significant difference was found with respect to PONV or length of stay; however, these findings suggest that guided imagery and music are effective strategies in improving pain management.

Rothrock (2007)

OTHER CONSIDERATIONS AFTER SURGERY

Postoperative nausea and vomiting

Postoperative nausea and vomiting (PONV) are anticipated postanaesthetic events that can be very distressing and potentially harmful to patients. PONV has multiple causes, which include patient movement, the side-effects of anaesthetic drugs such as opioids and nitrous oxide, surgical or vagal nerve stimulation, pain and hypotension. In many instances, nausea and vomiting are often independent phenomena. However, several factors place some patients at higher risk of developing PONV, including:

- female
- history of PONV and/or motion sickness
- non-smoker
- use of perioperative opioids
- age under 60, plus general anaesthesia for more than 60 minutes
- squint surgery (Tramèr, 2001).

A susceptible patient may suffer from PONV for several days after surgery, producing extreme discomfort. Patients with three or more risk factors should receive prophylactic antiemetic medication as part of their anaesthesia. Several antiemetics reliably prevent nausea and vomiting (Carlisle & Stephenson, 2006). The use of P6 acupuncture stimulation to prevent nausea should be considered, as it reliably reduces the incidence of nausea, with minimal side-effects, but not vomiting (Lee & Done, 2004).

The most serious medical complications associated with PONV are regurgitation, airway obstruction and aspiration of gastric contents. Once aspiration has occurred, 50% of patients suffer a major morbidity, and there is a 4% mortality rate (Australian Patient Safety Foundation, 2006).

Patients suffering PONV will be pale, clammy, tachycardic, restless, distressed, possibly in pain, dry reaching or actively vomiting and often have a decreased blood pressure.

Management of PONV includes:

- providing an emesis bowl, tissues or a moist cloth
- positioning patients on their side if unconscious or semi-conscious to prevent aspiration
- suctioning any vomitus from mouth and upper airway
- reassuring and providing distraction therapy (e.g. requesting patient to breath deeply)
- giving prescribed medication (e.g. ondansetron, droperidol, dexamethasone) or a combination (Board & Board, 2006)
- giving analgesia as indicated
- careful position change or patient transfer.

Persistent PONV requires medical review to assess and manage the other causes mentioned above.

CONSIDERATIONS FOR SPECIALTY SURGERY

As well as the routine observations carried out on every patient in the PARU, special observations will be carried out depending on the type of surgery the patient has undergone. Even though it is beyond the scope of this chapter to discuss in detail every type of surgery requiring special observations, some examples of observations that may be carried out for specialty surgery include:

- vascular—neurovascular observations of distal pulses (e.g. femoral, dorsal), skin colour and warmth
- orthopaedic—neurovascular observations as above, and close observations of limbs in plaster casts to ensure any signs of swelling, localised pain and evidence of circulatory insufficiency are addressed promptly
- neurological—use of Glasgow Coma Scale regularly to determine neurological status
- obstetrics and gynaecology—monitor vaginal blood loss and, post-Caesarean section, assess for presence of strong uterine contractions
- prostate—careful monitoring of bladder irrigation and urinary drainage.

Management of patients with diabetes mellitus

Patients suffering from diabetes mellitus are commonly encountered in the perioperative environment. These patients require regular checks of blood sugar levels, careful monitoring of fluid and electrolytes, and regular assessment of urine for evidence of glycosuria. This is because the stresses imposed by surgery and anaesthesia cause imbalances that may require active management to return blood sugar levels to within the normal range. Patients may require insulin given on a sliding scale during the perioperative period depending on the blood sugar results, and IV fluids to treat dehydration. Hyperglycaemia and coma may be difficult to ascertain in an unconscious patient, making regular blood sugar level monitoring a vital component of the overall monitoring of a diabetic patient (Drain & Odom-Forren, 2008).

Paediatric patients

Even though it is not within the scope of this text to provide a detailed discussion on the immediate postanaesthetic care of the paediatric patient, the following section provides an overview. PARU nursing of the paediatric patient has a number of similarities to that of the adult patient in relation to the close observation that is required. However, there are some specific areas to consider.

Patient safety, as with all patients, is paramount and the following must be taken into account with paediatric patients:

- postanaesthetic behaviour can be unpredictable and the child should never be left unattended
- a 1:1 nurse-to-patient ratio is required at all times
- children will often exhibit hyperactive behaviour, which requires constant nursing monitoring and modification of equipment to prevent injury (e.g. padded trolley rail covers to prevent head trauma if the child awakes suddenly).

A family-centred care approach is recommended to encourage parental contact as soon as practical to provide emotional support.

Clinical safety includes:

- medications—based on weight, not age
- careful fluid and electrolyte management—fluctuations in hydration are poorly tolerated
- regular temperature monitoring—babies are particularly sensitive to temperature extremes, which must be avoided
- hypoglycaemia—long periods of fasting are not well tolerated, so length of fasting time in recovery needs to be identified, addressed, and blood sugar levels monitored
- nourishment (e.g. ice blocks, breastfeeding, feeding bottles of glucose and water) can be provided
- blood pressure—not normally monitored except for specific procedures/interventions and patients with comorbidities.

Equipment must be specific for children of all ages. For example, the resuscitation trolley must be equipped with paediatric-sized airways.

Paediatric discharge criteria differs from adult discharge criteria in the parameters that are measured. Paediatric scoring systems include:

- airway
- breathing/oxygen saturation
- consciousness
- temperature
- pain.

Several paediatric discharge scoring systems are available; however, as with adult patients, clinical judgement must take precedence when deciding if a child is ready for discharge from the PARU (Landriscina, 2008; Sullivan, 2001; J. Wilkinson, RN, personal communication, 2008).

DOCUMENTATION AND DISCHARGE

Accurate and timely documentation of the condition of patients during their stay in the PARU is vital in order to monitor their progress, provide early detection of complications, assess their readiness for discharge from the PARU and facilitate continuation of care on discharge from the PARU (Fig 9-4).

There are several numerical scoring systems that provide a set of predetermined criteria against which the patient is scored each time a set of observations are taken. These systems provide an objective means to determine patient stability and suitability for discharge to a ward or the step-down (stage 2) recovery area. One system in common use is the Aldrete scoring system, which was developed in 1970 by Drs Aldrete and Kroulik. A score is allocated to a range of **discharge criteria**, including:

- activity
- respiration
- circulation

**Sydney Hospital &
Sydney Eye Hospital**

**POST ANAESTHESIA
CARE REPORT**

Title	Family Name	MRN
Given Names		V.M.O.
Address		D.O.B. Sex H.I.S.
Suburb	Postcode	Admission Date

10C

POST ANAESTHESIA CARE REPORT

(Post anaesthetic / surgery management
in Recovery and hand over to Ward)

Date:	Time of Arrival:	Admitting RN:	Anaesthetist:

PLEASE COMPLETE THIS TABLE BY PLACING INITIALS IN BOXES WHERE APPROPRIATE.

Anaesthesia:		Airway:		Time Out:	Special Observations:		Drains:	
General		Maintains own airway			Arterial Line		NG tubes	
Spinal		Guedel			CVP		Corrugated	
Epidural		Laryngeal			ECG monitoring		IDC	
Local		Nasal			Neurological		Varivac	
Regional		Endotracheal			Circulation		Stryker	
Sedation		Tracheostomy			FESS		Other:	
Nil		Jaw support			Others / N/A:		Nil	

USE THESE ABBREVIATIONS FOR COMPLETING THE OBSERVATION CHART BELOW

Dressing/Packs (nasal)		Peripheral IV Lines		Arterial Line Site		Peripheral IV Therapy	BSL (if applicable)
Dry	D	Yes / No		Yes / No		To continue - yes / no	Reading
Slight ooze	1	Site:		Site:			
Significant bleeding	2	Satisfactory	G	Leaking	L	Fluids ordered - yes / no	Time checked
Reinforced	R	Swelling	S	Disconnected	D		
Changed	C	Bleeding	B	Redness	R	Cannula removed time:	Bair Hugger
Nil	N	Pain	P	Not applicable	N/a		yes / no

POST ANAESTHESIA RECOVERY SCORE

Patient must achieve PARS of 12 before discharge to the ward. If less than 12 medical review is indicated.

Airway	Blood Pressure	Colour
0 – Obstructed airway	0 - Normal/+ - 50mm	0 – Cyanotic
1 – Artificial airway - clear airway	1 - Normal/+ - 20-50mm	1 - Pale, dusky, blotchy, jaundiced
2 – Breathing spontaneously	2 - Normal/+ -20mm	2 – Normal

Level of consciousness	Movement	Pain Score
0 – No response to verbal stimuli	0 - No voluntary movements	0 - severe pain 7-10
1 – Minimal response	1 - Minimal movement on command	1 - Moderate 4 – 6
2 – Respond verbally to command	2 - Lift head and arms or legs on command	2 - Mild or no pain 0 – 3
		(Ask patient to rate pain on a scale from 0-10)

Observation chart   **PAR Score**

TIME	O₂ L/min	Sa O₂	Pulse	BP	Resp	Temp	Arterial line	Dress -ing	Periph IV	Airway	BP	Colour	LOC	Move -ment	Pain Score	TOTAL	COMMENTS

Copyright Sydney Hospital & Sydney Eye Hospital August 2003 - Print Black Border Process Blue

Figure 9-4 PARU chart. (Sydney Hospital & Sydney Eye Hospital)

- neurological status
- oxygen saturation (DeFazio Quinn, 2008).

Table 9-2 shows both the Aldrete scoring system for patients in the PARU and also the Post Anaesthetic Discharge Scoring System (PADSS) used in ambulatory surgery to assess patients prior to discharge home.

Local policy will determine the total score that the patient must reach for discharge. Usually, a total score of less than 8 would require re-evaluation of the patient's condition by the anaesthetist and surgeon, whereas a total score of 10 would indicate readiness for discharge (DeFazio Quinn, 2008).

Although the scoring system is helpful in determining the patient's condition, it does not include detailed observations such as urinary output, pain management, temperature, wound stability or other observations required for specific types of surgery (e.g. extremity observations). These are important considerations when making decisions about patient discharge to less well staffed areas/wards. Clinicians' judgement always takes precedence

Table 9-2 Postanaesthetic scoring systems

Aldrete Scoring System	Postanaesthetic Discharge Scoring System (PADSS)
Respiration	*Vital signs*
• Ability to take deep breaths and cough = 2	• BP and pulse within 20% preoperative value = 2
• Dyspnoea/shallow breathing = 1	• BP and pulse within 20–40% preoperative value = 1
• Apnoea = 0	• BP and pulse within >40% preoperative value = 0
Oxygen saturation	*Activity*
• Maintenance of >92% on room air = 2	• Steady gait, no dizziness, or preoperative level met = 2
• Oxygen inhalation needed to maintain oxygen saturation >90% = 1	• Assistance needed = 1
• Oxygen saturation <90% even with supplemental oxygen = 0	• Inability to ambulate = 0
Consciousness	*Nausea and vomiting*
• Fully awake = 2	• Minimal or treated with oral medication = 2
• Arousable on calling = 1	• Moderate or treated with parenteral medication = 1
• Not responding = 0	• Severe or continues despite treatment = 0
Circulation	*Pain*

• Blood pressure (BP) ± 20 mmHg preoperative value = 2	• Controlled with oral analgesics and acceptable to patient:
	   • Yes = 2
	   • No = 1

• BP ± 20–50 mmHg preoperative value = 1	*Surgical bleeding*
• BP ± 50 mmHg preoperative value = 0	• Minimal or no dressing changes = 2
Activity	• Moderate or up to 2 dressing changes needed = 1
• Ability to move 4 extremities = 2	• Severe or more than 3 dressing changes needed = 0
• Ability to move 3 extremities = 1	
• Ability to move 0 extremities = 0	

Drain & Odom-Forren (2008)

over achievement of set criteria or guidelines and, wherever doubt exists about readiness for discharge and/or patient safety, discharge should be delayed and, if necessary, advice sought from appropriate medical personnel. In some PARUs, the anaesthetist will be required to review the patient prior to discharge, whereas in other PARUs, nurse-initiated discharge is permitted using collaboratively developed protocols.

Handover to ward/step-down staff

Once the patient's condition is stable and the discharge criteria have been met, local protocol will determine whether ward staff or PARU staff accompany the patient to the ward or stage 2 recovery area. Regardless of the local protocol, a full handover of the patient's care must take place between the nursing staff so that continuity of care is maintained. A final written report summarising the patient's progress in PARU will be made and included in the patient's medical record. This will form the basis of the handover report and it should include the following pertinent facts:

- surgical procedure and anaesthesia administered
- patient's general condition and progress while in PARU
- medications administered, particularly pain relief and current pain scores
- condition of the wound, drains and catheters
- fluid balance, including IV fluid currently in progress and urine output
- any specific postoperative orders (O'Brien, 2008).

The patient should be transferred on a trolley or bed accompanied by two people, one of whom should be a nurse, together with any equipment required to monitor the patient during transfer (e.g. ECG or pulse oximeter monitor).

CONCLUSION

The establishment of PARUs was predicated on the need to care for surgical patients in the immediate postoperative period, a time when they are high susceptible to adverse events. Decades of monitoring adverse events in anaesthesia, 50% of which were preventable, led to the creation of recovery areas within the perioperative suite. PARUs draw together the expertise of highly qualified, specialist nursing and medical staff, along with sophisticated technology, particularly equipment to monitor and manage patients with respiratory and haemodynamic instability. This chapter has provided an overview of the main features of a PARU, and explored the common complications of anaesthesia and surgery, along with their management. PARUs are high-dependency units that continue to evolve, and many now regularly care for patients who require mechanical ventilation.

CRITICAL THINKING EXERCISES

1. Case study

Mr Morgan has undergone an open radical prostatectomy under a general anaesthetic and has just arrived in the PARU accompanied by an anaesthetist and a nurse. Mr Morgan is unconscious and pale in colour, his breathing is shallow with an obstructed airway, and he has a moderate amount of blood in his urinary catheter.

During handover you are told your patient's medical history, indicating that Mr Morgan is a fit 60-year-old man who has oral medication for his diabetes, and has had a minor myocardial infarction 3 months prior to surgery, with some occasional angina following this event.

You are also informed that the surgery was uneventful and PCA has been commenced with morphine. Mr Morgan is receiving IV fluids of Hartmann's solution and an irrigating urinary catheter is in situ. His wife is waiting on the surgical ward.

- List the nursing interventions in order of priority required for Mr Morgan.
- What are the most likely causes for Mr Morgan's airway obstruction?
- Outline the initial interventions to manage his obstructed airway.
- List the observations and monitoring carried out on Mr Morgan during his stay in PARU.
- Outline the nursing assessment you will undertake to monitor the blood loss in Mr Morgan's catheter.
- How will you determine that Mr Morgan is ready to be discharged from the PARU and what information should be contained in your handover to the ward nurse?

RESOURCES

American Association of Nurse Anesthetists
    www.aana.com
American Society of PeriAnesthesia Nurses
    www.aspan.org
Association for Perioperative Practice
    www.afpp.org.uk
Australian College of Operating Room Nurses
    www.acorn.org.au
Australia & New Zealand College of Anaesthetists
    www.anzca.edu.au
British Anaesthetic & Recovery Nurses Association
    www.barna.co.uk
International Association for the Study of Pain
    www.iasp-pain.org
International Federation of Nurse Anesthetists
    www.aana.com
Perioperative Nursing College of the New Zealand Nurses Organisation
    www.pnc.org.nz

REFERENCES

ACORN. (2006a). *ACORN standards for perioperative nursing including nursing roles, guidelines, position statements and competency standards. NR6. Postanaesthesia recovery*. Adelaide: ACORN.

ACORN. (2006b). *ACORN standards for perioperative nursing including nursing roles, guidelines, position statements and competency standards. G4. Management of postanaesthesia recovery (PAR) Unit*. Adelaide: ACORN.

ACORN. (2006c). *ACORN standards for perioperative nursing including nursing roles, guidelines, position statements and competency standards. S19. Staffing requirements, standard statement 5*. Adelaide: ACORN.

Aitkenhead, A., Smith, G., Rowbotham, D. (Eds.). (2007). *Textbook of anaesthesia* (5th ed.). Edinburgh: Churchill Livingstone.

Australian and New Zealand College of Anaesthetists. (2006a). *Professional documents of the Australian and New Zealand College of Anaesthetists. PS4. Recommendations for the post–anaesthesia recovery room*. Retrieved April 11, 2008, from http://www.anzca.edu.au/resources/professional-documents/professional-standards/ps4.html.

Australian and New Zealand College of Anaesthetists. (2006b). *Professional documents of the Australian and New Zealand College of Anaesthetists. PS20. Recommendations on the responsibilities of an anaesthetist in the post–anaesthesia period*. Retrieved April 11, 2008, from http://www.anzca.edu.au/resources/professional-documents/professional-standards/ps20.html.

Australian and New Zealand College of Anaesthetists. (2007). *Professional documents of the Australian and New Zealand College of Anaesthetists. PS41. Guidelines on acute pain management*. Retrieved April 11, 2008, from http://www.anzca.edu.au/resources/professional-documents/professional-standards/ps41.html.

Australian and New Zealand College of Anaesthetists & Faculty of Pain Medicine (2005). *Acute pain management: scientific evidence* (2nd ed.). Melbourne: ANZCA.

Australian Patient Safety Foundation (2006). *Crisis management manual*. Sydney: APSF.

Ball, K. (2008). Transition from the operating room to the PACU. In C. Drain, & J. Odom-Forren (Eds.). *Perianesthesia nursing: acritical care approach* (5th ed.) (pp. 354–359). St Louis: Saunders.

Banks, A. (2007). Innovations in post operative pain management: continuous infusion of local anaesthetics. *AORN Journal, 85(5),* 904–914.

Board, T., & Board, R. (2006). The role of 5-HT$_3$ receptor antagonists in preventing postoperative nausea and vomiting. *AORN Journal, 83(1),* 209–211, 213–216, 219–220.

Boss, M. J., Ewing, P. H., Long, S. P. (2003). Pain management in the PACU. In C. Drain, & J. Odom-Forren (Eds.). *Perianesthesia nursing: a critical care approach* (5th ed.) (pp. 437–457). St Louis: Saunders.

Brown, D., & Edwards, H. (Eds.). (2008). *Lewis's medical–surgical nursing*. Sydney: Elsevier.

Bryant, B., & Knights, K. (2007). *Pharmacology for health professionals* (2nd ed.). Sydney: Elsevier.

Burden, N. (2008). Care of the ambulatory surgical patient. In C. Drain, & J. Odom-Forren. (Eds.). *Perianesthesia nursing: a critical care approach* (5th ed.) (pp. 652–664). St Louis: Saunders.

Carlisle, J. B., & Stephenson, C. A. (2006). Drugs for preventing postoperative nausea and vomiting. *Cochrane Database of Systematic Reviews, 3,* CD004125.

Centre for Health Assets Australasia. (2006). *Australasian healthcare facility guidelines*. Retrieved October 10, 2007, from www.healthfacilityguidelines.com.au.

Davis, T. (2008). Regional anesthesia. In C. Drain, & J. Odom-Forren (Eds.). *Perianesthesia nursing: a critical care approach* (5th ed.) (pp. 344–351). St Louis: Saunders.

Defazio Quinn, D. M. (2008). Management and policies. In C. Drain, & J. Odom-Forren (Eds.). *Perianesthesia nursing: a critical care approach* (5th ed.) (pp. 32–42). St Louis: Saunders.

DeLamar, L. (2007). Anesthesia. In J. C. Rothrock (Ed.). *Alexander's care of the patient in surgery* (13th ed.) (pp. 103–125). St Louis: Mosby.

Desborough, J. P. (2000). The stress response to trauma and surgery. *British Journal of Anaesthesia, 85(1),* 109–117.

Drain, C.D., & Odom-Forren, J. (Eds.). (2008). *Perianesthesia nursing: a critical care approach* (5th ed.). St Louis: Saunders.

Faber, P., & Klein, A. (2008). Theoretical and practical aspects of anaesthesia for thoracic surgery. *Journal of Perioperative Practice, 18(3),* 121–129.

Good, K., Verble, A., Secrest, J., Norwood, B. (2006). Post operative hypothermia—the chilling consequences. *AORN Journal, 83(5),* 1055–1066.

Hamlin, L. (2005). Perioperative concepts and nursing management. In M. Farrell (Ed.). *Smeltzer and Bare's textbook of medical-surgical nursing* (pp. 400–463). Sydney: Lippincott, Williams & Wilkins.

Hegedus, M. B. (2003). Taking the fear out of postanesthesia care in the intensive care unit. *Dimensions of Critical Care Nursing, 2(6),* 237–244.

Hockenberry M., & Wilson, D. (2007). *Wong's nursing care of infants and children* (8 ed.). St Louis: Mosby

Hughes, J. E. (1982). *A history of The Royal Adelaide Hospital* (2nd ed.). Adelaide: Griffin Press.

Iacono, M. (2004). Managing pain: an individual responsibility. *Journal of PeriAnesthesia Nursing, 19(3),* 217–219.

Klein, S., Evans, H., Nielsen, K., et al. (2005). Peripheral nerve block techniques for ambulatory surgery. *Anesthesia and Analgesia, 101(6),* 1663–1676.

Landriscina, D. (2008). Care of the paediatric patient. In C. Drain, & J. Odom-Forren (Eds.). *Perianesthesia nursing: a critical care approach* (5th ed.) (pp. 697–716). St Louis: Saunders.

Laurion, S., & Fetzer, S. J. (2003). The effect of two nursing interventions on the postoperative outcomes of gynaecologic laparoscopic patients. *Journal of PeriAnesthesia Nursing, 18(4),* 254–261.

Lee, A., & Done, M. (2004). Stimulation of the wrist acupuncture point P6 for preventing postoperative nausea and vomiting. Retrieved April 11, 2008, from http://www.cochrane.org/reviews/en/ab003281.html.

Lee, Y., Ngan Kee, W., Chang, H., So, C., Gin, T. (2007). Spinal ropivicaine for lower limb surgery a dose–response study. *Anesthesia and Analgesia, 105(2),* 520–523.

Lewis, S., Heitkemper, M., Dirksen, et al. (Eds.). (2007). *Medical-surgical nursing: assessment and management of clinical problems* (7th ed.). St Louis: Elsevier.

Liu, W., & Wu, C. (2007). The effect of analgesia technique on postoperative patient-reported outcomes including analgesia: z systematic review. *Anesthesia and Analgesia, 105(3),* 789–808.

Macintyre, P. E., & Ready, L. B. (2001). *Acute pain management: a practical guide.* (2nd ed.). St Louis: Saunders.

Mahajan, R. (2007). Postoperative care. In A. Aitkenhead, G. Smith, D. Rowbotham (Eds.). *Textbook of anaesthesia* (5th ed.) (pp. 484–509). Edinburgh: Churchill Livingstone.

Mitchell, M., Wilson, D., Wade, V. (2007). Psychosocial and cultural care of the critically ill patient. In D. Elliot, L. Aitken, W. Chaboyer, (Eds.). *ACCCN's critical care nursing* (pp. 153–185). Sydney: Elsevier.

O'Brien, D. (2008). Care of the perianesthesia patient. In C. Drain, & J. Odom-Forren (Eds.). *Perianesthesia nursing: a critical care approach* (5th ed.) (pp. 390–402). St Louis: Saunders.

Odom-Forren, J. (2007). Postoperative patient care and pain management. In J. Rothrock, & D. McEwen (Eds.). *Alexander's care of the patient in surgery* (13th ed.) (pp. 246–270). St Louis: Mosby.

Pasero, C. (2003a). Epidural analgesia for postoperative pain, Part 2. Multimodal recovery programs improve patient outcomes. *American Journal of Nursing, 103(11),* 43–45.

Pasero, C. (2003b). Multimodal balanced analgesia in the PACU. *Journal of PeriAnesthesia Nursing, 18(4),* 265–268.

Power, I., & Atcheson, R. (2007). Postoperative pain. In A. Aitkenhead, G. Smith, D. Rowbotham (Eds.). *Textbook of anaesthesia* (5th ed.) (pp. 510–525). Edinburgh: Churchill Livingstone.

Rathmell, J., Lair, T., Nauman, B. (2005). The role of intrathecal drugs in the treatment of acute pain. *Anaesthesia and Analgesia, 101(5S),* S30–S43.

Rodriguez, C., McMillan, S., Yarandi, H. (2004). Pain measurement in older adults with head and neck cancer and communication impairments. *Cancer Nursing, 27(6),* 425–433.

Rothrock, J. (2007). *Alexanders care of the patient in surgery* (13th ed.). St Louis: Mosby.

Sullivan, E. E. (2001). Family visitation in PACU. *Journal of PeriAnesthesia Nursing, 16(1),* 29–30.

Tramèr, M. R. (2001). A rational approach to the control of postoperative nausea and vomiting: evidence from systematic reviews. Part 1. Efficacy and harm of antiemetic interventions, and methodological issues. *Acta Anaesthesiologica Scandinavica, 45(1),* 4–13.

Windle, P. (2004). The challenges of pain management: adverse effects of analgesics. *Journal of PeriAnesthesia Nursing, 19(3),* 212–216.

Younker, J. (2008). Care of the intubated patient in the PACU: the 'ABCDE' approach. *Journal of Perioperative Practice, 18(3),* 116–120.

FURTHER READING

Gan, T. J., Meyer, T., Apfel, C. C., et al. (2003). Consensus guidelines for managing postoperative nausea and vomiting. *Anesthesia & Analgesia, 97(1),* 62–71.

Gazarian, P. (2006). Identifying risk factors for postoperative pulmonary complications. *AORN Journal, 84(4),* 616, 618–625.

Hatfield, A., & Tronson, M. (2003). *The complete recovery book* (3rd ed.). Oxford: Oxford University Press.

Macintyre, P. E., & Schug, S. (2007). *Acute pain management: a practical guide.* (3rd ed.). St Louis: Saunders.

Maloney, C. B., & Odom, J. (1999). Maintaining intraoperative normothermia: a meta-analysis of outcomes with costs. *AANA Journal, 67(2),* 155–164.

National Health & Medical Research Council. (1989). *Management of severe pain: report of the working party on the management of severe pain.* Canberra: NHMRC.

Oakley, M. (2003). Immediate postanaesthetic recovery: recommendations from the Association of Anaesthetists. *British Journal of Anaesthetic & Recovery Nursing, 4(1),* 17–19.

Osborne, S., Gardner, G., Gardner, A., et al. (2006). Using a monitored sip test to assess risk of aspiration in post operative patients. *AORN Journal, 83(4),* 908–912, 915–922, 925–928.

Pedersen, T., Dyrlund Pedersen, B., Moller, A. (2003). Pulse oximetry for perioperative monitoring. Retrieved April 11, 2008, from http://www.cochrane.org/reviews/en/ab002013.html.

Rowbotham, D. J. (2005). Recent advances in the non-pharmacological management of postoperative nausea and vomiting. *British Journal of Anaesthesia, 95(1),* 77–81.

Swatton, S. (2004). A discharge protocol for the post anaesthetic recovery unit. *British Journal of Perioperative Nursing, 14(2),* 74–80.

Tramèr, M. R. (2001). A rational approach to the control of postoperative nausea and vomiting: evidence from systematic reviews. Part 2. Recommendations for prevention and treatment and research agenda. *Acta Anaesthesiologica Scandinavica, 45(1),* 4–13.

10

Day surgery and endoscopy

Celia Leary and Lynn Rapley

LEARNING OBJECTIVES

After reading this chapter, you should be able to:

- describe the history and evolution of day surgery and endoscopy
- explain patient selection protocols and patient preparation for day surgery and endoscopy
- explore the patient's journey through day surgery, including endoscopy
- appreciate the complexity and management of equipment in endoscopy
- understand the importance of patient safety and risk management
- identify emerging roles for gastroenterology nurses.

KEY TERMS

ambulatory surgery	day surgery	nurse sedationist
bowel screening program	endoscopy	preoperative assessment
carer	nurse endoscopist	risk management

INTRODUCTION

This chapter provides an overview of the evolution of day surgery and endoscopy in Australia, the process involved in providing these services, and the benefits for the patient, the facilities and health care in general. Opportunities for day surgery to reach its true potential are also discussed. Flexible endoscopic procedures are a large and increasing component of throughput in a day surgery unit and unique considerations are associated with them. The associated technology enables doctors and surgeons to diagnose and treat many different disease processes, sparing patients from traditional surgical interventions. These are examined, along with new roles that are emerging for nurses working in these areas.

The Australian Day Surgery Council (ADSC) (2004) provides accurate and internationally accepted definitions of day surgery:

1. *Day surgery/procedure*: An operation/procedure, excluding an office or outpatient operation/procedure, where the patient would normally be discharged on the same day.
2. *Day surgery/procedure patient*: A patient having an operation/procedure, excluding an office or outpatient operation/procedure, who is admitted and discharged on the same day.
3. *Day surgery centre (facility)*: A registered centre (facility) designed for the optimum management of a day surgery/procedure patient.

HISTORY AND BACKGROUND

More than a century ago Dr James Nicoll, a Scottish surgeon working at the Sick Children's Hospital and Dispensary in Glasgow, published a paper in the British Medical Journal about his experiences of approximately 9000 paediatric surgical patients, most of whom he operated on alone in an outpatient setting (Jarrett, 1999). Nicoll believed that much inpatient treatment was a waste of hospital resources because the results obtained in the outpatient department were equally as good but at a fraction of the cost. He believed that carefully selected children recovered better at home, in the care of their family, provided that they were given the necessary education and information to care for their child postoperatively. He also believed that outpatient surgery was cost-effective and, that by removing children from inpatient beds, their treatment and recovery would be of a higher quality. Nicoll could not have realised then the impact that his practice would make in the mid-to-late 20th century, when the rising costs of health care created a trend to the performance of more surgery on an outpatient or day surgery basis. Nicoll is regarded as establishing the foundations for modern **day** or **ambulatory surgery**.

Like the impact that is attributed to Nicoll's work, Hippocrates is noted to be one of the first people who attempted to see inside the gastrointestinal tract by inspecting the rectum with a candle. In 1795 Bozzini used a rigid sigmoidoscope. By the 1870s, Kussmaul was attempting to visualise the stomach with a rigid tube; however, it was not until 1932, when a semi-flexible instrument was designed by Rudolph Schindler to inspect the stomach, that flexible **endoscopy** began to move into its own domain. Hirschowitz, Curtiss, Peters and Pollard enhanced the design of these instruments in 1958 with their new fibrescope, using fibreoptic bundles to transmit the image. From this point, gastroenterology has evolved into what it has become today (Mays, 2003).

The advent of rapid development in endoscope design, along with procedural advancements, has created a demand for skilled personnel who can manage not only the patient but also care of the equipment. Specialised endoscopy units have developed as free-standing entities as well, as in hospitals, and practice within all of them is under-pinned by clinical guidelines, professional standards and specific health department policies. These have been developed collaboratively and some of them are now mandated (Mays, 2003).

DEVELOPMENT OF DAY SURGERY

In the 1950s some day surgery was being performed internationally but the concept of a purpose-designed day surgery unit was not taken up until 1962, with the development of a hospital-based ambulatory surgery unit at the University of California, followed by the first free-standing 'surgicenter' opened in 1969 in Phoenix, Arizona (Jarrett & Staniszewski, 2006). In Australia, the first purpose-designed, free-standing day surgery centre was built in Dandenong, Victoria, in 1982, and the first free-standing centre on the campus of a public hospital at Campbelltown, New South Wales, in 1984 (Roberts, 2004). These were followed quickly by the development of other units around Australia.

Initially, this new concept generated little enthusiasm for changing the way health care was provided, as there was no incentive to change at that time. However, since the late 1980s and 1990s, a slow but steady growth of day surgery units has occurred in both the public and private sectors. These units have demonstrated their efficiency, combining good postoperative outcomes with high levels of patient satisfaction. Factors contributing to the growth of day surgery have included: the continuing need to reduce extensive hospital waiting lists; the rising costs of health care in general; an increasing and ageing population demanding more surgical interventions; advances in surgical and non-surgical techniques and technology; the development of new, shorter-acting anaesthetic agents and drugs; and the commencement of national cancer screening programs.

The advantages offered by day surgery are listed below.

- Day surgery is cost-effective because the unit functions Monday to Friday, and staff normally only work regular morning and afternoon shifts. Units usually close over the weekend and on public holidays.
- Expensive inpatient beds are not required.
- Organised day surgery lists have a high turnover and cases are rarely cancelled.
- When self-contained or free-standing, day surgery frees up valuable operating time in the main perioperative environment.
- There is a reduced risk of hospital-acquired infections.
- Early ambulation reduces the risk of thromboembolism.
- Patients, particularly the elderly, are less anxious, knowing that they can recover in the comfort of their own home.
- Day surgery is associated with less anxiety in paediatric patients (Davidson & Sale, 2006).

For most patients, spending minimal time in hospital is a great advantage and day surgery has become accepted as an alternative to lengthy hospital stays. Despite the obvious advantages of day surgery, there has been little encouragement from federal or state governments to increase activity rates. Roberts (2004) estimated that the potential for day surgery had increased from 50% to 75% (possibly more) of all operations/procedures. However, statistical information from the Australian Institute of Health and Welfare (AIHW) (2007) shows that, in 1996–97, the rate of same-day activity, for all separations, was 44.7%. The rise in activity over the last 10 years has been approximately 1% per annum, as current statistics show (Table 10-1).

Table 10-1 Current activity, all separations, 2005–06

State/Territory	Day surgery activity
Victoria	58.8%
Queensland	56.9%
Western Australia	55.2%
South Australia	52.2%
New South Wales	51.8%
Tasmania	not published
Northern Territory	not published
Australian Capital Territory	not published
Average	55.3%

AIHW (2007)

The driving force to increase utilisation of day surgery principles in Australia is the Australian Day Surgery Council (ADSC), which is a multidisciplinary body of experts who have been responsible for setting standards and introducing clinical indicators, and who are involved with federal and state government on all aspects of day surgery (ADSC, 2004). The Australian Day Surgery Nurses Association (ADSNA) and the Gastroenterological Nurses College of Australia (GENCA) have also been instrumental in promoting best practice guidelines for ambulatory surgery and procedures, as well as providing educational opportunities for nurses working in day surgery and endoscopy settings. However, notwithstanding the utility of professional guidelines, they are not without limitations, as a systematic review described in Box 10-1 demonstrates.

Box 10-1 Systematic reviews of day surgery

Richardson-Tench, M., Pearson, A., Birks, M. (2005). The changing face of day surgery: using systematic reviews. *British Journal of Perioperative Nursing, 15(6),* 240–246.

This paper discusses the systematic reviews that resulted in the ADSNA publishing its best practice guidelines for:

- staffing models in day surgery units
- pre-admission procedures for day surgery units
- care of patients while in the day surgery unit.

The article highlights the lack of quantitative evidence to ensure best practice, noting instead that expert opinion underpinned many professional standards. Richardson-Tench et al (2005) strongly recommend the need for primary research in the above areas; it is not only relevant for day surgery practice but also for perioperative practice in general.

A steady increase in day surgery has been carried out internationally; however, this varies between countries, between and within regions, and in the types of procedures performed. Developed countries have performed better than developing countries as there are fewer barriers. Table 10-2 presents data on selected procedures extracted from a survey carried out by Toftgaard and Parmentier (2006) for the International Association for Ambulatory Surgery (IAAS). Table 10-2 shows that there are opportunities for growth in day surgery for some procedures in Australia, whereas for other procedures the limits appear to have been reached.

Table 10-2 Percentage of selected cases completed in day surgery settings by country

Country	Arthroscopic menisectomy	Laparoscopic cholecystectomy
Australia	81%	2%
England	70%	3%
Germany	32.5%	0.5%
United States	96.7%	49.8%
Canada	97.7%	43.9%

GROWTH OF DAY SURGERY AND ENDOSCOPY

Advances in surgical techniques and technology

The availability of endoscopes has been instrumental in changing the face of day surgery, and has required surgeons/proceduralists to learn new skills. Similarly, surgeons have developed techniques of operating via smaller incisions. These techniques have led to less tissue trauma, less postoperative pain and quicker overall recovery from surgery. Advances in wound drainage systems allow the patient to be discharged with a small drain in situ (to be removed the next day). Diagnostic and therapeutic laparoscopy and other forms of endoscopy, removal of simple skin growths/cancers, repair of varicose veins, hernia repair, cataract removal, cystoscopy and in-vitro fertilisation are some examples of procedures commonly performed in day surgery settings.

The development of flexible endoscopes, along with the use of cameras that can be attached to them (resulting in the visualisation of the internal operative site on large-screen monitors), has resulted in a new range of procedures subsequently evolving. Flexible endoscopes are complex, long-lumened instruments that can be used to visualise the lungs, upper and lower intestinal tracts, biliary, gynaecological and urological systems. The small bowel has been difficult to visualise due to its length but this is improving as new technologies evolve, such as the double-balloon endoscope. There is also an ingestible capsule which, during its 8-hour transit through the small bowel, is able to take thousands of photographs. Although most endoscopic procedures are completed within the day surgery or endoscopy unit, lengthy procedures may require an extended or overnight stay for the patient to facilitate the process of monitoring that is required for patients undergoing small bowel investigations.

Another influence on the growth in day surgery procedures is exemplified by the National Bowel Cancer Screening Program. This screening initiative is a preventive measure to improve patient outcomes and to lessen health care costs by diagnosing bowel cancers earlier via a faecal occult blood test. This program evolved because of the development, firstly, of an effective, easy to administer, population-based faecal occult blood test. Subsequently, the Australian government implemented the National Bowel Cancer Screening Program in 2006 (MacLellan, 2006). It is anticipated that this will result in greater numbers of patients undergoing flexible colonoscopy to identify the cause of the bleeding from the bowel previously detected via faecal occult blood test.

De Jong et al. (2006) discuss the role of day surgery in a variety of surgical specialties for frequently performed procedures, and recommend that more complex procedures be introduced in the near future. However, careful patient selection remains the key to success.

Advances in anaesthesia

Over the last two decades, significant improvements in anaesthetic techniques have been made owing to the availability of more refined, shorter-acting anaesthetic agents with minimal side-effects. Volatile inhalational agents, such as sevoflurane, desflurane and isoflurane, are popular, and propofol is now commonly used because its properties are such that patients recover rapidly following its use. Total intravenous anaesthesia (TIVA) is ideal for some procedures (Raeder, 2006) and local infiltration, with or without peripheral or regional nerve blocks, may be used and provide good pain relief intra- and postoperatively. Fentanyl is another drug with a rapid onset and short duration, making it ideal intraoperatively as well as postoperatively, where it provides excellent analgesia (Gupta, 2006). The variety of antiemetic drugs currently available allows for more effective control of postoperative nausea and vomiting than previously (Bustos et al., 2006; Langton & Gale, 2007).

Equipment used by the anaesthetist has also markedly improved. The laryngeal mask airway has replaced the endotracheal tube for the majority of patients having a general anaesthetic. More sophisticated monitoring equipment records all events and data throughout the anaesthetic and allows for early warning of untoward events, facilitating early intervention. Raeder (2006) states that, 'The most important aspects of quality in an optimum anaesthetic technique are rapid and clear headed emergence, no postoperative pain, no postoperative nausea or vomiting and absence of any perioperative side effects or discomfort' (p 186).

Patient acceptance

Patient acceptance of and satisfaction with day surgery is consistently high, providing that their expectations of the experience are met, namely:

• a smooth and trouble-free preoperative admission process
• a successful surgical intervention
• no or minimal postoperative side-effects
• able to go home on the same day with the confidence to cope and recover at home.

The ideal facilities are specifically designed to provide a relaxed, non-threatening, hotel-like ambience where patients receive individualised care. Day surgery is particularly suited to children, who are separated from their parents for as short a time as possible. Given a choice, most paediatric patients and their families would choose day surgery over an inpatient stay (Davidson & Sale, 2006).

However, expectations can be problematic to manage if patients are not given the correct information and explanations during the preoperative consultation. The day surgery experience can seem like a 'production line' and patients can feel they are being rushed through the system (Richardson-Tench et al., 2005). Adequate education and care will alleviate these problems, and must be combined with good communication between day surgery and/or perioperative/endoscopy staff, and patients and their families/carers.

Even though patient acceptance of the day surgery experience is mainly positive, acquiescence with the bowel preparation for lower endoscopic procedures can be problematic. Many patients inform staff on admission to the day surgery unit that they were unable to complete the bowel preparation. This is due to its unpalatable nature and/or quantity of medications to be consumed, combined with the (frequent) onset of headache, hunger and diarrhoea caused by the preparation. This, together with the perceived embarrassment associated with the procedure, prevents a number of patients attending for colonoscopy. It is important to educate patients adequately about these matters and their subsequent management prior to the event. This education enhances their overall experience and improves compliance with the necessary preparation. It is often the gastroenterological specialist who gives this information to private patients, which nursing staff reinforce when telephoning the patient on the day before to confirm admission time the following day. Adequate bowel preparation is vital to the success of the procedure and, if this is not completed as directed, then patients need to be aware that the procedure may produce suboptimal results or even be cancelled (Dix, 2007).

PATIENT SELECTION AND ASSESSMENT

Careful selection and assessment is paramount to successful day surgery and endoscopy, and many factors need to be taken into account in making a decision. It is strongly advised that each facility adopt a team approach to establishing written criteria for patient assessment and selection. This means that all who may be involved in the care of the patient—surgeons, doctors, anaesthetists, nurses, social workers, diabetes educators, pain management consultants, physiotherapists—should be involved. Ensuring this involvement results in all stakeholders taking ownership of the criteria developed, and consequently abiding by them. The criteria should address, but not be limited to, suitability of the procedure, significance of medical history, the minimal physical and anaesthetic assessments to be undertaken, and how the evaluation of social circumstances will be determined. The criteria are then used throughout the selection and assessment process, allowing those patients who do not meet the criteria to be referred for treatment as an inpatient.

Traditionally, patients have been selected following the American Association of Anesthesiologist's (ASA) physical status classification system, whereby patients classified as ASA 1 and 2 were deemed appropriate for day surgery. This classification is presented in Table 2-2.

However, Gudimetia and Smith (2006) noted that the ASA classification is a simple, albeit crude, evaluation of chronic health and further add that patients with a ranking of ASA 3 do not experience more complications in the medium-to-late recovery period or problems after day surgery. They therefore recommend that patients who are classified as ASA 1–3 should be considered suitable for day surgery unless they have other contraindications, and that some patients classified as ASA 4 may also be acceptable for day surgery under local anaesthetic.

The assessment process

A variety of models are available for preoperative patient assessment. The most commonly used model internationally is one that utilises a nurse who is experienced in all aspects of day surgery practice using a well-structured medical/health questionnaire, following completion by the patient of a physical and social questionnaire at least 1 week prior to surgery. The ideal interview is a face-to-face meeting with the patient and carer (if possible), which also provides the opportunity for physical assessment, and preoperative diagnostic and other tests to be carried out, and for information sharing and education to occur. An anaesthetist should be available for referral or advice as necessary. Where distance is a problem, the assessment may be carried out by telephone, followed by a mail-out of written information. The **preoperative assessment** needs to ensure that:

- the patient agrees to be a day patient and that the procedure is suitable
- a responsible adult is available to act as **carer** and understands the responsibilities of the role
- the patient is medically fit for surgery and anaesthesia, and any necessary investigations are carried out

- the patient understands the procedure to be performed and the anaesthetic to be given, as well as the side-effects and alternative treatments
- verbal and written information covering all aspects of the day surgery experience are given
- preoperative preparation is explained and education is completed; this includes fasting instructions, medications or other preparations to be taken or withheld, and includes special instructions for insulin-dependent diabetic patients and patients undergoing a colonoscopy or capsule endoscopy
- postoperative instructions are understood (e.g. controlling pain, how soon driving can be resumed following anaesthesia, possible side-effects, and where and when to seek help)
- the patient and carer are given the opportunity to ask and receive answers to their questions
- discharge planning is implemented as required (e.g. community support for the elderly or infirm is organised).

This information, once gained, and following the proscribed criteria, enables identification of those patients who are suitable, those who may be suitable following further assessment, and those who are unsuitable and must be referred for inpatient admission.

Investigations and other screening tests

Routine screening tests are expensive and of no clinical benefit. Investigations should be based on the findings of the preoperative patient assessment and evaluation (Gudimetia & Smith, 2006). This assessment and evaluation may have already been conducted by the medical specialist prior to the day of the procedure and the appropriate tests ordered as relevant to the patient's current medical history. It is therefore necessary to ascertain which, if any, tests have been completed and to ensure that the results are made available once the patient arrives at the hospital/facility and prior to the surgery or procedure.

Factors affecting the selection and assessment process

Whether patients are interviewed/assessed face to face or via telephone, several details needs to be ascertained.

Demographic details, which include confirming the patient's name, home address and other relevant details, must be obtained. *Age* may be a factor as some facilities have either upper and/or lower age limits. A *consent form* that indicates the correct procedure must be completed. An incomplete consent form should not be accepted and steps must be taken to rectify this before the day of surgery. If this is not possible, it must be rectified prior to the surgery or procedure.

Recording of baseline observations should occur where possible. Recording of *weight and height* should occur if pertinent, and always for children. Obesity is an increasing problem in Australian society and the decision to apply a weight limit (calculated on body mass index or BMI) is a matter to be decided by the team and subsequently included in the criteria for admission to the individual facility. Obesity is a predictor of adverse events in day surgery, specifically, respiratory events (along with smoking and asthma) (Langton & Gale, 2007).

A review of the list of the *patient's current medications* should take place and include identifying the use of herbal and complementary medicines, as these are now commonly used and can cause adverse effects in patients undergoing anaesthesia and surgery. It is imperative that patients undergoing an endoscopic procedure (like many other procedures) and taking aspirin, anticoagulants or non-steroidal anti-inflammatory drugs are asked to cease these several days prior to the procedure (Robertson, 2005).

A *medical history* is important as many patients have chronic or concurrent medical conditions, such as cardiac disease, liver disease, pulmonary disease, hypertension, diabetes mellitus or latex allergy. In these cases a specific clinical pathway should be initiated, indicating the necessary preoperative tests and patient management throughout their surgical experience. Those patients with an artificial heart valve or other prosthesis may also require prophylactic antibiotic therapy (Robertson, 2005).

Anaesthetic evaluation is particularly important in patients identified as having previous or family problems with anaesthesia and includes patients who have a known (or possible) difficult airway, a history of malignant hyperthermia, sleep apnoea or those with drug and egg allergies. The anaesthetist should always be consulted for specific advice, although few of these difficulties will preclude day surgery (Gudimetia & Smith, 2006). Recommendations provided by the Australian and New Zealand College of Anaesthetists (ANZCA) on the pre-anaesthesia consultation indicate that all patients must be seen by an anaesthetist prior to anaesthesia and surgery to ensure that the patient is in an optimal state of health, and to facilitate the planning of anaesthesia along with appropriate discussion and consent for the anaesthesia, and related procedures (ANZCA, 2003, PS7). This consultation may be at the initial patient interview following referral by the nurse but prior to the day of surgery or on the day of surgery but prior to the patient going to the operating or procedure room. The final decision on patient suitability for day surgery is made by the anaesthetist.

Social factors are also important. Patients who are unable to make satisfactory arrangements for travel and/or do not have a responsible carer to accompany them, take them home after surgery or their endoscopic procedure, and provide care postoperatively, are deemed unsuitable for day surgery. Other factors to be considered include the distance that patients have to travel from home, the times at which they need to travel (e.g. the elderly driving at night), the availability of help locally (e.g. a nearby hospital) and access to a telephone. If distance is an issue, local motel accommodation may be an option as it is much cheaper than an overnight hospital bed. Special consideration must be given to elderly and infirm patients as they may require community health services post discharge. If they are to undergo colonoscopy, they may also need hospitalisation prior to the event to assist with bowel preparation. Many elderly patients experience dizziness and weakness during this period and are susceptible to falls. Closer monitoring is reassuring to these patients and allows them to relax and attend the procedure in an unstressed state.

In some cases, carer support will be required for more than 24 hours post discharge. For example, a mother of pre-school children who has undergone a laparoscopy will almost certainly need someone to assist with the daily tasks of caring for her family beyond the first postoperative day. Patient compliance with the requirement for a carer is greatly enhanced when the reasons for this are explained. Generally, the majority of patients will have someone who can provide care and support; however, alternative arrangements must be considered when patients themselves are also the sole carer of another reliant person, for example, those with a spouse who has dementia. It is important that these patients are given any additional assistance to enable them to attend the hospital and then be supported while resuming their own role once they have returned to the home environment.

Information and education are essential. Patients have a right to be fully informed on all aspects of the day surgery process and this should be done both verbally and in a written, easy-to-understand format. Information may also be provided by video and through internet access. Use of an interpreter may be required and written information may need to be provided in several languages. Most units now have well-developed patient information brochures. In many cases, carers must also be privy to and fully understand this information. Failure to provide information, particularly related to pain management, personal hygiene and emergency contacts, are among the most significant sources of patient dissatisfaction with day surgery (Richardson-Tench et al., 2005).

Castoro et al. (2006) recommend four different information leaflets. These are outlined in Boxes 10.2–10.5. The information contained in brochures needs to be specific to the individual day surgery unit and requires regular review to ensure that it is current and written in a format that is easily understood. It should not include jargon or medical terminology and should be aimed at the level of an average reader. Regular patient satisfaction surveys should be conducted and used to improve the quality of the day surgery service, including the quality of the information given.

Box 10-2 Booklet construction: Day surgery general information leaflet

Day surgery

An introductory section may address questions frequently asked by patients such as:

- What is day surgery?
- Why should I have day surgery?
- Is it safe?
- Can I have day surgery?
- What happens after day surgery?
- What would I need at home?

Day surgery unit

A second section provides the following:

- Description of the facilities and services offered.
- Address, telephone numbers and operating hours of day surgery unit.
- Description of the nature and quality of service.
- Explanation of the referral to day surgery process.
- Map of the location of the day surgery unit, directions for public and private transport, parking details and brief hospital details (if appropriate).

Castoro et al. (2006). Reproduced with permission.

Box 10-3 Booklet construction: Day surgery unit instructions and procedures

Welcome to the day surgery unit

- Describes the day surgery unit.
- Introduces the staff, facilities and services.
- Provides contact information.
- Gives a brief description of each step of the patient's journey through day surgery:
  - pre-assessment examination
  - preoperative examination
  - the day of surgery

(contd)

- discharge from day surgery
- recovery at home.

The information provided should answer questions about patient expectations and requirements, including what to wear and items to bring in, such as diversionary materials. Pre-assessment instructions and procedure checklists should also be included.

Castoro et al. (2006). Reproduced with permission.

Box 10-4 Booklet construction: Procedure-specific information

Medical information

- Describes the medical condition and rationale for surgery.
- Describes the surgical procedure and informed consent.
- Describes the surgical itinerary:
  - preoperative fasting, medications and other preoperative preparations
  - anaesthesia
  - complications
  - discharge
  - recovery.
- Addresses a range of issues pertinent to the specific procedure, such as:
  - normal/abnormal conditions and responses
  - pain relief and medications
  - wound management
  - role of the caregiver
  - anticipated mental state
  - personal hygiene issues
  - return to normal activity (including work, driving, operating machinery, physical and sexual activity)
  - diet
  - postoperative procedures and examination.

The brochure may also include:

- space for handwritten, patient-specific instructions
- space for appointment dates and times
- contact information.

Castoro et al. (2006). Reproduced with permission.

Day of surgery

On the day of surgery, the patient should be well-prepared and undergo routine admission procedures as per unit/facility and surgeon-specific protocols. This includes establishing that the patient has fasted appropriately (Tudor, 2005). Staggered admissions are the ideal but may not be possible in some facilities. Immediate preoperative preparations may need to be carried out, such as the instillation of local eye drops or wicks for ophthalmic patients (Kirby, 2005) and the use of antiseptic solution on the operative site of patients undergoing orthopaedic surgery. Clipping of the body hair may also be necessary and should occur either immediately prior to

---

Box 10-5 Booklet construction: Information for caregivers

Key points to include:

- Role of the caregiver in day surgery
- What is expected of caregiver before, during and after surgery
- Parking arrangements—map and costs
- Availability of refreshments, shops and other amenities
- The routine in the facility, including the usual timing of admission and discharge
- Contact information

It should also provide any specific information the caregiver needs to know regarding a specific procedure, such as:

- an approximate length of time care is likely to be needed
- information regarding prescribed medications and other postoperative requirements.

Castoro et al. (2006). Reproduced with permission.

---

or on entry to the operating/procedure room. Allergy bands must be securely placed, as needed. Sedative premedication is rarely given in day surgery, and in many units patients walk into the operating/procedure room.

Where appropriate, assessment of the colonoscopy patient's completion of the bowel preparation is crucial because inadequate preparation may compromise visualisation and identification of relevant pathology. In this case, it is probable that further attempts will be made to clean the bowel, which may include the use of one or two small enemas or a bowel washout if the patient is still passing formed faeces. The patient may also need some form of rehydration, as many complain of headaches, which are due to dehydration and electrolyte imbalance caused by some types of bowel preparation (Dix, 2007). These patients, anecdotally, usually feel much better with this treatment. Fasting is essential for patients having gastroscopy or similar, upper gastrointestinal procedures. These patients are often being assessed for reflux problems and the incidence of aspiration can be much higher with this cohort of patients (Grant et al., 2007).

Intraoperative care

Management procedures and care of the patient intraoperatively must follow recommended nursing and health department standards, and best practice guidelines for perioperative nursing. In addition to the standards of ACORN (2006) and the Perioperative Nurses College (NZNO) (2005), endoscopy nurses follow the GENCA guidelines (2003), together with the relevant Australian and New Zealand Standards, such as those that apply to cleaning, sterilisation and disinfection methods (Standards Australia, 2003, AS/NZS 4187). These documents govern practice for endoscopy patient care and reprocessing of endoscopic equipment, and form the basis of risk management in endoscopy and all perioperative settings.

Explanation of the procedure to reinforce information given previously, along with reassurance and clear directions about positioning, monitoring and other procedural events, will alleviate patient anxiety and improve intraoperative compliance. This applies to many types of surgery, especially when procedures are completed under local anaesthesia. Some public hospitals do not use the services of an anaesthetist during endoscopy when drugs such as fentanyl and midazolam are used for sedation. These are administered by the registered nurse under the guidance of the proceduralist.

Postoperative care

The same safety standards apply for postoperative care as for inpatient surgery throughout each stage of the recovery process.

Stage 1 recovery

In stage 1 recovery, the patient is unconscious and requires one-to-one nursing care. Close monitoring is required (see Ch 9). Before transferring to stage 2, the patient must have regained consciousness, have stable vital signs and be able to obey verbal commands. Medication for pain and postoperative nausea and vomiting is given either intravenously or intramuscularly. Patients need to be observed for temperature changes, haemorrhage, distension or a rigid abdomen, breathing difficulty and excessive pain following endoscopic procedures, as these could indicate an adverse event, such as bowel perforation. Other, procedure-specific observations must also be instigated.

Stage 2 (step-down) recovery

During stage 2 recovery, the patient is awake and oral medication can be taken to control pain and postoperative nausea and vomiting. The blood pressure is 20 mmHg above or below the pre-anaesthetic level and oxygen saturation is over 92% on room air (Awad & Chung, 2006).

With the improvements in anaesthesia management and the ability of the anaesthetist to eliminate postoperative complications (particularly pain and postoperative nausea and vomiting) a new concept of 'fast tracking' is now being explored. This allows patients to bypass stage 1 recovery and proceed directly to stage 2 recovery provided they meet certain criteria. This concept has merit but requires further research and validation to ensure patient care is not compromised (Awad & Chung, 2006).

Stage 3 recovery

During stage 3 recovery, the patient is ambulant and meets the criteria for discharge home. The modified 'postanaesthesia discharge scoring system' (PADS), introduced by Chung in 1995, is the most commonly used criteria for assessing 'home readiness'. This system is based on giving a score to each of five major criteria, namely, vital signs, activity level, presence of nausea and vomiting, pain and surgical bleeding. A patient with a score of 9–10 is considered to be ready for discharge home (Awad & Chung, 2006).

Discharge

Before final discharge, a simple checklist should be completed (Table 10-3). Discharge of the patient may be nurse initiated providing there are agreed protocols in place.

Table 10-3 Patient discharge checklist
• Patient alert and orientated.
• Patient ambulant with no dizziness.
• Carer present.
• Intravenous cannula removed.
• Script provided if necessary.
• Medical certificate given if required.
• Follow-up appointment arranged.
• Letter to local doctor provided if required.
• All belongings returned to patient.
• Contact telephone numbers supplied.
• The patient 'happy to go home'.

Follow-up

It is normal procedure for follow-up telephone calls to be made to patients the day after discharge to check that they are recovering and coping well, that they are satisfied with the treatment they received and so that they have an opportunity to ask any further questions. Many facilities also telephone patients again 3–4 days postoperatively to check on progress. All follow-up calls should be documented and evaluated as part of the unit/facility quality improvement and risk management program.

CARE OF ENDOSCOPIC EQUIPMENT

A key aspect of **risk management** in day surgery and endoscopic settings is prevention of nosocomial infections. While most aspects of sterilising and disinfection have been dealt with in Chapter 5, this section deals with the unique considerations of endoscopic instruments. These may be reprocessed within the endoscopy or day surgery unit or they may go to a separate sterilising department. Technical staff involved in this specific activity need to be adequately trained and deemed competent prior to engaging in this work. Irrespective of the location of the day surgery or endoscopy unit, nursing staff employed there must be conversant with all aspects of patient care, and have an understanding of instrument cleaning, maintenance, reprocessing and infection control issues. In endoscopy units, it is important to have dedicated personnel to work with the medical specialists/proceduralists because of the highly specialised and often complex nature of the procedures and equipment (Mays, 2003).

Flexible endoscopic instruments are complex and expensive. Some of their numerous accessories are also expensive and many of these are designed for single use, adding further to costs, both financial and environmental. When purchasing the equipment used in the endoscopy unit, patient safety as well as the best possible equipment affordable or available are often key determinants. Consequently, care of that equipment is of the utmost importance.

The equipment required for endoscopy includes:

* a range of appropriate endoscopes
* a processor—provides light, air/water
* a monitor—provides an image on a screen
* accessories that are passed through the endoscope to perform diagnostic tests or therapeutic intervention (e.g. biopsy forceps, polypectomy snares, stents and dilators)
* accessories that are attached to the endoscope to enable it to function and prevent damage during reprocessing.

General care

All facilities benefit from having written policies, procedures and protocols in place. This assists in ensuring all equipment is properly cared for and maintained, and in accordance with the manufacturers' recommendations. Broadly, it will include the following activities.

* Daily inspections of endoscopes should be made to check for tears, ridging and wear to the external surfaces.
* Angulation of the operative head of the endoscope, which is controlled by the rotatable knobs at the top, needs to be checked to ensure functionality of the internal wires so that they do not fail inside the endoscope during use.
* The lens needs to be checked for cracks and the air/water flow assessed for adequacy to ensure good vision throughout a procedure.

- Checks must be made to see if corrosion is evident. This can occur on the pins at the point where they enter the light source processor and, if present, reduces the clarity and brightness of the image on the monitor.
- The globe in the processor lamp should be changed as soon as it begins to dim.
- The equipment needs to be professionally tested and serviced on a regular basis in accordance with manufacturers' recommendations, and it is inadvisable to circumvent this or wait until an endoscope fails.

Cleaning after use

Many chemicals are involved in the reprocessing of endoscopes and it is important that they are handled correctly and in the manner and concentration for which they were designed. Usually a detergent/enzymatic agent is used in the 'pre-clean' phase and a biocide during the disinfection/sterilisation period. As noted earlier, technical staff responsible for reprocessing flexible endoscopes (in fact, all surgical instrumentation) must be adequately trained in the care and handling of equipment and understand the importance of high-level chemical disinfection. The provision of ongoing education, particularly when newer endoscopes and other instrumentation are introduced, is necessary.

Storage

Flexible endoscopes need to be hung at full length to allow for excess moisture to drain away. When not in use, they require storage in purpose-built, well-ventilated cabinets that allow for good air flow. They should never be stored within a box or suitcase while still wet. Some hospitals have designed and installed systems that force air through the endoscope continuously when it is not in use.

Documentation

Documentation is a crucial aspect of endoscope care. All stages of the process that each endoscope undergoes during cleaning, reprocessing and sterilisation must be recorded, and a copy of this record included in the patient's medical record. This data must also be retained at unit level. This is essential to facilitate tracking in the event that a look-back review is required by the health department. This will occur if routine microbial testing reveals a contaminated endoscope, in which case it becomes essential to identify all patients on whom the contaminated endoscope has been used (see below).

Infection control breaches

Endoscope reprocessing is an activity that must only be completed by personnel who are adequately trained. Most breaches of infection control have been attributed to inadequate manual cleaning of these instruments (GENCA, 2003). As there is no way to visualise the effectiveness of the cleaning of internal endoscopy channels, it is imperative that personnel adhere to the manufacturer's recommendations, and the guidelines and recommended practices developed by organisations such as the Gastroenterological Society of Australia (GESA), GENCA and the pertinent Australian and New Zealand standards. Additionally, certain measures provide validation for this process. These measures include completing routine, periodic microbiological testing of endoscopes, which will alert endoscopy personnel to the presence of microorganisms (or biofilm) within the instrument's channels. This process is very specific and, if testing shows the presence of microorganisms, the potential for cross-contamination and infection in patients exists (GENCA, 2003). If this occurs, the state or national health department is contacted, and patients may be recalled and tested for hepatitis B and C, and human immunodeficiency virus (HIV), if necessary (GENCA, 2003). This is traumatic for patients, their families and the personnel involved in the reprocessing of the equipment; however, it is crucial to the effective management of any potential acquired infection.

QUALITY ACTIVITIES AND RISK MANAGEMENT

As part of the accreditation process it is essential that day surgery and endoscopy facilities constantly monitor performance, clinical outcomes and patient satisfaction. Clinical indicators for day surgery recommended by the ADSC and endorsed by the Australian Council on Healthcare Standards (ACHS) (2006) include monitoring the incidence of:

- cancellation of booked procedures
- unplanned return to the operating room
- unplanned transfer (or overnight admission)
- delayed discharge.

Other indicator sets that may also be used are related to anaesthesia, endoscopy, ophthalmology and oral health (ACHS, 2006). Frequent evaluation and continuous improvement on all aspects of day surgery and endoscopy are essential to ensure a first-class service to the community.

EMERGING NURSING ROLES WITHIN ENDOSCOPY

A number of new, advanced roles are emerging within perioperative settings, most of which are addressed in Chapter 12. Two roles, however, are specific to endoscopy and day surgery settings, and are already in evidence. These roles are those of the **nurse endoscopist** and **nurse sedationist**. These roles have evolved because, like other countries (Sprout, 2000), Australia does not have enough gastroenterologists or surgeons to cope with the amount of work generated by national **bowel screening programs** and growth in the range of endoscopic procedures available.

The role of nurse endoscopist is an important, nurse-led development and encompasses diagnostic endoscopy (Smith & Watson, 2005). Careful selection of nurses for this training is vital; only a small number of nurses will wish to develop such skills and/or have the necessary aptitude. The nurse endoscopist is an autonomous, Nurse Practitioner level role with a minimum academic requirement of a Masters degree. This is a relatively new role in Australia, with only one nurse known to be practising currently. Overseas, where the role developed more than a decade ago, it initially involved the incumbent performing an accurate endoscopic examination while maintaining patient safety and comfort, and conducting patient education within a cost-effective framework (Sprout, 2000). However, within a decade in the United Kingdom nurse endoscopists were also providing interventional procedures, such as oesophageal dilatation, percutaneous endoscopic gastrostomy (PEG) tube insertions, variceal injections, banding and endoscopic ultrasounds. They also complete full colonoscopic procedures and are not limited to flexible sigmoidoscopy only.

In Australia and New Zealand, Nurse Practitioner legislation provides the framework for the development of the nurse endoscopist role. Additionally, as Waters (1998) noted, collaborative relationships with medical colleagues are necessary so that this specialised role can evolve. Mutual responsibility for patient care within the framework of the different disciplines is essential and can only occur through trust, confidence and respect for all areas of expertise. This will only happen when current beliefs about discipline boundaries are revoked, and all stakeholders are open to working in unity to the common goal of achieving positive patient outcomes.

This is also the case in point for the emerging role of the nurse sedationist. Halliday (2006) identifies new tasks and responsibilities for those nurses who take on this role within the endoscopy unit. Advanced assessment skills, a greater understanding of the relevant pharmacology and advanced life-support techniques are critical for this nursing role, and these should be acquired via formal training. Currently, endoscopy units within New South Wales and other parts of Australia use appropriately qualified and prepared perioperative nurses who give the sedation and subsequently manage the patients (Jones et al., 2006). Nurse sedationists work within various guidelines and clinical protocols and their outcomes of care are consistent with the data from the United States and Switzerland (Rex et al., 2005). Within the Australasian context, the role will require an extensive number of hours of advanced practice working with a mentor, such as an anaesthetist or gastroenterologist, along with the other requirements needed to be a Nurse Practitioner, if it is to evolve fully. Additionally, the varying perspectives of several key stakeholders and the guidelines each produce to support (or countermand) the role and activities of the nurse sedationist will need reconciling (ANZCA, 2007; Jones et al., 2006). This work is ongoing.

In summary, the nurse endoscopist and nurse sedationist are examples of the nursing profession developing its identity and forging new career paths. These roles are also necessary for the retention of highly skilled registered nurses who might otherwise travel overseas to expand their knowledge and skills. Issues such as formal training programs, reimbursement and recognition need to be addressed.

CONCLUSION

It is clear that the future for increased day surgery and endoscopy in Australia, with or without extended recovery capabilities, has a major role to play in the delivery of health care services in the future. The Australian government (2006), as part of its 'broader health cover' legislation, has introduced a new *Private Health Insurance Act* (2007) and the distinction between day surgery facilities and private hospitals has been removed. Further, accreditation will become compulsory, at least in Australia.

NSW Health (2007) and the Victorian Department of Human Services (2007) are two examples of state departments that outline reasons for, and supply toolkits to assist in, implementation of extended day surgery services. These policies will actively encourage an increase in day surgery and enable performance of more complex procedures in the future. For many reasons, variations exist in clinical practice among specialists, hospitals and states, and benchmarking would assist to promote greater consistency on a national basis. Those surgeons, proceduralists and anaesthetists performing more complex procedures need to monitor, evaluate and publish outcomes as encouragement to others, and all facilities should have a responsibility to undertake research to improve patient outcomes continually and ensure best practice. The lack of formal training in day surgery and clinical education for medical students in day surgery should be a priority for medical schools as students have little exposure to surgical conditions being treated as day cases. Learning in this environment is essential for clinical skills development (Roberts, 2004).

Dedicated and free-standing facilities totally committed to day surgery, including endoscopy, are the best performers and should be encouraged in future planning or redevelopment projects. Day surgery will continue to increase because it is a safe and financially viable alternative to inpatient treatment, and the rising costs of health care alone will force acceptance of it as one of the solutions to increasing surgical demand.

CRITICAL THINKING EXERCISES

1. Preoperative education

You are working in the preoperative assessment clinic and Mrs Schmidt, age 45 years, presents as a stable, insulin-dependant diabetic for a diagnostic laparoscopy the following week.

- What preoperative information/education would you give to her?

2. Discharge criteria

Mr Williams, age 32 years, has undergone a repair of a left inguinal hernia under general anaesthetic and is getting dressed. He meets the discharge criteria and tells you he feels 'great'. You are unable to contact his carer and realise that Mr Williams's car is parked outside. He firmly declares that there is nobody else who can pick him up. You now suspect that Mr Williams has no carer and intends to drive himself home. This is a problem that has previously occurred in your unit.

- What action would you take in this situation?

3. Bowel preparation

Mr Moroni, a young fit man, attends the endoscopy unit and informs you he has not taken all of his bowel preparation. Further, he states he is still passing formed stools.

- What actions (if any) are required prior to performing a colonoscopy on this patient?

4. Patient support

Mrs Crane has had a colonoscopy today following a positive faecal occult blood test, which she underwent recently as part of the National Bowel Cancer Screening Program. The gastroenterologist has advised her that a suspicious lesion was found in her sigmoid colon and biopsies have been taken for pathology testing. Mrs Crane is very distressed by this news and, further, has no family with her.

- What information and support could you give this patient?

RESOURCES

Ambulatory Surgery Journal
    ambulatorysurgery.org
American Society of Anesthesiologists
    www.asahq.org
Australian Day Surgery Nurses Association
    http://www.adsna.info
Australian national cancer screening programs
    www.cancerscreening.gov.au
British Association of Day Surgery
    www.bads.co.uk
Endonurse
    www.endonurse.com
Gastroenterological Nurses College of Australia (GENCA)
    www.genca.org
Joanna Briggs Institute
    www.joannabriggs.edu.au
Society of Gastroenterology Nurses and Associates (SGNA)
    www.sgna.org
Society for Ambulatory Surgery (SAMBA)
    www.sambahq.org

REFERENCES

ACORN. (2006). *ACORN Standards for perioperative nursing including nursing roles, guidelines, position statements and competency standards*. Adelaide: Australian College of Operating Room Nurses.

Australian Council on Healthcare Standards. (2006). *Day surgery indicators, clinical indicator users' manual, version 4*. Retrieved December 3, 2006, from http://www.achs.org.au.

Australian Day Surgery Council. (2004). *Day surgery in Australia: report and recommendations*. Retrieved August 23, 2007, from www.surgeons.org.

Australian Department of Health and Ageing. (2006). *Private health insurance: directions for broader health cover products* (PHI 49/06). Retrieved October 3, 2007, from http://www.health.gov.au.

Australian Institute of Health and Welfare. (2007). *Australian hospital statistics, 2005–2006.* Retrieved October 8, 2007, from http://www.aihw.gov.au/datadevelopment/index.cfm.

Australian and New Zealand College of Anaesthetists. (2003). *Professional documents of the Australian and New Zealand College of Anaesthetists. PS7. Recommendations on the pre-anaesthesia consultation.* Retrieved July 12, 2004, from http://www.anzca.edu.au/publicationa/profdocs/profstandards/ps7_2003.htm.

Australian and New Zealand College of Anaesthetists, Gastroenterological Society of Australia and Royal Australasian College of Surgeons. (2007). *Professional documents of the Australian and New Zealand College of Anaesthetists. PS9. Guidelines on sedation and/or analgesia for diagnostic, interventional medical or surgical procedures.* Retrieved February 4, 2008, from http://www.anzca.edu.au/publications/profdocs/profstandards/sp9 2007.htm.

Awad, I., & Chung, F. (2006). Discharge criteria and recovery in ambulatory surgery. In P. Lemos, P. Jarrett, B. Philip (Eds.). *Day surgery development and practice* (pp. 241–255). London: International Association for Ambulatory Surgery.

Bustos, F., Semeraro, C., Lopez, S., Giner, M. (2006). Management of postoperative nausea and vomiting in ambulatory surgery. In P. Lemos, P. Jarrett, B. Philip (Eds.). *Day surgery development and practice* (pp. 229–240). London: International Association for Ambulatory Surgery.

Castoro, C., Drace, C. A., Baccaglini, U. (2006). Patient information and preparation of day cases. In P. Lemos, P. Jarrett, B. Philip (Eds.). *Day surgery development and practice* (pp.157–184). London: International Association for Ambulatory Surgery.

Davidson, A., & Sale, S. (2006). Predicting and preventing pre-operative anxiety in children. *Day Surgery Australia, 5(2),* 5–12.

De Jong, D., Rinkel, P. M., Marin, J., et al. (2006). Day surgery procedures. In P. Lemos, P. Jarrett, B. Philip (Eds.). *Day surgery development and practice* (pp. 89–123). London: International Association for Ambulatory Surgery.

Dix, K. (2007). *Bowel preps: a primer on what's right for your patients.* Retrieved 8 April, 2008, from http://www.endonurse.com/ebooks/aug06_bowel.html.

Gastroenterological Nurses' College of Australia. (2003). *Infection control in endoscopy* (2nd ed.). Sydney: Gastroenterological Society of Australia.

Grant, I., Nimmo, G., Nimmo, S. (2007). Intercurrent disease and anaesthesia. In A. Aitkenhead, G. Smith, D. Rowbotham (Eds.). *Textbook of anaesthesia* (5th ed.) (pp. 533–539). Edinburgh: Churchill Livingstone.

Gudimetia, V., & Smith, I. (2006). Pre-operative screening and selection of adult day surgery patients. In P. Lemos, P. Jarrett, B. Philip (Eds.), *Day surgery development and practice* (pp. 125–137). London: International Association for Ambulatory Surgery.

Gupta, A. (2006). Analgesia techniques for day cases. In P. Lemos, P. Jarrett, B. Philip (Eds.). *Day surgery development and practice* (pp. 209–227). London: International Association for Ambulatory Surgery.

Halliday, A. B. (2006). Shades of sedation. *Nursing, 36(4),* 36–41.

Jarrett, P. (1999). James H. Nicoll (1864–1921). *Ambulatory Surgery,* 7(2), 63–64.

Jarrett, P., & Staniszewski, A. (2006). The development of ambulatory surgery and future challenges. In P. Lemos, P. Jarrett, B. Philip (Eds.). *Day surgery development and practice* (pp. 21–34). London: International Association for Ambulatory Surgery.

Jones, B., Bourke, M., McCann, E. (2006). *Sedation for gastrointestinal endoscopic procedures.* Draft discussion paper prepared by the Greater Metropolitan Clinical Taskforce, Sydney.

Kirby, H. (2005). Report on use of eye wicks with ophthalmic medication for dilation of pupils before cataract surgery at Mackay Day Surgery. *Day Surgery Australia, 4(2),* 6–7.

Langton, J., & Gale, T. (2007). Day case anaesthesia. In A. Aitkenhead, G. Smith, D. Rowbotham (Eds.). *Textbook of anaesthesia* (5th ed.) (pp. 533–539). Edinburgh: Churchill Livingstone.

Mays, M. (2003). The gastroenterology nurse and associate. In The Society of Gastroenterology Nurses and Associates (Eds.). *Gastroenterology nursing: a core curriculum* (3rd ed.) (pp. 3–11). Chicago: The Society of Gastroenterology Nurses and Associates.

MacLellan, D. (2006). *Colonoscopy provision in NSW—meeting demand through redesign.* Paper presented at The Cancer Council of Australia's 'Moving forward on bowel cancer screening in Australia' forum for health professionals, Melbourne, Australia.

NSW Health. (2007). *Extended day only (EDO) admission policy directive.* (PD2007_065). Retrieved October 16, 2007, from http://www.health.nsw.gov.au/policies.

Perioperative Nurses College of New Zealand Nurses Organisation. (2005). *Recommended standards, guidelines and position statements for safe practice in the perioperative setting.* Wellington: PNCNZNO.

Raeder, J. (2006). Anaesthetic techniques for ambulatory surgery. In P. Lemos, P. Jarrett, B. Philip (Eds.). *Day surgery development and practice* (pp. 185–208). London: International Association for Ambulatory Surgery.

Rex, D. K., Hues, L. T., Walker, J. A. (2005). Trained registered nurses/endoscopy teams can administer propofol safely for endoscopy. *Gastroenterology, 126,* 1384–1361.

Richardson-Tench, M., Pearson, A., Birks, M. (2005). The changing face of day surgery: using systematic reviews. *British Journal of Perioperative Nursing, 15(6),* 240–246.

Roberts, L. (2004). Day surgery: national and international. From the past to the future. *Day Surgery Australia, 3(3),* 22–23.

Robertson, D. J. (2005). Preprocedure assessment of patients undergoing gastrointestinal procedures. In D. Drossman, N. Shaheen, I. Grimm (Eds.). *Handbook of gastroenterologic procedures* (4th ed.) (pp. 3–9). Philadelphia: Lippincott, Williams & Wilkins.

Smith, G., & Watson, R. (2005). *Gastrointestinal nursing*. Oxford: Blackwell Publishing.

Sprout, J. (2000). Nurse endoscopist training: the next step. *Gastroenterology Nursing, 23(3),* 111–114.

Standards Australia. (2003). AS/NZS 4187. *Cleaning, disinfecting and sterilizing reusable medical and surgical instruments and equipment and maintenance of associated environments in health care facilities.* Sydney: Standards Australia.

Toftgaard, C., & Parmentier, G. (2006). International terminology in ambulatory surgery and its worldwide practice. In P. Lemos, P. Jarrett, B. Philip (Eds.). *Day surgery development and practice* (pp. 35–59). London: International Association for Ambulatory Surgery.

Tudor, G. (2005). How long is too long—a fasting issue. *Day Surgery Australia, 4(3),* 12–17.

Victorian Department of Human Services. (2007). *Extended day surgery. Guidelines for the implementation and evaluation of 23-hour service models in Victoria.* Retrieved March 1, 2007, from http://www.health.gov.au/electivesurgery.

Waters, T. (1998). The role of the nurse practitioner in the gastroenterology setting. *Gastroenterology Nursing, 21(5),* 198–206.

FURTHER READING

Berry, M. (2007). Herbal medicines: considerations for the perioperative setting. *Day Surgery Australia, 6(2),* 10–16.

Burden, N., DeFazio Quinn, D., M., O'Brien, D., Gregory Dawes, B. S. (2000). *Ambulatory surgical nursing.* Philadelphia: Saunders.

Cameron, T. (2007). Diabetes in day surgery. *Day Surgery Australia, 6(2),* 6–8.

Drossman, D., Shaheen, N., Grimm, I. (Eds.). *Handbook of gastroenterologic procedures* (4th ed.). Philadelphia: Lippincott, Williams & Wilkins.

Griffin, V. (Ed.). (2003). *Gastroenterology nursing: a core curriculum* (3rd ed.). Chicago: The Society of Gastroenterology Nurses and Associates.

Mitchell, M. (2006). Nursing knowledge and expansion of day surgery in the United Kingdom. *Ambulatory Surgery, 12,* 131–138.

Thompson, P., Fletcher, I., Downey, C. (2004). Nurses versus clinicians—who's best at pre-operative assessment? *Ambulatory Surgery, 11(1–2),* 33–36.

Watkins, A. C., & White, P. F. (2001). Fast-tracking after ambulatory surgery. *Journal of PeriAnesthesia Nursing, 16(6),* 379–387.

Williams, C., & Jarman, H. (2006). Uncovering caring aspects of perioperative nursing practice: Caring in perioperative nursing. *Journal of Advanced Perioperative Care, 2(3),* 75–84.

CHAPTER 11

Medicolegal aspects of perioperative nursing practice

Lois Hamlin and Menna Davies

LEARNING OBJECTIVES

After reading this chapter, you should be able to:

- understand the regulatory framework that governs nursing practice
- explore the scope of practice of nurses and the decision-making framework that underpins it
- review the role of health policies and professional standards in guiding perioperative practice
- discuss the legislation and common law cases that support issues related to informed consent to treatment, as well as negligence and privacy
- examine patient safety, risk management and quality activities as they relate to the perioperative environment.

KEY TERMS

adverse event	negligence	risk management
coroners' courts	patient safety	scope of practice
electronic health record	professional standards	sentinel events
informed consent		

INTRODUCTION

This chapter focuses on medicolegal and ethical topics as they relate to care delivery in the perioperative setting. It addresses issues that are central to safe practice and patient care delivery in terms of their legal, ethical or moral underpinnings. Nursing practice is informed and guided by legislation and common law decisions, by various codes of professional conduct and practice standards, and by state and federal health department or national ministry policies. At a time of strong public and professional interest in safety and quality in health care, patient safety, risk management and quality improvement remain central to the delivery of surgical care in the operating suite.

THE REGULATORY ENVIRONMENT

Nursing practice, like the practice of other health professionals, is regulated to protect the public. In Australia and New Zealand this happens via the enactment of variously titled Nurses' Acts, which enable the establishment of statutory bodies, such as nurse regulatory authorities (NRAs), to administer the Acts. In Australia, nurses are registered by individual state and territory NRAs; however, the *Mutual Recognition Act 1993* eliminates unnecessary restrictions on worker mobility between states, including nurses. The *Trans-Tasman Mutual Recognition Act 1996* and its New Zealand counterpart extend this privilege (Staunton & Chiarella, 2008). Notwithstanding the current arrangement, a national nurse registering authority in Australia is anticipated in 2009 (Council of Australian Governments, 2006; NSW Nurses and Midwives Board, 2007). In New Zealand, nurses, like all health practitioners, are registered in accordance with the requirements of the *Health Practitioners Competence Assurance Act 2003*, which also addresses scope of practice and fitness for practice, and provides mechanisms to ensure ongoing competency of nurses.

For nurses, the obvious advantage to a single, national NRA is the ability to practice across jurisdictions without any impediment. A national NRA will facilitate the work of the Australian Nursing and Midwifery Council (ANMC), the peak body in Australia established more than a decade ago to bring a national approach to the regulation of nursing (and midwifery). The ANMC works with state and territory NRAs to evolve national standards for practice and for the accreditation of courses, as well as codes of conduct, which are reviewed and updated regularly (ANMC, 2007). The Nursing Council of New Zealand serves the same purpose and function as an NRA; the Council also publishes a code of conduct for nurses.

Codes of conduct

Perioperative nursing practice in Australia is further informed by national codes of conduct, which are developed and revised by the ANMC (2008; Australian Nursing Council, 2004). In New Zealand, the code of conduct for nurses published by the Nursing Council of New Zealand (NCNZ) (2006) is the pertinent code (Table 11-1). These Australasian organisations also publish standards for registered and enrolled nurses, Nurse Practitioners, and other information that guides practice (ANMC, 2007; NCNZ, 2005, 2006, 2007).

The Australian code of ethics and code of professional conduct is based on contemporary research evidence. It is designed to:

- provide distinct professional codes for the discipline of nursing and the discipline of midwifery
- communicate to consumers the codes of ethics and professional conduct that can be applied to the care that nurses and midwives provide within the Australian health profession context

Table 11-1 New Zealand code of conduct for nurses
Four principles with criteria form the framework for the Code. The nurse:
1. complies with legislated requirements
2. acts ethically and maintains standards of practice
3. respects the rights of patients/clients
4. justifies public trust and confidence.

Nursing Council of New Zealand (2006)

- assist nursing and midwifery regulatory authorities with matters of professional ethics or conduct in relation to nurses' and midwives' practice
- inform overseas nurses and midwives wishing to practice within Australia of the standards required in relation to professional practice
- enhance recognition of the contribution of the ANMC to the professions of nursing and midwifery and the Australian community (ANMC, 2008).

Accountability

In all of their activities, individual perioperative nurses remain accountable for their practice and, as necessary, advocate on behalf of their patients; these are enshrined in the various codes of conduct. Box 11-1 provides the ANMC definition of accountability. Accountability and advocacy are further explored under scope of practice (p 265), as well as via an exploration of several legal cases involving perioperative nurses.

Box 11-1 ANMC definition of accountability/accountable

Accountability means that nurses and midwives must be prepared to answer to others, such as health care consumers, their nursing and midwifery regulatory authority, employers and the public for their decisions, actions, behaviours and the responsibilities that are inherent in their roles. Accountability cannot be delegated. The registered nurse or midwife who delegates an activity to another person is accountable, not only for their delegation decision, but also for monitoring the standard of performance of the activity by the other person, and for evaluating the outcomes of the delegation (ANMC, 2007, p 14).

Advocacy

Advocacy can be considered a process whereby nurses provide patients with information to help them make certain decisions, or it can be a nurse pleading for better care of a patient. Acting as the patient's advocate has legal and ethical implications, which the perioperative nurse must consider. There are few better examples of acting on behalf of the patient than doing so in the perioperative environment where patients are either sedated or anaesthetised and unable to look after themselves. As patient advocate, the perioperative nurse works to ensure the patient's physical, emotional and ethical needs are met, and must be ready to intervene to protect the patient's safety. This may include speaking up if correct policies or procedures are not being adhered to or when potential exists for injury without intervention. Ensuring the patient's safety while they are in the perioperative environment is a clear example of patient advocacy (Schroeter, 2002).

Acting as a patient advocate is not without its challenges, especially if acting on behalf of the patient brings the perioperative nurse into conflict with co-workers, some of whom may be close colleagues. It may be easier to turn a blind eye to incorrect or inappropriate behaviour than to speak up and risk the consequences that confronting the person concerned may bring. However, such inaction may result in harm to the patient and is in conflict with codes of ethics and conduct and the New Zealand Code of Rights. It may also place the perioperative nurse at risk of legal proceedings and professional scrutiny. If faced with this type of situation, the perioperative nurse must either confront the person concerned or seek advice from more senior colleagues who can advise on an appropriate course of action.

Scope of nursing practice

In 2007, the ANMC published a national framework for decision-making by nurses about their **scope of practice** with the purpose of fostering consistency across jurisdictions. It was developed in the context of national workforce strategies to promote diversity, flexibility and responsiveness in the workforce, and reflects a whole-of-health workforce perspective. The decision-making framework consists of a set of principles that form the foundations for the development and evaluation of decision-making tools (ANMC, 2007). This framework is significant because it will facilitate the development of advanced perioperative roles, as well as other health care provider roles that may be relevant to patient care in perioperative settings. The Nursing Council of New Zealand has similar mechanisms for the development of advanced nursing roles.

Influences for change in nursing practice arise for several reasons, which include:

- legislative or technological change
- community expectations
- professional development
- changes in education
- resource changes, including availability of health care workers and an ageing workforce
- work practice changes, which may include changing models of care initiated by organisations or professional groups; changes in other health professionals or emergent new health care roles (ANMC, 2007; NZ Ministry of Health, 2006).

Nurse Practitioners can now practice in Australia and New Zealand following the progressive introduction of the necessary legislation and processes of authorisation by the relevant NRAs. Even though there are over 100 Nurse Practitioners now authorised across Australia and 26 in New Zealand, very few are in perioperative settings (Michael & Williamson, 2006; NZ Ministry of Health, 2006). One example of Nurse Practitioners in the operating suite is shown in Box 11-2. Advanced roles are explored further in Chapter 12.

Decision-making related to new, evolving or advanced roles in the perioperative environment should occur within a sound **risk management**, professional, regulatory and legislative framework, as is spelt out by the ANMC (2007). Such a thoughtful process enables nurses to work to their full and/or potential scope of practice. This also enables appropriate delegation. Perioperative nurses, like all others, must practice within the scope of practice of the nursing profession; that is:

'… the full spectrum of roles, functions, responsibilities, activities and decision-making capacity that individuals within that profession are educated, competent and authorised to perform' (ANMC, 2007, p 4).

This definition highlights that they must practice within their own scope of practice as an individual. Thus, as individuals, nurses necessarily have their scope of practice more specifically defined than that of the profession as a whole. The relevance of this

---

Box 11-2 Nurse Practitioners in the operating suite

A small number of perioperative registered nurses are practising at an advanced level and in advanced roles; for example, there are experienced instrument and circulating nurses in one NSW public hospital who are in transitional Nurse Practitioner positions. Part of their role involves seeing (potential) surgical patients in the emergency department and admitting them to expedite their care and management. They do this by assessing and preparing them for surgery, ordering necessary diagnostic tests and arranging their inpatient bed postoperatively.

These roles have the potential to improve patient care because perioperative Nurse Practitioners expedite care in the situation of limited availability of surgical registrars. They also provide continuity of care/assistance more effectively than that provided by rotating junior medical officers. Equally importantly, they have evolved because of an identified local need to improve the surgical patients' experience and from a nursing perspective (Ward & Hamlin, 2006). However, much work remains to be done to establish perioperative Nurse Practitioner positions in Australasia.

---

notion becomes apparent when considering, for example, requests made to individual nurses to scrub for cases where they may have no prior experience, knowledge and/or support; the result may be that the individual is performing outside her or his scope of practice. The same must be borne in mind when consideration is given to the delegation of activities to other health care workers, such as those roles or activities traditionally completed by registered nurses. When delegation is being considered, the following must be taken into account:

- The motivation for any decision about patient care should be based on meeting patients' needs.
- Nurses are accountable for making professional judgements about when an activity is beyond their capacity or scope of practice.
- Nurses are also accountable for determining who is the most appropriate person to perform nursing care.
- Nursing practice decisions are made collaboratively, and in the context of planning, risk management and evaluation.

Thus, any decision about care activities that a perioperative nurse might make must involve:

- careful planning
- incorporation of patient wishes whenever possible
- collaboration with the multidisciplinary health care team
- comprehensive patient assessment
- identification of potential risks and hazards, and strategies to avoid them (ANMC, 2007).

An example of the use of such a process, which was used to change enrolled nurses' scope of practice, is highlighted in Box 11-3.

Professional perioperative standards

Perioperative practice is also informed directly by **professional standards**, including those that are developed and revised by professional associations, such as the Australian College of Operating Room Nurses (ACORN, 2006a) and the Perioperative Nurses College of the New Zealand Nurses Organisation (PNCNZNO, 2005). These standards provide guidance for care delivery and management within perioperative settings and are used by a number of national accreditation agencies (ACORN, 2006a). The evolution,

---

Box 11-3 Developing an educational pathway for the enrolled instrument nurse

In 2002 a meeting of perioperative nurse managers from one area health service in New South Wales was held to address the issue of inadequate numbers of registered nurses working in the operating suite, by proposing a new model of role allocation. This was prompted by the view that nurses urgently needed to be engaged in workforce design, rather than be sidelined by it, with subsequent limited influence on its outcomes.

The managers knew that enrolled nurses were being allocated successfully to the instrument nurse role in some private facilities in New South Wales and in other states and countries. The advantage of this allocation was that it had the potential to create a more flexible and self-reliant registered nurse/enrolled nurse workforce, whereby the circulating nurse alternates roles with the instrument nurse. When these roles are interchangeable, the nurses can share the workload more equitably, match skills and knowledge more effectively and relieve each other for meal breaks more efficiently.

The managers believed that the time had come to explore this enrolled nurse model in the operating suites and, from the beginning of the proposal, were encouraged and supported by the Area Director of Nursing and Midwifery (Sutherland-Fraser, 2006); they followed a process similar to that found in the ANMC guidelines. So began the journey from a pilot course in one area health service, which was successful, to the implementation of a perioperative education program for enrolled nurses state-wide, which is now a formally recognised certificate course for endorsed, enrolled nurses.

---

development and ongoing revision of perioperative nursing standards are a key activity of professional perioperative nursing associations worldwide. Perioperative nurses have a role that many other nurses see as highly technical and task-focused (Kuiper, 2004; Riley & Peters, 2000), orientated towards the physical, rather than psychological, aspects of care (McGarvey et al., 2000), and not necessarily even a real nursing role (Fitzgerald & Bull, 2004). Yet perioperative nurses in Australia and New Zealand govern their own practice and, as a group of specialist nurses, act to construct knowledge that informs practice on a wider professional level (Gillespie et al., 2006; Riley & Manias, 2002), which they have done for a significant length of time. The disciplined practices and knowledge that guide perioperative nursing practice and which aid **patient safety** are underpinned by professional standards. These, among other things, help distinguish perioperative nurses from other categories of health care workers in the operating room, as well as demonstrate the commitment of perioperative nurses to direct patient care and safe patient outcomes (Hamlin, 2005). Much of this knowledge is constructed within the framework of professional standards of practice. One such standard, ACORN's A3 *Handling of accountable items* ('the count'), is now the legal benchmark for perioperative nursing practice in Australia (Hamlin, 2005; Staunton & Chiarella, 2008).

Perioperative competency standards

Perioperative nursing competency standards are aligned with standards for practice. The significance of competency for practice has already been highlighted on page 265. For nurses working in the perioperative environment, the relevant competency standards that guide individual nursing practice are those developed by the two perioperative nursing colleges. In Australia during the course of a 6-year research project, which commenced in 1993, the ACORN competency standards for perioperative nurses were identified and validated (Hilbig, 1999). They have since been reviewed and updated

(Williamson & Hill, 2007). These are now used to underpin performance development activities in many perioperative workplaces, and form the framework of the clinical component of some postgraduate perioperative courses (University of Technology, Sydney & Sydney South West Area Health Service, 2007). ACORN does not offer an accreditation service, which is another potential use of competency standards; however, the Perioperative Nurses College (2003) does so on a voluntary, user-pays basis (PNCNZNO, 2003).

STATUTE AND COMMON LAW

A number of statutes (Acts of Parliament) nationally in New Zealand, and in each state, territory and/or the Commonwealth (Cth) in Australia, directly concern perioperative nurses and nursing practice. They include those associated with privacy and confidentiality, such as national Privacy Acts: Australian *Privacy Act 1988* (Cth) and NZ *Privacy Act 1993*. The states and territories of Australia also have variously titled legislation governing information privacy, such as the *Health Records and Information Privacy Act 2002* (NSW), the *Health Records Act 2001* (Vic.) and the *Information Act 2002* (NT).

Another group of statutes include those that address poisons and drugs regulation, such as the *Health (Drugs and Poisons) Regulation 1996* (Qld) and the *Poisons and Drug Act 1978* (ACT). Other legislation to bear in mind includes the *Therapeutic Goods Act 1989* (Cth) and various occupational health and safety statutes enacted in each state. In New Zealand, the *Health and Disability Commissioner Act 1994* and *Health and Disability Commissioner Amendment Act 2003* incorporate The Code of Health and Disability Services Consumers' Rights (known as the 'Code of Rights'), which is wide and extends to any person or organisation providing a health service to the public. The Code of Rights also covers all health professionals, and an obligation under the Code is to take reasonable actions in the circumstances to give effect to the rights, and comply with the duties. No such bill or code of rights exists in Australia, although a National Patient Charter of Rights is currently at the draft stage (Australian Commission for Safety and Quality in Health Care, 2008).

Common law decisions also have a direct bearing on practice, such as those related to **negligence**, which is a civil wrong (or tort), and to consent to treatment. Failure to gain consent from patients before treating them constitutes part of the civil wrong of trespass to the person, specifically assault and battery; it should not be confused with the civil wrong of negligence. The underpinning legal principles associated with all civil wrongs are well-established common law principles developed by the courts over several centuries (thereby establishing precedents) and sometimes referred to as case law. Some of the principles addressing the law of civil wrongs or torts have been extended by national, state or territory legislation, all of which vary somewhat (Forrester & Griffiths, 2005; Staunton & Chiarella, 2008). In each Australian state and New Zealand, legislation covers the adult who is incompetent to give consent (Forrester & Griffiths, 2005).

Additionally, state, territory or national health department/ministry policies have a direct bearing on perioperative practice; for example, the NSW Department of Health has a policy related to the conduct of the surgical count, which is mandatory in public hospitals (NSW Health, 2005). Another example is infection control policies, which all states, territories and the Commonwealth have (as well as enshrined in legislation), and which have great relevance to perioperative nursing practice.

Negligence

Negligence is the most widely known civil wrong or tort. Although there is no one accepted definition of negligence, the cardinal principle is that the party complaining (the plaintiff) is owed a duty of care by the party complained of (the defendant), that this duty of care has been breached and, as a consequence of that breach, the party complaining suffered damage (Staunton & Chiarella, 2008).

The roles that perioperative nurses undertake while caring for surgical patients requires diligence and discipline, as there are numerous areas where the potential for injury to the patient can occur within the perioperative environment. This is because of the vulnerability of individuals undergoing surgical intervention and the nature of the surgical environment itself. Some examples of the mishaps that surgical patients may experience, although this list is by no means complete, include:

- incorrect positioning
- inadvertently retained surgical items
- lost tissue specimens
- incorrect operation or operative site
- medication error
- equipment failure (Institute of Medicine, 1999; Wilson et al., 1995).

When entering the operating suite, patients are at one of the most vulnerable periods of their hospitalisation. They place their trust in the surgical team to ensure that no harm will be done. Unfortunately, sometimes events occur that result in patients being harmed. Patients who experience injury or harm may decide to bring an action against those whom they believe are responsible for that harm. A civil case for negligence can be brought by patients who believe that they have been injured as a result of health professionals' care falling below the required or accepted standard of care; that is, the acts (or omissions) were not those expected of the ordinary, reasonable health professional. Nurses can and do become involved in legal proceedings, resulting in their practices being examined; however, it should be noted that it is rare for nurses to have an action brought against them directly (i.e. be sued individually).

In an action of negligence, a patient, or plaintiff, has to prove a number of elements to establish that, on the balance of probabilities, negligence has occurred. These elements include establishing that:

- the nurse owed the patient a duty of care; this is usually unequivocal.
- there was a breach of the duty of care (i.e. the nurse failed to act according to accepted practice standards)
- there was damage to the patient, which can be physical or psychological
- there was a direct link between the breach of the duty of care and the damage suffered by the patient (Staunton & Chiarella, 2008).

All these elements are exemplified in the Australian negligence case, *Langley & Another v Glandore Pty Ltd (in Liq) & Another* (1997), which is outlined in Box 11-4.

The elements of negligence from this case were as follows:

- The surgical team owed a duty of care to the patient during surgery.
- The nurses breached their duty of care by failing to follow accepted standards in relation to counting (this was determined to be the ACORN standard, A3 *Handling of accountable items*).
- The sponge left inside the patient caused damage, pain and suffering.
- The sponge inadvertently left inside the abdomen was the direct cause of the damage to the patient.

> **Box 11-4** *Langley & Another v Glandore Pty Ltd (in Liq) & Another* (1997)
>
> A patient underwent a hysterectomy in a Queensland hospital. After suffering symptoms over a period of months, investigations revealed that a surgical sponge had been inadvertently left in her abdomen. This was removed in a second operation 10 months after the first procedure. She sued the surgeons and hospital, as the latter was vicariously responsible for the perioperative nurses. The judge at the first hearing found the surgeons negligent for leaving the sponge inside the patient, but the nurses were found not to be negligent. The surgeons appealed the judgement on the basis that the circulating and instrument nurses played a crucial role in accounting for the sponges used in the procedure. At the appeal hearing. the judge agreed with the surgeons and, in a significant judgement for perioperative nurses, made it clear that both of the nurses were 'primarily responsible' for the count. Neither nurse could provide an explanation as to how a counting error occurred or why the count sheet from the original operation was shown to be complete (Staunton & Chiarella, 2008).

Significant points highlighted by this case were the use of the ACORN Standards in court in order to establish the standard of care expected when handling accountable items (ACORN Standard A3 *Handling of accountable items*). Another significant point made by the judge in the appeal hearing was to place 'primary responsibility' for the count in the hands of the circulating and instrument nurses. It should be noted that the count sheet produced in evidence in this case was complete, with no indication of a counting error evident. This Queensland case, and others that have since arisen (e.g. *Elliot v Bickerstaff* [1999]), highlight the need for vigilance when conducting and recording counts, and handling accountable items intraoperatively.

Consent to treatment

All patients undergoing surgery must understand and give **informed consent** to the procedure. This is the same for any health care treatment, which patients may accept or decline (Staunton & Chiarella, 2008). Health department and local policies set out the requirements for consent that are considered to be valid based on common law decisions, which vary from state to state (see Box 11-5 on *Rogers v Whitaker*). In New Zealand, the Code of Rights enshrines patients' rights related to consent, which must be fully informed and given freely. Although it is not the role of perioperative nurses to obtain the patient's consent for a surgical intervention, they do have a responsibility to check that patients have given consent to treatment, and that the consent is informed. This is usually evidenced by the presence of a signed consent form.

For patient consent to be valid:

- it must be freely and voluntarily given
- the patient must be of the correct age, which varies from state to state/territory, and have the mental capacity to understand the intended procedure
- the consent form must cover the procedure to be performed
- the patient must be provided with information about the procedure, its benefits, side-effects, complications and alternate treatments, and have their questions answered (Staunton & Chiarella, 2008).

The final point was significant in the case of *Rogers v Whitaker* (1992) 175 CLR 479, which is outlined in Box 11-5.

It must be understood that the responsibility for providing information about proposed surgery and for obtaining the patient's consent remains with the surgeon performing the procedure or a delegated deputy. However, the perioperative nurse, as part of the

---

Box 11-5 The case of *Rogers v Whitaker* (1992) 175 CLR 479

Mrs Whitaker, a lady in her 60s, was blind in her right eye following a penetrating eye injury when she was 9 years old. Despite this, she had led a normal life, was married and had raised four children. In 1983 she decided to rejoin the workforce and went for a pre-employment health check. Her general practitioner suggested that she might investigate the possibility of a corneal graft to her damaged right eye and referred her to Dr Rogers, an expert in this area. Over the next few months, Mrs Whitaker and Dr Rogers had several consultations and treatment options were discussed. Dr Rogers felt that surgery could significantly improve her sight and Mrs Whitaker agreed to undergo surgery.

Surgery proceeded uneventfully, but complications developed in the postoperative period. Significantly, the left eye (the eye that had vision) developed 'sympathetic ophthalmia', a serious, although rare, inflammatory condition. Despite intensive treatment, Mrs Whitaker lost the sight in her left eye and, unfortunately, had little improvement in the right eye. She was, effectively, left blind. Mrs Whittaker sued Dr Rogers for negligence on the grounds that he had failed in his duty of care by not warning her of the possibility of sympathetic ophthalmia. She won her case and was awarded compensation. Dr Rogers appealed the decision against him in a case that went all the way to the High Court of Australia. In a majority judgement, the High Court upheld the decision of the lower court and, in doing so, made several significant statements, which have influenced policy development in the area of informed consent (Staunton & Chiarella, 2008).

---

checking procedure that the patient undergoes during their perioperative experience, will sight the consent form and ask the patient to verify the surgery they are about to undergo. The perioperative nurse should be alert to any signs of the patient lacking understanding of the procedure. In such a situation, the perioperative nurse should discuss this with the surgeon in charge of the patient's care to follow up with the patient prior to surgery commencing. Taking this action is an example of the perioperative nurse acting as an advocate for the patient.

Coroners' courts

Even though the outcome of the vast majority of surgical cases is positive for the patient, occasionally patients die on the operating table, or within 24 hours of surgery. This is naturally a devastating event for all concerned, and, as well as the emotional aftermath, legal requirements must be adhered to which fall within the jurisdiction of the coroner. The role of the coroner and **coroners' courts** in Australia has been inherited from English common law, where it has existed for hundreds of years. The main role of the coroner is to 'detect unlawful homicides' and investigate deaths that have occurred in unusual, unexpected, violent or unnatural circumstances to ensure that no foul play was involved (Staunton & Chiarella, 2008). Each Australian state/territory has it own Coroners' Act and in New Zealand there is the *Coroners Act 2006*. Under these Acts, the coroner must hold inquests into deaths that occur under certain circumstances. It is beyond the scope of this text to discuss these in detail; however, the circumstance that has direct implication for perioperative nurses is the death of a patient who has (for example):

'… died while under, or as a result of, or within 24 hours after the administration of, an anaesthetic administered in the course of a medical, surgical or dental operation or procedure or an operation or procedure of a like nature, other than a local anaesthetic administered solely for the purpose of facilitating a procedure for resuscitation from apparent or impending death' (*Coroners' Act 1980* [NSW]).

Even though responsibility for the actual documentation related to the death of a patient on the operating table rests with the surgeon, perioperative nurses must be aware of certain requirements related to the care of the patient after death. These policies are well documented within individual units, but are essentially concerned with leaving the body undisturbed; this means leaving in place drains, cannulae and other such items until a post-mortem examination is completed. Items such as a patient's clothing or belongings may also be required for forensic examination, and local policies will provide guidance on the correct handling of these items (NSW Health, 2005).

Organ transplantation

The coroner is also involved in cases where the patient has consented to donating their organs for transplantation. In Australia, legislation governing organ and tissue donation is state- or territory-based, although all have followed the Commonwealth's proposed legislation (developed by the Australian Law Reform Commission), adopting parts or sections of it as they considered relevant or necessary. However, the result is a piecemeal body of case law and legislation (Staunton & Chiarella, 2008). Solid organ (e.g. liver, kidneys) donation agencies based in each state coordinate the retrieval of organs, and separate tissue banks facilitate the retrieval of other tissue (e.g. eyes, skin) from around Australia. In New Zealand, legislation is national and the donor agency, Organ Donation New Zealand, coordinates all organ and tissue retrieval from deceased donors (Currey et al., 2007).

Legislation in both countries takes the form of Acts addressing the retrieval and use of human tissue before and after death. The legislation gives individuals or their next of kin the choice to 'opt in' and give specific consent to be a donor (Staunton & Chiarella, 2008). Organ donation can subsequently proceed unless that consent is revoked by the donor or the next of kin. If the deceased's wishes are not apparent, consent for organ donation rests with the next of kin. Most (but not all) Australian state and territory Human Tissue Acts (howsoever named) define death (e.g. as in the Tasmanian *Human Tissue Act 1985*, s 27A) as:

• irreversible cessation of all function of the brain of the person
• irreversible cessation of circulation of blood in the body of the person (Staunton & Chiarella, 2008).

Note: South Australia and Western Australia have not adopted the proposed definition of death (Staunton & Chiarella, 2008).

Likewise, in New Zealand the *National Human Tissue Act 1964* does not provide a definition of death, but it is defined in the NZ Ministry of Health's (1987) code of practice for the transplantation of cadaveric organs. Both countries have processes for organ and tissue retrieval and transplantation governed by the Joint Agency for the Regulation of Therapeutic Products. This agency, together with numerous professional bodies in both countries, is responsible for the education of health professionals, the process of potential donor identification, the regulation of donor criteria and organ allocation (Currey et al., 2007).

Donation after brain death

Although the diagnosis of brain death is now widely accepted in Australia and New Zealand, it remains controversial (Staunton & Chiarella, 2008). The most common cause of brain death has changed from traumatic head injury to spontaneous intracranial haemorrhage, which has implications for the organs and tissues retrieved as the donors are older and often have cardiovascular and other comorbidities (Australian and New Zealand Organ Donation Registry, 2005; Streat & Silvester, 2001). Clear, specific and incontrovertible policies and protocols regarding the confirmation of brain death are necessary; however, it is beyond the scope of this text to explore this in detail. Information on this subject can be obtained from the references listed on page 282.

Donation after cardiac death

Prior to brain death legislation, donation after cardiac death (DCD) was the only source of cadaveric kidneys for transplantation. However, DCD programs are being re-established globally (Staunton & Chiarella, 2008) and successfully, and these increase the availability of transplant material. DCD, also referred to as non-beating heart donor, provides a solid organ and tissue donation option for the person who has not and is not likely to proceed to brain death (Currey et al., 2007). For further information, particularly related to ethical issues associated with transplantation, the National Health and Medical Research Council has draft guidelines available on its website (see Resources, p 281).

All potential donor families will be informed that retrieval may not take place because of a number of variables, including the length of time from treatment withdrawal to cardiac standstill (American College of Critical Care Medicine Ethics Committee, 2001). Should the time frames be exceeded, the potential retrieval process is aborted and end of life care continues. Otherwise, withdrawal of treatment and confirmation of death occurs within the intensive care unit (Currey et al., 2007).

The procurement process

Throughout the processes regarding confirmation of death and pre-transplantation requirements, the operating suite is kept fully informed as it will be necessary to have a fully equipped operating room and experienced staff on standby for the procurement process. The donor is transferred to the operating suite and the routine preoperative checks are carried out and documentation completed, including death confirmation and consent for the removal of organs and tissue. Thereafter, the donor is treated intraoperatively in the same manner as any other surgical patient (i.e. counting, intraoperative care plans and other documentation are completed). Following surgery, the patient may remain in the operating room or be returned to the intensive care unit for post-mortem preparation prior to transfer to the mortuary, depending on local policy.

The transplant coordinator plays a vital role in providing support for both the families of the donor and the staff who have been involved in the organ retrieval. Bereavement counselling and information on recipient outcomes are proven aspects of successful transplant programs (Beard et al., 2002; Rodrigue et al., 2003).

Documentation

Documentation is an integral part of the work of the perioperative nurse, providing a record of continuity of patient care for use by colleagues when the patient returns to the ward postoperatively. The patient notes can also form important evidence for use in lawsuits or disciplinary proceedings (Staunton & Chiarella, 2008). Much of the documentation used in the perioperative environment involves charting aspects of the patient's care, namely patient assessment, nursing and other interventions, and the evaluation of the care delivered. This information is recorded on documents such as anaesthetic records, fluid balance charts, the 'count' sheet, intraoperative care plans and patient observation/assessment charts used in the postanaesthesia recovery unit. The potential for documentation errors in the perioperative environment is highlighted in research conducted by Butler et al. (2003), which is presented in Box 11-6. The circulating nurse, in particular, is involved in a large amount of documentation, which may be paper-based, although increasingly this information is being captured electronically.

Box 11-6 Documentation errors in counting

A pilot study conducted in 2003 (Butler et al., 2003) sought to determine the influences on count errors and documentation errors. The study revealed that:

- the most frequent error was one of documentation rather than lost or otherwise unaccounted for surgical items
- these errors occurred more commonly during 'routine' cardiovascular and general procedures
- these errors occurred on the first three days of the week
- these errors involved needles.

Lengthy cases, inexperienced staff, more than one instrument nurse and two procedures conducted at the same time were also believed to be influential. Further research, building upon these preliminary findings, continues.

Many operating suites now enter data related to the patient's care directly onto an electronic record via computer terminals and this method of 'documentation' will increase in the future (Cubitt, 2007; Weaver, 2006). The advent of the **electronic health record** (EHR) has the potential to provide all nurses, including the perioperative nurse, with an even better medium to outline the care they deliver and its effectiveness in a transparent format that can be understood by those outside nursing (Kerr, 2006; Saba & Taylor, 2007). Many countries, including New Zealand, have adopted the EHR as a means of facilitating an efficient flow of information related to the patient's care across hospital departments at a local level to state and national boundaries (Westbrooke & Fogarty, 2006). This has the potential to benefit the continuity of patient care, particularly in populations that travel or move around for work or family reasons.

An electronic record does not require the reader to decipher handwriting and possibly misunderstand, providing a safer method of communication, although it does require a level of computer literacy to enter the data. A number of hospitals have introduced customised software that allows the capture of specific patient information by those involved in the patient's care. Electronic record keeping can be a fast and efficient method of documenting care, as well as allowing hospitals to generate data that can assist with allocating resources, monitoring patient care and demonstrating the attainment of key performance indicators. However, issues related to privacy and patient confidentiality, as well as the secure transmission of data, remain. Some of these can be addressed by the introduction and use of a 'unique' or individual, password-protected sign-on process (Cook & Conrick, 2006). Even though most perioperative records may become electronic in the future, the 'count sheet' is likely to remain paper-based for practical reasons. Regardless of whether documentation is electronic or on paper, the principles of accuracy and completeness remain foremost (Weaver, 2006).

An example of nursing information currently entered electronically in the operating suite is the intraoperative nursing care plan. The nursing care plan captures information about the nursing care carried out on the patient and includes information on patient positioning, placement of electrosurgery equipment, skin preparation solutions used, specimens taken, the placement of drains and/or catheters, the patient's skin condition (before and after surgery) and pressure care measures utilised. All this information (often more, depending on local policy) provides a clear picture of the intraoperative nursing care provided to the patient, helping dispel the notion held by some that very little nursing care takes place during the perioperative period.

Specimen collection

During the course of a surgical procedure the surgeon may remove tissue from the patient, which will be forwarded to pathology for examination. The handling of specimens is an important part of the instrument and circulating nurses' role and must be carried out with diligence and accuracy. To ensure patient safety, correct handling and labelling is vital and the surgeon, instrument and circulating nurses must work together to ensure this occurs. The perioperative nurse must recognise that the patient's diagnosis and future treatment is dependent on the correct handling of specimens.

The methods for handling and labelling specimens have been discussed in Chapter 4. Placing a specimen in an unlabelled container can be a dangerous practice as it can result in unlabelled or incorrectly labelled specimens being sent to the pathology department, which in turn could lead to a significant adverse event, such as patients undergoing unnecessary surgery, or other inappropriate interventions. A case for negligence could be made if a patient were to undergo an unnecessary procedure as a result of an incorrectly labelled specimen. All operating suites require policies and procedures to ensure safe handling of specimens, which are important patient safety and risk management strategies.

Occasionally, patients seek to have certain surgical tissue, such as gallstones, or explanted items, such as orthopaedic plates and screws, returned to them. In Australia, these requests are generally denied based on the infection risk that such items pose; each hospital should have a policy related to the disposal of explanted tissue. When such requests are made of perioperative nurses, they must respond according to this policy, which may include the requirement that patients sign a disclaimer form accepting responsibility for the items (ACORN, 2006b). However, the situation in New Zealand regarding the return of patient tissue is different, with such requests for the return of body parts/tissue addressed within a cultural context. This was discussed in Chapter 1.

PATIENT SAFETY AND RISK MANAGEMENT IN THE PERIOPERATIVE ENVIRONMENT

Health care workers, including perioperative nurses, strive to ensure patient safety and provide quality care. Notwithstanding this, mishaps occur, and the incidence of errors and adverse events documented over the last decade or so is significant. Worldwide, there is much activity at regulatory, governmental and local levels to address increasingly complex and diverse systems, as well as cultural issues that affect patient outcomes negatively (Aspden, 2004; Barraclough, 2001; Degeling et al., 2004; Institute of Medicine, 1999). Further, there is increasing public interest in, and knowledge of, health care and its standards, and an expectation that the health care system will achieve better standards of safety and quality (Australian Council for Safety and Quality in Health Care (ACSQHC, 2004; NZ Ministry of Health, 2003). Aligned with this is the need to foster a transparent and just culture, one that acknowledges that health care workers can and do make errors, and that, on occasions, patients suffer unanticipated and unintentional harm (ACSQHC, 2003, 2004).

Both Australia and New Zealand have mechanisms to address quality and safety in health care. In Australia, the Australian Commission (formerly Council) for Safety and Quality in Health Care (ACSQHC) has responsibility for these issues. Within New Zealand, this is embedded within the New Zealand health strategy that:

'… embraces a culture of continuous quality improvement … which:
• is system-wide

- uses a risk management approach to reduce preventable harm
- fosters consistency of practice through shared learning, benchmarking and clinical governance within a standards framework
- takes account of community and health service users' views on quality of care' (NZ Ministry of Health, 2003, p 25).

Quality is a multifaceted concept that is difficult to define (ACSQHC, 2003). One way to conceive it is 'doing the right thing the first time, in the right way and at the right time' (NSW Health, 2002). However, before a high-quality, safer health care system can be designed, the magnitude of the problem must first be determined. This is an extraordinary challenge, particularly across multiple jurisdictions, because it requires multiple but consistent data collections and methodologies (ACSQHC, 2003, 2004), and these are still being developed. By using techniques from other high-risk industries where safety is paramount, such as the aviation industry, the health sector is developing techniques to identify risks, and investigate and analyse incidents, and to use the knowledge gained to improve practice.

The incidence of adverse events

Australia was the first country to undertake a nationally representative study of **adverse events** in hospital patients (Wilson et al., 1995; Wilson et al., 1999), which revealed a 16.6% incidence of adverse events, half of which were associated with a surgical procedure. Of these adverse events, 51% were considered preventable. Even higher levels of adverse events (21.9%) have been reported among one cohort of surgical patients, of which 48% were preventable; of these patients, 13% suffered a permanent disability and 4% died (Kable et al., 2002). In New Zealand, the first national report on adverse events was published in 2001. The New Zealand results identified a rate of incidence of adverse events comparable with other studies, and noted that systems errors featured prominently in the analysis of areas for prevention of recurrence (NZ Ministry of Health, 2001).

The incidence and causes of sentinel events

Several states, including Victoria, Queensland and New South Wales, have published data about adverse and/or **sentinel events** for several years, with the Victorian Department of Human Services (DHS) being the first to do so (Victorian DHS, 2004). The first national report of sentinel events in Australian public hospitals was published in 2007 (Australian Institute of Health and Welfare [AIHW], 2007). To date, there is no equivalent (published) New Zealand data. Of the 130 events identified by the AIHW, and of particular concern for perioperative nurses, the single type of sentinel event that accounted for the greatest number (53 cases) was 'procedures involving the wrong patient or body part'. The second most commonly occurring event (27 cases) was 'retained instruments or other material after surgery requiring reoperation or further surgical procedure'. Although this is not the sum total of sentinel events, these two types of sentinel events are focused on because they concern perioperative nurses directly. Of the 53 cases involving the wrong patient or body part, 10 cases involved the wrong patient undergoing an invasive procedure, a further 10 cases were an invasive procedure on the wrong body part and five cases were patients given anaesthetics/blocks to the wrong area of the body (AIHW, 2007). Following analysis, the contributing factors associated with these sentinel events mainly related to 'rules, policies and procedures', 'documentation' and 'communication'. Table 11-2 lists all of the contributing factors, which are further explored in the case study presented in Box 11-7.

Table 11-2 Contributing factors reported for procedures involving the wrong patient or body part, 2004–05

Contributing factors	Number of cases
Lack of, problems with or breakdown in:	
Rules/policies/procedures	36
Information/documentation	17
Communication	18
Patient factors	1
Staff factors	0
Equipment	2
Work environment	6
Patient assessment	1
Coordination	3

AIHW (2007)

Box 11-7 Case study of a procedure involving the wrong patient or body part

Event description

Two non-English-speaking patients, with a common surname, each presented themselves for a colonoscopy. Each was accompanied by an interpreter. A doctor called the full name of patient 1 but was answered by patient 2 and went ahead with the procedure. The identification error was discovered when patient 1 approached clinic staff after waiting 3 hours to be called. Patient 2 was then correctly identified. Both patients had been awaiting the same procedure.

Contributing factors

- *Communication:* The coincidence of two non-English-speaking patients having a common surname contributed to communication problems associated with identification of the correct patient. Absence of signage in languages other than English could have contributed to patient 2 not checking into the clinic reception.
- *Policies and procedures:* Lack of a formal process by which staff was required to positively identify each patient contributed to the incorrect patient undergoing the procedure.

Risk reduction

After the analysis of contributing causes, action was taken by the hospital to assess all of its ambulatory clinics for the adequacy of signage, in English and relevant community languages, clearly instructing patients to register at the clinic's reception. Management also actively implemented the 'correct patient, correct site, correct procedure' policy and reinforced to all staff the need to use available resources, including interpreters, to ensure correct patient identification.

AIHW (2007)

It can be seen from the case study in Box 11-7 that communication between patients and staff, and the organisation (notwithstanding the presence of an interpreter) was unsatisfactory or absent. Additionally, it appears that there was inadequate (or non-existent) implementation of a policy designed specifically to manage this risk. Both of these contributing factors are examples of system factors, and are those factors most commonly identified in all sentinel events, along with inadequate or absent 'information/ documentation' (AIHW, 2007; Victorian DHS, 2004). A more detailed understanding of these issues is beyond this text and readers are directed to the Resources on page 281.

The second most frequently reported sentinel event was 'retained instruments or other material after surgery requiring reoperation or further surgical procedure', of which there were 27 cases. Again, this is significant because of the important role perioperative nurses play in preventing such events. The contributory causes of retained items are presented in Table 11-3. The contributing factors of note are 'rules/policies/procedures', 'staff', 'equipment' and 'information/documentation'. These are further explored in the case study presented in Box 11-8, which emphasises the interplay of contributing causes, and includes the solutions offered following root cause analysis. Nursing research into the role and effectiveness of perioperative nursing standards aimed at preventing the inadvertent retention of surgical items identified similar issues (Hamlin, 2005). This research also noted the need to take a systems approach to managing the risk.

Table 11-3 Contributing factors reported for retained instruments or other material after surgery requiring reoperation or further surgical procedure, 2004–05

Contributing factors	Number of cases
Lack of, problems with or breakdown in:	
Rules/policies/procedures	7
Information/documentation	4
Communication	2
Patient factors	0
Staff factors	6
Equipment	6
Work environment	0
Patient assessment	1
Coordination	0

Note: Events for which no information on contributory factors could be extracted (1) are not included.
AIHW (2007)

A systems approach to managing risk

Commonly, sentinel events have their genesis in systems factors, which Reason (1990, 2001) has described as recurrent error traps in the workplace and the organisational processes that give rise to them. This has been clearly demonstrated in the data and case studies presented here. By acknowledging, analysing and reporting these incidents in this transparent fashion, the opportunity is created to change systems (and cultures) and subsequently to develop and implement policies to reduce or prevent them. This approach is also an example of a move away from a blame culture, which focuses on punishing individual health professionals for their mistakes and errors, to a systems-based approach to manage and prevent adverse events (ACQSHC, 2003).

In relation to the sentinel event of 'procedures involving the wrong patient or body part', the Australian Commission for Safety and Quality in Healthcare recommended that all public hospitals adopt the 'correct patient, correct site, correct procedure' protocol

Box 11-8 Case study of a retained instrument or other material after surgery requiring reoperation or further surgical procedure

Event description

A surgical sponge was reported missing after peritoneal suturing was complete and wound closure was underway. The patient had undergone a lumbar spinal fusion procedure. Sponges were inserted into the wound during a nursing shift changeover that occurred during the operation. The patient had begun to awaken from the anaesthetic when a postoperative X-ray confirmed retention of the sponge in the patient's abdomen. Immediate retrieval of the sponge was not feasible. It was removed during an uneventful return to theatre on the following day.

Contributing factors

- *Work environment:* Staff was under pressure to begin a tightly scheduled afternoon operating suite list during which lengthy procedures were to be undertaken.
- *Staff factors:* Although experienced in a wide range of surgery, it was the instrument nurse's first operation of this type. The surgeon left the operating room after peritoneal suturing was complete, leaving wound closure to the registrar.
- *Policies and procedures:* Incorrect set-up of the operating lists due to pressure to start. The registrar was unaware of a policy requiring an immediate X-ray check of the patient when a count discrepancy arose. Instead, an earlier, intraoperative X-ray that had been enhanced for a different purpose was reviewed in the first instance, with inconclusive results.
- *Communication:* The surgeon had placed sponges inside the patient during changeover, without the instrument nurse's knowledge. Once the sponge count discrepancy was realised, communication of the situation to the registered nurse coordinator was not immediate.

Risk reduction

A general review of the operating room set-up process was recommended. Specific matters for attention included the scheduling of potentially long cases and scheduled list times, the method of allocating cases and changeover strategies. A review of appropriate policy/procedures was performed to ensure that:

- the instrument nurse was notified of surgical sponges placed in cavities
- surgeons remain in the operating room until verification of the count
- discrepancies be communicated to all members of the surgical team.

The appropriateness of viewing X-ray material for other than its primary purpose was also recommended for review. The hospital is to develop strategies to ensure policy procedure compliance for all disciplines.

AIHW (2007)

to reduce the possibility of patients undergoing the wrong procedures (ACSQHC, 2003). Senior perioperative nurses and surgeons were (and remain) involved in its evolution, implementation and evaluation (Davies, 2004). As far as sentinel events in the category of 'retained instruments or other material after surgery requiring reoperation or further surgical procedure', the development of a standardised method to account for all surgical instruments, enshrined in professional standards, has a much longer history, and has always been led by perioperative nurses (Richardson, 2003). Thus, it is clear that perioperative nurses have a significant role, at all levels of the health system, to ensure that surgical care of the patient is safe and of a high quality.

CONCLUSION

This chapter examined a range of medicolegal and ethical topics as they relate to care delivery in the perioperative setting. As well as exploring the regulatory framework that governs nurses' practice, the evolving nature of that practice is also acknowledged, as are the mechanisms that have developed to accommodate the shifts. Additionally, codes of professional conduct and practice standards, and state/federal or national health ministry policies have been overviewed, with emphasis on those pertinent to perioperative settings.

At a time of intense public scrutiny and professional interest in safety and quality in health care, ways to ensure patient safety in the high-risk setting of the operating suite remain paramount. The nature of some surgical adverse events and risk management strategies to prevent them has consequently been addressed.

CRITICAL THINKING EXERCISES

1. Scope of practice

You are allocated to an operating room caring for patients undergoing procedures with which you are unfamiliar. You are working with a new graduate registered nurse, who is the anaesthetic nurse, and an endorsed, enrolled nurse, who has some experience caring for the patients in this operating room.
- What are your responsibilities here?
- How will you demonstrate your accountability?

2. Consent for surgery

You are checking a patient, Mr Papadopoulos, into the operating suite. Mr Papadopoulos is scheduled to have a transurethral resection of prostate gland and this is stated on his consent form, which he has signed and the signature witnessed. However, when you ask Mr Papadopoulos to verify the nature of the operation, his response indicates that he is unsure of the operation he is about to undergo.
- What are your responsibilities as a patient advocate in this situation? Identify the actions you would take.

3. The surgical count

You are the circulating nurse for a procedure and are working with an experienced registered nurse, who is the instrument nurse. During the course of the initial count you note that the instrument nurse is not counting items according to practices set out in your operating suite's policy manual, which is based on professional standards.
- How would you handle this situation?
- What are your professional responsibilities in relation to conducting the count of accountable items?

4. Working in the postanaesthesia recovery unit

You are working in the postanaesthesia recovery unit. It is a very busy day with several patients already in the unit, stretching your resources to the limit. Another patient arrives accompanied by the anaesthetist and the anaesthetic nurse. However, neither you nor your colleagues are able to attend to the new arrival as you cannot leave your current patients without compromising their care.
- What action should you take in this situation?

RESOURCES

Australian Bureau of Statistics
  www.abs.gov.au
Australian Capital Territory Department of Health and Community Care
  http://www.health.act.gov.au/c/health
Australian Capital Territory Nursing and Midwifery Board
  www.actnmb.act.gov.au
Australian College of Operating Room Nurses (ACORN)
  www.acorn.org.au
Australian Commission for Safety and Quality in Health Care
  www.safetyandquality.org
Australian Department of Health and Ageing
  www.health.gov.au
Australian Government Attorney General
  http://www.comlaw.gov.au/ComLaw/legislation
Australian Government—Health Insite
  www.healthinsite.gov.au
Australian Institute of Health and Welfare (AIHW)
  www.aihw.gov.au
Australian Nurse Practitioner Association
  www.nursepractitioners.org.au
Australian Nursing and Midwifery Council
  www.anmc.org.au
College of Nurses Aotearoa (NZ) Inc.
  www.nurse.org.nz
College of Nursing (NSW)
  www.nursing.aust.edu.au
Council of Australian Governments (COAG)
  www.coag.gov.au
Department of Health, Western Australia
  http://www.health.wa.gov.au/home
Department of Human Services, Victoria
  www.health.vic.gov.au
Enrolled Nurse Professional Association
  www.enpansw.org.au
Health Care Complaints Commission (NSW)
  www.hccc.nsw.gov.au
Health Practitioners Competence Assurance Act 2003 (NZ)
  www.legislation.govt.nz
Health Workforce Advisory Committee (NZ)
  http://www.hwac.govt.nz/default.htm
International Council of Nurses
  www.icn.ch
Māori Health (NZ)
  www.Māori health.govt.nz
Ministry of Health (NZ)
  www.moh.govt.nz
National Council of Māori Nurses
  http://www.ngangaru.co.nz/ncmn/resources/index.cfm?fuseaction=
  resources&fusesubaction=links

National Health and Medical Research Council
www.nhmrc.gov.au
NSW Health
www.health.nsw.gov.au
New Zealand Government—Health and Disability Commissioner
http://www.hdc.org.nz/theact/theact-thecode
New Zealand Government—legislation
http://www.legislation.govt.nz/browse_vw.asp?content-set=pal_statutes
Nurse Practioners in New Zealand
http://www.moh.govt.nz/nursepractitioner Nurse Practitioners in New Zealand
Nurses and Midwives Board, NSW
www.nmb.nsw.gov.au
Nurses and Midwives Board of Western Australia
www.nmbwa.org.au
Nurses Board of South Australia
www.nursesboard.sa.gov.au
Nurses Board of Victoria
www.nbv.org.au
Nursing Council of New Zealand
www.nursingcouncil.org.nz
Nursing and Midwifery Board of the Northern Territory
www.nt.gov.au/health/org_supp/prof_boards/nurse_midwifery/board.shtml
Nursing Board of Tasmania
www.nursingboardtas.org.au
Northern Territory Health Services
http://www.nt.gov.au/health
Perioperative Nurses College of New Zealand Nurses Organisation
http://www.nzno.org.nz/Site/Sections/Colleges/Perioperative/default.aspx
Queensland Health
www.health.qld.gov.au
Queensland Nursing Council
www.qnc.qld.gov.au
Royal College of Nursing Australia
www.rcna.org.au
South Australia Department of Human Services
http://www.dhs.sa.gov.au/index.htm
Tasmania Department of Health and Human Services
http://www.dhhs.tas.gov.au

REFERENCES

ACORN. (2006a). *ACORN standards for perioperative nursing including nursing roles, guidelines, position statements and competency standards.* Adelaide: Australian College of Operating Room Nurses.

ACORN. (2006b). *ACORN standards for perioperative nursing including nursing roles, guidelines, position statements and competency standards. S4. Disposal of surgically removed human tissue and explanted items.* Adelaide: Australian College of Operating Room Nurses.

American College of Critical Care Medicine Ethics Committee. (2001). Recommendations for non-beating organ donation. *Critical Care Medicine, 29,* 1826–1831.

ANMC. (2007). *National framework for the development of decision making tools for nursing and midwifery practice.* Retrieved August 9, 2007, from http://www.anmc.org.au/projects/current_projects.php#dmf.

ANMC. (2008). *Current projects: review of the Code of Ethics for Nurses (2002), Code of Professional Conduct for Nurses (2003).* Retrieved March 1, 2008, from http://www.anmc.org.au/projects/current_projects.php#codes.

Aspden, P. (2004). *Patient safety: achieving a new standard for care.* Washington, DC: National Academies Press.

Australian and New Zealand Organ Donation Registry. (2005). *ANZOD Registry report.* Adelaide: ANZOD.

Australian Commission for Safety and Quality in Health Care (ACSQHC). (2008). *Draft National Patient Charter of Rights.* Retrieved February 3, 2008, from: http://www.safetyandquality.org/internet/safety/publishing.nsf/Content/PriorityProgram-01.

Australian Council for Safety and Quality in Health Care (ACSQHC). (2003). *Patient safety: towards sustainable improvement. 4th report to the Australian Health Ministers' Conference.* Canberra: Department of Communications, Information Technology and the Arts.

Australian Council for Safety and Quality in Health Care (ACSQHC) and the National Institute of Clinical Studies (NICS). (2004). *Charting the safety and quality of health care in Australia.* Report presented to the Australian Health Ministers' Conference, 29 July, 2004. Retrieved August 2, 2007, from http://www.safetyandquality.org/internet/safety/publishing.nsf/Content/charting.

Australian Institute of Health and Welfare (AIHW) and the Australian Commission on Safety and Quality in Health Care (ACSQHC). (2007). *Sentinel events in Australian public hospitals 2004–05.* Canberra: AIHW. Retrieved August 23, 2007, from http://www.aihw.gov.au/publications/index.cfm/criteria/Sentinelevents.

Australian Nursing Council. (2004). *Codes of conduct and ethics.* Canberra: ANC.

Barraclough, B. (2001). Safety and quality in Australian healthcare: making progress. *Medical Journal of Australia, 174,* 616–617.

Beard, J., Ireland, L., Davis, N., et al. (2002). Tissue donation: what does it mean to families? *Program Transplant, 12,* 42–48.

Butler, M., Boxer, E., Sutherland-Fraser, S. (2003). The factors that contribute to count and documentation errors in counting: a pilot study. *ACORN Journal, 15(1),* 10–14.

Cook, R., & Conrick, M. (2006). Case study 29B Australia's Health*Connect*: delivering value for nurses and their patients. In C. Weaver, C. White Delaney, P. Weber, R. Carr (Eds.). *Nursing informatics for the 21st century: an international look at practice, trends the future* (pp. 457–462). Chicago: Healthcare Information and Management Systems Society.

Council of Australian Governments. (2006). *Health workforce.* Retrieved September 26, 2007, from http://www.coag.gov.au/meetings/140706/index.htm#health.

Cubitt, J. (2007). NSW Operating Theatre Association: President's report. *ACORN Journal, 20(1),* 46–47.

Currey, J., Dimovski, S., Treloggen, J. (2007). Organ donation and transplantation. In D. Elliott, L. Aitken, W. Chaboyer (Eds.). *ACCCN's critical care nursing.* Sydney: Elsevier.

Davies, M. (2004). NSW Operating Theatre Association: President's message. *ACORN Journal, 17(3),* 44–45.

Degeling, P., Maxwell, S., Iedema, R., Hunter, D. (2004). Making clinical governance work. *British Medical Journal, 329,* 679–681.

Fitzgerald, M., & Bull, R. (2004). The invisible nurse—behind the scenes in an Australian OR. *AORN Journal, 79(4),* 810–823.

Forrester, K., & Griffiths, D. (2005). *Essentials of law for health professionals* (2nd ed.). Sydney: Elsevier.

Gillespie, B., Wallis, M., Chaboyer, W. (2006). Clinical competence in the perioperative environment: implications for education. *ACORN Journal, 19(3),* 19–26.

Hamlin, L. (2005). *Setting the standard: the role of the Australian College of Operating Room Nurses.* Unpublished doctoral thesis, University of Technology, Sydney.

Hilbig, J. (1999). Validation of the ACORN Competencies research project report. *ACORN Journal,* 12(3), 18.

Institute of Medicine. (1999). *To err is human: building a safer health system.* Washington, DC: National Academy Press.

Kable, A., Gibberd, R., Spigelman, A. (2002). Adverse events in surgical patients in Australia. *International Journal for Quality in Healthcare, 14(4),* 269–276.

Kerr, K. (2006). Nursing and the EHR in Asia, Australasia and the South Pacific. In C. Weaver, C. White Delaney, P. Weber, R. Carr (Eds.). *Nursing informatics for the 21st century: an international look at practice, trends the future* (pp. 443–450). Chicago: Healthcare Information and Management Systems Society.

Kuiper, R. (2004). Nursing reflections from journaling during a perioperative internship. *AORN Journal, 79(1),* 195–218.

McGarvey, H., Chambers, M., Boore, J. (2000). Development and definition of the role of the operating department nurse: a review. *Journal of Advanced Nursing, 32,* 1092–1100.

Michael, R., & Williamson, C. (2006). The perioperative nurse practitioner: reality or myth? A western and eastern states' perspective. *ACORN Journal, 19(4),* 24–27.

NSW Nurses and Midwives Board. (2007). National registration update. Retrieved July 23, 2007, from http://www.nmb.nsw.gov.au/National-Registration/default.aspx.

NSW Health. (2002). Easy guide to clinical practice improvement: a guide for healthcare professionals. Sydney: NSW Health.

NSW Health. (2005). Operating suite & other procedural areas—handling of accountable items—standard procedures: PD2005_571. Retrieved July 29, 2007, from http://www.health.nsw.gov.au/policies/pd/2005/PD2005_571.html.

NZ Ministry of Health. (1987). *A code of practice for transplantation of cadaveric organs.* Wellington: NZ Ministry of Health.

NZ Ministry of Health. (2001). *Adverse events in New Zealand public hospitals: principal findings from a national survey.* Retrieved September 4, 2007, from http://www.moh.govt.nz/publications/adverse events.

NZ Ministry of Health. (2003). *The New Zealand health strategy.* Retrieved August 30, 2007, from http://www.moh.govt.nz/quality.

NZ Ministry of Health. (2006). *Nurse practitioners in New Zealand.* Retrieved September 4, 2007, from http://www.moh.govt.nz/nursepractitioner.

Nursing Council of New Zealand. (2005). *Competencies for the registered nurse scope of practice.* Retrieved July 29, 2007, from http://www.nursingcouncil.org.nz/contcomp.html#Comps.

Nursing Council of New Zealand. (2006). *Code of conduct for nurses.* Retrieved July 29, 2007, from http://www.nursingcouncil.org.nz/pub.html.

Nursing Council of New Zealand. (2007). *Competencies for the nurse practitioner scope of practice.* Retrieved July 19, 2007, from http://www.nursingcouncil.org.nz/contcomp.html#Comps.

Perioperative Nurses College New Zealand Nurses' Organisations. (2003). *Accreditation for perioperative nurses.* Retrieved July 30, 2007, from http://www.nzno.org.nz/Site/Sections/Colleges/Perioperative/Professional.aspx.

Perioperative Nurses College New Zealand Nurses' Organisations. (2005). *Standards and educational manual.* Retrieved August 20, 2007, from http://www.nzno.org.nz/Site/Sections/Colleges/Perioperative/Standguide.aspx.

Reason, J. (1990). The contribution of latent human failure to the breakdown of complex systems. *Philosophical Transactions of the Royal Society, London, 32,* 473–484.

Reason, J. (2001). Understanding adverse events: the human factor. In C. Vincent (Ed.). *Clinical risk management: enhancing patient safety* (pp. 9–30). London: BMJ Publishing.

Richardson, M. (2003). *The history of ACORN: from little acorn's grow.* Unpublished report commissioned by Australian College of Operating Room Nurses. Adelaide: ACORN.

Riley, R., & Manias, E. (2002). Foucault could have been an operating room nurse. *Journal of Advanced Nursing, 39(4),* 316–324.

Riley, R., & Peters, G. (2000). The current scope and future direction of perioperative nursing practice in Victoria, Australia. *Journal of Advanced Nursing, 32(3),* 544–553.

Rodrigue, J. R., Scott, M. P., Oppenheim, A. R. (2003). The tissue donation experience: a comparison of donor and nondonor families. *Program Transplant, 113,* 258–264.

Saba, V., & Taylor, S. (2007). Moving past theory: use of a standardized, coded nursing terminology to enhance nursing visibility. *CIN Computers, Informatics, Nursing, 25(6),* 324–331.

Schroeter, K. (2002). Ethics in perioperative practice—patient advocacy. *AORN Journal, 75(5),* 941, 943–944, 947, 949.

Staunton, P., & Chiarella, M. (2008). *Nursing and the law* (6th ed.). Sydney: Elsevier.

Streat, S., & Silvester, W. (2001). Organ donation in Australia and New Zealand: ICU perspectives. *Critical Care and Resuscitation 3,* 48–51.

Sutherland-Fraser, S. (2006). It's time to examine alternatives to the traditional staffing mix and role allocation in the perioperative environment. *ACORN Journal, 19(4),* 22–23.

University of Technology, Sydney & Sydney South West Area Health Service. (2007). *Clinical Accreditation Program (CAP) for perioperative nurses.* Unpublished curriculum document. Sydney: UTS.

Victorian Department of Human Services. (2004). *Sentinel event program.* Melbourne: VDHS. Retrieved September 13, 2007, from http://www.health.vic.gov.au/clinrisk.

Ward, K., & Hamlin, L. (2006). Lead or be led: are we ready to face the challenge? *ACORN Journal, 19(4),* 14–23.

Weaver, C. (2006). Introduction. In C. Weaver, C. White Delaney, P. Weber, R. Carr (Eds.). *Nursing informatics for the 21st century: an international look at practice, trends the future* (p. 3). Chicago: Healthcare Information and Management Systems Society.

Westbrooke, L., & Fogarty, A. (2006). The New Zealand approach to the electronic health record. In

C. Weaver, C. White Delaney, P. Weber, R. Carr (Eds.). *Nursing informatics for the 21st century: an international look at practice, trends the future* (pp. 457–462). Chicago: Healthcare Information and Management Systems Society.

Williamson, C., & Hill, V. (2007). Review of the competency standards for perioperative nursing. *ACORN, 20(2)*, 22–33.

Wilson, R., Runciman, W., Gibberd, R., Harrison, B., Newby, L., Hamilton, J. (1995). The quality in Australian health care study. *Medical Journal of Australia, 163*, 458–471.

Wilson, R., Harrison, B., Gibberd, R., Hamilton, J. (1999). An analysis of the cause of adverse events from the quality in Australian health care study. *Medical Journal of Australia, 170*, 411–415.

FURTHER READING

Barnard, A., & Locsin, R. (Eds.). (2007). *Technology and nursing practice concepts and issues.* Basingstoke, UK: Palgrave Macmillan.

Chiarella, M. (2002). *The legal and professional status of nursing.* Sydney: Elsevier.

E-Health Research Centre (E-HRC). *Annual report 2005–2006.* Retrieved September 20, 2007, from http://e-hrc.net/pubs/corporate.htm.

Hansen, D. (n.d.). *Trends in health data integration. Report of the health data integration Project, E-Health Research Centre (E-HRC).* Retrieved September 20, 2007, from http://e-hrc.net/hdi.

International Health Terminology Standards Development Organisation (IHTSDO). (n.d). *SNOMED CT FAQs.* Retrieved September 20, 2007, from http://www.ihtsdo.org/our-standards/snomed-ct.

Knight, S. (2004). The feasibility of developing interprofessional education within the perioperative setting. *Journal of Advanced Perioperative Care, 2(2)*, 41–45.

Lindwall, L., von Post, I., Eriksson, K. (2007). Caring perioperative culture: its ethos and ethic. *Journal of Advanced Perioperative Care, 3(1)*, 27–34.

Schwartz, L. (2002). Is there an advocate in the house? The role of health care professionals in patient advocacy. *Journal of Medical Ethics, 28*, 37–40.

Smith, A., Kane, M., Milne, R. (2006). Prospects for the introduction of non-physician anaesthetists in the United Kingdom: a qualitative analysis of interviews and case studies. *Journal of Advanced Perioperative Care, 2(3)*, 123–130.

Smith, J. (2003). Organ donation: what can we learn from North America? *Nursing and Critical Care, 8(4)*, 172–178.

12

Professional development and future roles and practice

Jennifer Rabach and Sally Sutherland-Fraser

LEARNING OBJECTIVES

After reading this chapter, you should be able to:

- discuss the opportunities available to nurses for entry to perioperative practice
- identify the need for ongoing professional development
- outline the role of professional perioperative nursing organisations
- discuss the importance of evidence-based nursing research for practice
- define advanced practice and opportunities for expanded scope of practice.

KEY TERMS

advanced practice	orientation programs	research
competencies	professional associations	standards for practice
evidence-based practice	professional development	

INTRODUCTION

This chapter explores perioperative nursing knowledge development and its application to perioperative patient care, as well as the professional development required of the perioperative nurse. Educational opportunities that exist from entry to practice through to postgraduate programs are identified and discussed. The development of nursing organisations is outlined, with particular emphasis on the development of international and national specialist perioperative nursing organisations and their activities. Their role in the development of standards and competencies for practice is discussed in detail. The use of evidence in providing nursing care based on research findings is highlighted. The influences on the perioperative workplace are identified and, finally, a range of advanced practice perioperative roles are described.

ENTRY TO THE PERIOPERATIVE ENVIRONMENT

There are two divisions of nurse in the Australian health care system. The first division is the registered nurse (RN) (Division 1 in Victoria and Western Australia), who, since the mid 1980s, is university prepared at the bachelor degree level. The second division is the enrolled nurse (EN, or RN Division 2, Victoria and Western Australia, hereafter referred to as EN), who is vocationally prepared at Certificate IV or diploma level. The EN provides care to patients in a model of delegation and supervision by the RN. The Australian perioperative nursing workforce includes both RNs and ENs, who do not require specialist qualifications to gain entry to this practice environment, even though perioperative nursing is recognised as an area of specialty nursing practice (Australian Health Workforce Advisory Committee [AHWAC], 2006).

Continuing education providers, such as technical and further education (TAFE) institutions, and the College of Nursing (formerly the NSW College of Nursing) offer short, introductory programs in perioperative nursing for both RNs and ENs, which do not require employment in a perioperative setting. Courses such as these can only provide an overview of the perioperative specialty; however, participation in them can demonstrate to potential employers the nurse's interest in perioperative nursing care and their desire to enter the specialty. In New Zealand, District Health Boards (DHBs) are funded to support nursing entry to practice (NETP) programs for newly graduated RNs (NZ Ministry of Health, 2006).

The registered nurse

Like many specialty areas of nursing practice that were once part of hospital-based training, perioperative nursing is no longer a core component of the undergraduate curriculum in Australia (AHWAC, 2006) or New Zealand (P. Hames, personal communication, 2007). Consequently, the newly qualified RN may have little knowledge or experience in the care of the unconscious patient during general anaesthesia and surgery, the principles of aseptic technique or the management of a patient's recovery from anaesthesia and surgery. An undergraduate curriculum that does not offer perioperative experience affects graduates as well as perioperative nurse managers. For example:

- graduates may not develop an interest in a perioperative nursing career
- graduates may have limited knowledge and inadequate perioperative nursing skills to prepare them for a role in the operating suite
- managers may be reluctant to recruit graduates to the operating suite because of their limited experience.

The international experience is similar in as much as the current perioperative recruitment issues in the United States have been linked to the loss of perioperative nursing from the undergraduate curriculum in the 1980s (Gutierrez et al., 1989; Happell, 2000; Jones & Sorrell, 1989). This is compounded by the ageing of the nursing workforce (Australian Institute of Health & Welfare [AIHW], 2005).

Opportunities for undergraduates

For undergraduate nurses in Australia and New Zealand, entry to the perioperative environment may be possible during a rotation or clinical placement on a surgical ward. Astute perioperative managers and educators will encourage these short, observational visits during undergraduate clinical placements (P. Hames, personal communication, 2007) as a means of attracting nurses to consider the specialty on graduation (NSW Operating Theatre Association, 2007).

In recent years, universities in Australia (e.g. University of Technology, Sydney) have begun to offer the perioperative specialty as an elective in second or third year nursing curricula, while others offer it as a core subject (e.g. Notre Dame University). The Australian Catholic University (ACU) has offered a perioperative elective in the final year nursing practicum since 2005, when 25 students were enrolled. This number has increased almost four-fold in the 2 years since, with 95 students enrolled in 2007 (Frotjold et al., 2007).

This growing interest in perioperative nursing at the undergraduate level echoes the findings of a US study (Gutierrez et al., 1989) and supports the inclusion of the perioperative specialty in the nursing curriculum in Australia. Effective collaborations between nursing faculties and operating suites have many benefits for potential employers. The ACU students' evaluations of the perioperative elective indicate the program's success as a recruitment strategy; 88% of students indicated that they would consider employment in the operating suite on graduation as a direct result of their positive experiences during the clinical placement. Indeed, the hospitals participating in the ACU elective have reported an increasing number of graduates recruited to the perioperative specialty since the inception of the undergraduate elective (Frotjold et al., 2007).

Clearly, undergraduate programs with outcomes such as this can have a positive impact on the graduate workforce. This is borne out by recent research in the United Kingdom (Andrews et al., 2002), which investigated the impact of clinical placements on 650 past and present nursing students. The research was carried out in two large, metropolitan universities, using questionnaires, focus groups and interviews. A key finding from the research was that the organisations that provided a supportive learning environment for the nursing students during their clinical placements became the nurses' preferred employers on graduation. The authors concluded that employers will attract and retain more nurses by creating a positive workplace—one in which learning is encouraged and supported (Andrews et al., 2002).

Opportunities for graduates

Newly graduated registered nurses also have opportunities to enter the perioperative specialty. New graduate transition programs may include a placement in (or rotation to) the operating suite; these rotations vary in duration from weeks to months, with some employers offering an entire year of specialist perioperative nursing practice. These latter 'dedicated stream' models, which include rotations to each of the perioperative roles, are suitable for graduates who have a strong desire for perioperative nursing practice as a career choice, or for those who have perioperative experience as an enrolled nurse and have subsequently completed a Bachelor of Nursing conversion course.

The shorter, 3–4 month rotation of most new graduates to the operating suite provides time beyond orientation for the nurse to explore the practice of a single perioperative role only. By the end of a 4-month rotation in anaesthetics, for example, the new graduate nurse should be able to manage the care, within a limited range of elective patients, at induction and emergence from anaesthesia with minimal direction and support. Similarly, the new graduate circulating and instrument nurse should have developed the knowledge and skills to prepare the environment, patient and equipment for a limited range of elective procedures under the guidance of an experienced nurse. During the short rotation, neither of these nurses would have developed the knowledge or skills of the other roles; however, they should have developed an understanding of the relationship between the nursing roles and the teamwork required to provide effective patient care in the perioperative environment. Longer rotations, such as the 'dedicated stream' models, do allow movement within the full range of perioperative roles.

The enrolled nurse

The educational preparation of the EN in Australia has undergone intensive review in recent years in response to the National Review of Nursing Education (Australian Department of Education, Science and Training [DEST], 2002). A key recommendation was the development of a national qualification that would incorporate the EN competencies of the Australian and Nursing Council (ANC), now known as the Australian Nursing and Midwifery Council (ANMC). This has culminated in the development of the Health Training Package HLT07 (Certificate IV, Diploma and Advanced Diploma in Enrolled Nursing/ Division 2 Nursing), which is available for delivery across Australia (Community Services & Health Industry Skills Council [CS&HISC], 2007). New Zealand does not have an EN category; the entry level for all nurses is registration via a 3-year bachelor degree program (NZ Ministry of Health, 2007).

The availability of the health training package in Australia means that the EN qualification will be delivered by a greater number of providers. Previously, the largest provider of the EN qualification in Australia has been TAFE institutions, which are the vocational arms of the state and territory departments of education and training. Some, but not all, of the TAFE pre-enrolment programs have included employment in a hospital setting with the potential for a clinical rotation to the operating suite. The benefit of such a rotation is that trainee ENs can observe and practise the beginning skills of the perioperative nurse in preparation for permanent employment in a perioperative setting.

ENs may work in the anaesthetic nurse role with or without a post-enrolment qualification, such as the Certificate IV in Anaesthetic Technology (CS&HISC, 2007). Those ENs who posses this qualification are able to function in the role of anaesthetic technician. A smaller number of perioperative ENs may work in the circulating and instrument nurse role; however, there are fewer post-enrolment qualifications for this specialised role, which has most often been performed by the RN within Australian jurisdictions (NSW Health, 2007b). As opportunities increase for advanced practice roles for RNs, so too, will opportunities increase for ENs. This is explored further under advanced practice on pages 301–302.

ORIENTATION AND CLINICAL PROGRAMS

Without exposure to the perioperative environment, the majority of nursing graduates, be they RNs or ENs, will have received little theory or clinical practice in the care of the perioperative patient during their initial education. Operating suites that do attract graduates to specialty practice must, therefore, provide comprehensive **orientation** and clinical programs to equip these new recruits for a role in the perioperative environment. Table 12-1 lists activities that are appropriate for inclusion in an orientation program.

Table 12-1 Sample content of a 5-day orientation program
Perioperative roles

1. Medicolegal principles and policy
  • Consent for surgery
  • Patient identification and 'time out'
  • Documentation and the surgical count
  • Negligence and examples of case law

2. Patient and environmental safety
3. Principles of asepsis and infection control
4. Sterilisation and sterile supplies

5. Patient care during anaesthesia
  • Airway management
  • General and regional anaesthesia
  • Pharmacology and preparation of equipment for anaesthesia

6. Patient care during surgery
  • Positioning
  • Sterile technique, skin preparation and draping
  • Electrosurgery

7. Postoperative patient care
  • Patient assessment and postoperative complications
  • Pain management
  • Preparation for discharge

South Eastern Sydney Illawarra Area Health Service (2006)

The Association of periOperative Registered Nurses (AORN) in the United States offers the 'Perioperative Curriculum 101', which was first developed in 1999 and is now available as an online educational resource (AORN, 2007). Members of the Perioperative Nurses College (PNC) of the New Zealand Nurses Organisation (PNCNZNO) are able to purchase a perioperative education manual, which has been approved by the New Zealand Nurses Organisation (Marenzi, 2006). A key goal of the PNC is the establishment of a national perioperative education program and, to this end, the College structure includes an education subcommittee.

Currently, there is no equivalent program offered by the Australian College of Operating Room Nurses (ACORN). Orientation to specialty practice, therefore, is provided by individual healthcare facilities in Australia (ACORN, 2007) and, in some cases, centralised orientation and clinical programs are provided across an organisation or health service. The duration of these programs ranges from a few days orientation to 6-month or 12-month extended clinical programs. These extended programs may supplement the content of new graduate RN rotations, or they may provide an alternative pathway to specialty practice as part of an organisational recruitment strategy (South Eastern Sydney Illawarra Area Health Services, 2007).

In addition to a structured orientation, extended programs offer a theoretical framework of regular study days, as well as supported clinical practice and assessment. Extended programs may also be recognised for subject credit in tertiary-level graduate programs. This relationship exists between Deakin University and Barwon Health in Victoria, Adelaide University and the Royal Adelaide Hospital in South Australia and, in New South Wales, the ACU and St Vincent's Hospital, as well as the Wollongong University and Wollongong Hospital, to name just a few examples.

ONGOING PROFESSIONAL DEVELOPMENT

Progress along the nursing career pathway requires a commitment to ongoing education and **professional development**. This commitment is even more important in specialty areas such as perioperative nursing, where technology, health policy and nursing practice are continually developing and changing (Senate Community Affairs References Committee, 2002). The knowledge and skills that the beginning RN or EN develops during the orientation period are the foundation upon which specialty practice is built. Ongoing perioperative nursing practice requires the acquisition of further qualifications and/or work experience. The role that training and education plays in the elevation of the profession's status is explored on page 293.

Formal development

Australian and New Zealand universities and colleges provide a range of postgraduate programs for perioperative nurses, including graduate certificates, graduate diplomas, masters and doctoral programs. Historically, hospital-based certificates were the mainstay of professional development courses for perioperative nurses (AHWAC, 2006). Even though certificates were available for anaesthetic and postanaesthesia recovery unit (PARU) nurses, there were many more for instrument and circulating nurses. These certificates were routinely of 12 months' duration, during which time the students were required to rotate through the major surgical specialties, as well anaesthetics and PARU.

Since the transition of nursing education to the tertiary sector in the mid 1980s, these certificates have disappeared from hospitals; however, some have re-emerged (in somewhat smaller numbers) as graduate certificate courses in the tertiary sector. There are some notable exceptions as a few facilities continue to offer hospital-based programs, including the Fremantle Hospital in Western Australia, the Queen Elizabeth Hospital in South Australia, and the Liverpool Hospital in New South Wales (AHWAC, 2006). In New Zealand, the DHBs fund postgraduate nursing studies based on local need, as well as providing clinical learning placements (NZ Ministry of Health, 2007).

In a survey of Australian course coordinators in 2005, the Australian Health Workforce Advisory Committee (AHWAC, 2006) identified 16 providers of postgraduate programs for perioperative nurses. This figure included the three hospitals mentioned above, 12 universities and the College of Nursing. At the time, students enrolled in perioperative specialisations outnumbered anaesthetic and PARU students by 3:1, echoing the trend seen in hospital-based certificates (AHWAC, 2006).

The AHWAC noted that, at the time, there were no providers of postgraduate perioperative programs in the Australian Capital Territory, Northern Territory or Tasmania. Residents of these jurisdictions would, however, be able to access distance (online) programs, such as those offered by Curtin University in Western Australia or the distance education courses offered by the College of Nursing. In New Zealand, the Auckland University, Massey University and the Whitireia Community Polytechnic offer postgraduate education for perioperative nurses (P. Hames, personal communication, 2007).

Informal or continuing education

In 2002, the Senate Inquiry into Nursing reported that continuing education for perioperative nurses was:

... essential for the ongoing maintenance of professional expertise and therefore professional standards. With the rapid development of new technologies in the operating room environment, nurses need access to professional development programs on a regular basis (Senate Community Affairs References Committee, 2002, p 192).

The Senate Inquiry made a number of suggestions, including the need for more opportunities for specialist nurses, in particular, to maintain knowledge and skills. At much the same time, another review into the nursing profession was underway in Australia. Not surprisingly, similar themes emerged. The National Review of Nursing Education also recommended that nurses undertake lifelong learning as a means of maintaining competence (Australian DEST, 2002).

Even though nurses may recognise the need to maintain their competence to practise, they may not recognise the broad range of continuing education activities that are available in the perioperative environment. Informal teaching and learning activities are no less valid than formal courses as a demonstration of the nurse's commitment to lifelong learning. Such activities might include participation in:

- professional associations, particularly perioperative organisations
- informal tutorials by colleagues
- clinical instruction and demonstrations
- journal clubs or engaging with audiovisual material
- short courses, and attendance at seminars and conferences.

Professional portfolios can be used to record these activities and will, more importantly, provide an effective mechanism for the nurse to reflect on practice. In fact, self-reflection is vital because it ensures that the individual nurse's portfolio is more than a list of activities completed, but rather it enables the nurse to demonstrate what has been achieved through participation in the activities (McMullan et al., 2003).

A commitment to lifelong learning is not simply valued by the nursing profession; nursing and midwifery registering authorities have begun to stipulate continuing education hours as a requirement for annual licence renewal (ANMC, 2006a; National Nursing and Nursing Education Taskforce [N3ET], 2006). The ANMC's position is articulated in its Continuing Competence Framework (ANMC, 2007b). This framework comprises the elements of:

- self-assessment
- continuing professional development
- practice hours.

The professional portfolio is recognised here as one of the best methods for nurses to document their maintenance of competence (ANMC, 2007b; Davies & Hamlin, 2003). Certainly, then, the professional portfolio can serve many purposes for the perioperative nurse.

PERIOPERATIVE NURSES AS PROFESSIONALS

The division of labour is also a division of knowledge, with consequential implications of reciprocal dependence and vulnerability between participants (Dingwall & Lewis, 1983, p 12).

In Australia in the 1880s, assisting surgeons during operations was fundamental to the work of all nurses because they attended operations in the home, hospital ward and operating suite. Initially, all nurses were trained to meet the skill requirements of this role: to prepare patients, the environment, the necessary equipment and dressings, and then assist patients to recover from their operation. As with any occupation, it was important for nursing to gain recognition as a profession because it carried with it status and security; furthermore, as with any occupation, professional status provides a basis for protection from occupational competition (Freidson, 1983).

As medical specialties developed, nursing specialties emerged alongside to meet gaps in skills and knowledge. Training was important in elevating nursing's professional status (Bessant & Bessant, 1991). Freidson (1994) argued that the division of labour is specialisation and that (former) operating suite nursing is an example of a dynamic nursing specialty that continues to evolve into super-specialty areas of skills and knowledge that are not constrained by geographical boundaries. For example, within perioperative nursing, nurses may specialise and work exclusively in areas such as cardiothoracic surgery or neurosurgery, or they move into day surgery settings and work across the continuum of ambulatory patient care.

As nursing evolved from a service to a trained practice, and scientific and technological advances developed in medicine, nurses were measured not only by their character but increasingly by their technical skills and knowledge, which gave them portability to practice in the hospital or to work privately. Perioperative nurses, as with other specialist nurses, are identified not only by the geographical locus of work (in this case operating suites, perioperative units, outpatient clinics and day surgery units) but also by their specialist skills and knowledge. That is, their specialist skills and knowledge admit them into a world of specialist practice as a professional and differentiate them from generalist nurses (Heartfield, 2006).

There has been much debate among nurses (and others) about whether nursing has achieved professional status (Schwirian, 1998). Although there is no universally accepted definition, the term 'profession' refers to an occupation that controls its own boundaries of work, is organised by a set of institutions and is informed by a particular ideology of expertise and service. While the line between nursing and domestic service could hardly be drawn in the mid-19th century (Rosenberg, 1987) and the term 'quintessential domestic scientists' was used to describe nurses at this time (Bashford, 2000), operating room nurses made sense of germ theory and incorporated this knowledge into their practice to make it more scientific. As anaesthesia advanced and the complexity of surgery increased, so too did the range of the nurse's skills, and an occupational gap was created for a worker with specialised knowledge and skills to care for patients, but mainly to assist surgeons during operations. Technical virtuosity was inextricably related to status for institutions as well as individuals (Rosenberg, 1987).

Control over the labour market is one of the defining characteristics of a profession and this may be achieved by giving credentials to members of the profession (Leicht & Fennell, 2001). Individually, most nurses have limited control over their work, and the role of the perioperative nurse is constantly being renegotiated by policy makers, nurses and employers. Because of this renegotiation, specialist nurses are never secure in their role. The renegotiation is played out in the contest for physical and professional space in the operating room, where medical and nursing hierarchies are often reinforced (Lingard et al., 2002).

PROFESSIONAL ASSOCIATIONS

The role of professional associations

Professional associations may be defined as those whose primary purposes are to protect, enhance and advance the common interests of the organisation, and their professional and non-professional members. They operate at local, state, national and international levels, and perform a number of functions, including gaining support through political lobbying, providing education, and developing standards for practice, care-givers, resources and the environment. These activities may also include establishing and enforcing a code of ethics, stimulating and promoting the professional development of practitioners, and ensuring members' financial and general welfare (Brooks & Berman Brown, 2002). For nurses, they also provide an opportunity to develop a bigger picture of nursing and health care overall (Frank, 2005).

From a sociological perspective, professional organisations are a convenient way of mobilising practitioners' allegiance to the profession (Freidson, 1983, 1994). The nursing profession is no exception and the role of one of the earliest Australian organisations, the Australasian Trained Nurses' Association, which was formed in 1899, was to protect the public from ignorant and incompetent nurses, to improve and standardise general nurse training and to promote the professionalisation of trained nurses (Hamlin, 2005).

In Australia and New Zealand, more than 60 professional nursing organisations represent clinical, managerial, educational, research-based and industrial interests. Most have small membership numbers, and this proliferation of organisations can be counterproductive to the overall aims and goals of nursing. In Australia, the two most significant national nursing organisations are the Royal College of Nursing, Australia (RCNA), which is affiliated with the International Council of Nurses (ICN), and the Australian Nurses Federation (ANF), which is an industrial body. Both have state branches or chapters. Many of the state and national specialist organisations are part of a coalition, the National Nursing Organisations (NNO). Formed in 1991, the NNO acts as a lobby group and provides a forum for discussion about future directions in nursing. Importantly, recent work conducted by an NNO workgroup and funded through the National Nursing and Nursing Education Taskforce (NNO, 2006), resulted in the publication of a toolkit on governance standards for nursing and midwifery organisations. The toolkit is in the process of being implemented by several national specialist nursing organisations and should result in an improvement in the governance of them, and better accountability to members.

In New Zealand, there is one coalition of all nurses' organisations, called the New Zealand Nurses Organisation (NZNO), which is affiliated with the ICN. It is the largest union and professional organisation of nurses, midwives and caregivers in that country and, in serving both the professional and industrial needs of nurses, is similar to the Royal College of Nursing (RCN) in the United Kingdom.

However, specialist organisations, such as those of interest to perioperative nurses, generally better meet the interests of their membership because they are focused largely on the specialty of interest (Hamlin, 2005). Contemporary nurses must be committed to lifelong learning in order to maintain their nursing registration and to practise safely. Although few of the specialist professional organisations offer formal education programs, they meet a need for ongoing development in the specialist nursing community by providing continuing education for their members. This is through their national, state or regional member groups, which organise study days, seminars and conferences, and via publication of journals and newsletters. These activities also provide opportunities for networking with specialist colleagues. Perioperative organisations are examined in closer detail below.

Perioperative nursing associations

As well as writing standards for practice and conducting conferences and educational meetings, most specialist nursing organisations, including perioperative associations, publish journals or newsletters and have established websites. The opportunities provided by professional associations include:

- networking opportunities
- mentoring opportunities
- opportunities to learn about specialist practice
- point of contact for government for policy consultation
- opportunities to input into policy-making and represent the profession
- provision of standards for practice in an area of specialist practice
- educational activities
- journals and newsletters
- scholarships for study
- research grants
- clinical education
- accreditation of members
- accreditation of education programs.

Australia

In Australia, there are six state- or territory-based perioperative nursing organisations, which (with the exception of the NT Perioperative Nurses group) evolved independently during the 1950s and 1960s. They subsequently joined forces to form the Australian College (formerly the Confederation) of Operating Room Nurses in 1977 (Hamlin, 2005). The state/territory groups that are branches of ACORN include the:

- Victorian Perioperative Nurses Group (VPNG)
- NSW Operating Theatre Association Inc. (NSWOTA) (which incorporates the ACT)
- Perioperative Nurses Association of Queensland (PNAQ)
- Tasmanian Operating Room Nurses (TORN)
- Operating Room Nurses Association (ORNA) of Western Australia
- SA Perioperative Nurse Association (SAPNA)
- NT Perioperative Nurses (NTPN).

As with many clinically oriented professional associations, ACORN is focused on improving and standardising nursing care, and educating and supporting nurses. In ACORN's case, the focus occurs within perioperative settings. The formation of ACORN was deemed necessary because of a wide variety in practice in operating suites at the time and, in many areas, no written standards (Hamlin, 2005). This was believed by perioperative nurse leaders to be a significant deficit in perioperative nursing care. Of particular concern at that time was the need to standardise the way the surgical count was conducted (Richardson, 2004). Another key driver was organising and conducting a national conference every 3 years to bring operating room nurses together nationally to discuss perioperative nursing issues.

In the early 1990s, ACORN funded a 6-year research project, which identified and subsequently validated the ACORN competency standards for perioperative nurses (the **competencies**) (Hilbig, 1999). These were published in 1999 (ACORN, 1999) and a research project to revalidate them was completed in 2006 (Williamson & Hill, 2007). However, ACORN has previously rejected the development of an accreditation service. ACORN has also funded the development, writing and introduction of a curriculum to prepare nurses for the extended role of perioperative nurse surgeon's assistant (PNSA) in conjunction with the Southern Cross University (NSW) (Richardson, 2004). However, it has no formal relationship with this university currently.

Although ACORN is a member of the NNO, it remains an independent, limited company. The state/territory perioperative nursing associations, even though they are branches of ACORN, are themselves independently incorporated entities (with the exception of VPNG). Neither state branches nor ACORN itself meet perioperative nurses' industrial needs.

Two or three of ACORN's state or territory member organisations previously had a relationship with the ANF, an industrial organisation. This remains the case for VPNG, which is a special interest group of ANF (Victorian Branch). Consequently, although VPNG is a member of ACORN, it is more closely associated legally with ANF (Victorian Branch).

New Zealand

In contrast to ACORN, the PNC is an affiliated NZNO. The PNC has a membership of 680 nurses across nine member regions (Marenzi, 2006). These are Auckland, Central North Island, Hawke's Bay, Ruahine/Egmont, Wellington, Nelson/Marlborough, Canterbury/West Coast, Otago and Southland.

The PNC is closely associated legally with the NZNO. It has similar goals to that of most national perioperative organisations, which include:

- provision of leadership in perioperative matters
- development of standards for perioperative nursing
- publication of a journal, *Dissector*, on a quarterly basis
- national and international representation and promotion of perioperative nursing
- provision of education programs—an annual conference on perioperative issues and an education manual for perioperative nurses (PNC, n.d.).

The PNC provides a national perioperative nursing education program and offers endorsed modules, which give successful students advanced standing when completing further studies in some NZ tertiary institutions. PNC also offers an accreditation process for perioperative nurses. The PNC model for accreditation was developed during 2000–01 and the first perioperative nurses were accredited in 2003. These processes were recently re-endorsed by the Board of the NZNO (Board of Directors, 2007). The PNC appears to be proactive on many professional issues and, at an annual conference in Invercargill in 2006, concern was raised by members about roles not being performed by nurses in the operating room; a working party was formed to address this issue (Nelson, 2006).

International perioperative organisations

Globally, the International Federation of Perioperative Nurses (IFPN) is an organisation of national perioperative nursing organisations. The IFPN promotes education and research for nurses in perioperative settings to provide best practice based on the latest and best available evidence. The member associations of IFPN include:

- Association for Perioperative Practice, UK (AfPP)
- Association of periOperative Registered Nurses, USA (AORN)
- Australian College of Operating Room Nurses (ACORN)
- European Operating Room Nurses Association (EORNA)
- Japan Operative Nursing Academy (JONA)
- Korean Association of Operating Room Nurses (KAORN)
- National Nurses Association of Kenya—Theatre Nurses Chapter
- Operating Room Nurses Association of Canada (ORNAC)
- Papua New Guinea Perioperative Nurses Association
- Perioperative Nurses College New Zealand (PNCNZ)
- South African Theatre Nurses (SATS)
- Thailand Operating Room Nurses (TORN).

The IFPN is particularly committed to improving standards of patient care in developing countries, and its activities are focused on providing universally applicable guidelines for practice, which IFPN Board members develop. Some of the IFPN guidelines, which are available on their website (see Resources), include:

- surgical counts
- general hand washing
- surgical hand washing
- surgical site skin preparation
- sterilisation and disinfection
- use of protective eyewear
- use of masks in the perioperative environment.

The IFPN is a member of the International Council of Nursing (ICN), a global federation of national nurses' associations. The ICN works globally and the focus of its activities is to ensure quality nursing care, sound health policies globally and the advancement of nursing knowledge (ICN, n.d.).

Many other organisations represent nurses working in a diversity of roles in perioperative settings. The European Operating Room Nurses Association (EORNA) is another international specialist nursing organisation that represents perioperative nurses and is now a member of IFPN.

Other professional associations, such as the Association of periOperative Registered Nurses (AORN) in the United States, the Association for Perioperative Practice (AfPP) in the United Kingdom and the Operating Room Nurses Association Canada (ORNAC), also provide a variety of educational opportunities and other benefits. An important difference between the AfPP and other national nursing organisations is that the AfPP represents non-nurses working in the perioperative setting. This is a critical issue for the specialist nursing organisations, as well as much more widely, because, as the nursing workforce ages, members will retire and membership numbers will start to decline.

STANDARDS FOR PRACTICE

The ANMC provides competency standards for Nurse Practitioners, RNs and ENs, as well as codes of practice and conduct; the NZ Nursing Council performs a similar role in New Zealand. More recently, the ANMC published a decision-making framework (ANMC, 2007a), which has subsequently informed the activities of the state- and territory-based nurse regulatory authorities in Australia. Standards for practice, including competency standards (hereafter called standards for practice and/or competency), have also been developed by many of the specialist nursing organisations over the last decade. They both inform and underpin specialty nursing practice.

Practice standards

Many professional nursing organisations now view the development of **standards for practice** as part of their role and in Australia this has led to the development of a plethora of standards by the clinical specialty organisations. This includes ACORN, which has been involved in the publication of standards for use in perioperative settings since its inception, and the PNC, which publishes standards and guidelines for safe practice for perioperative nurses in New Zealand (2005).

ACORN's standards for perioperative nursing, including nursing roles, guidelines, position statements and competencies (the ACORN standards), were first published in 1980 (without competency standards) by the (then) Australian Confederation of

Operating Room Nurses and have since been regularly reviewed, revised and updated (Richardson, 2004). Although initially published every 3 years, they are now published biennially, which is a reflection of the dynamic perioperative environment. Table 12-2 provides a summary overview of the ACORN standards.

Table 12-2 An overview of the ACORN Standards	
ACORN Standard	**Summary**
Standards (24)	These incorporate: • seven direct clinical care standards (e.g. S2 'Aseptic technique') • two standards that are specific to controlling or managing the perioperative environment (e.g. S6 'Environmental management') • nine standards that address both direct patient care and environmental management issues (e.g. S22 'Use of high level disinfection in the perioperative environment') • two standards that relate to nursing staff, and their management and development (e.g. S10 'Performance management') • four standards that address quality management, patient safety and risk management (e.g. S17 'Risk management').
Nursing roles (7)	Seven perioperative nursing role descriptions (e.g. NR4 'The instrument nurse').
Guidelines (4)	Each of the four guidelines has a management focus and addresses management of the perioperative environment and the PARU, planning and design of the perioperative environment, and budget preparation.
Position statements (11)	• Two position statements address direct patient care (e.g. PS6 'Ensuring correct patient, correct site, correct procedure'). • Two statements address staff support (e.g. PS3 'Bullying and harassment'). • Two statements are about legal or documentation issues (e.g. PS7 'Legal implications'). • One statement is about nursing research. • Two statements address roles in the perioperative environment (e.g. PS1 'Advanced practice nurse and nurse practitioner roles'). • Two standards are about nurse education (e.g. PS9 'Postgraduate nursing').
Competency standards (11)	Each of the competency standards, which include criteria and elements, address all aspects of contemporary perioperative nursing practice.

Competency standards

The term 'competency' may be defined as 'the ability to perform the activities within an occupation or function to the standard expected in employment' (Heywood et al.,

1992, p 99). Competency standards specify the level of achievement expected, and the tasks and contexts of professional practice in which competency may be demonstrated (Gonczi et al., 1990). In a nursing context, and for the purposes of this discussion, competency is defined as, 'The combination of skills, knowledge, attitudes, values and abilities that underpin effective and/or superior performance in a profession/occupational area' (ANMC, 2006c, p 8).

RN and EN competency standards were first published by the ANMC in the 1990s, and most of the specialist colleges, including ACORN and PNC, have now published their own competency standards for specialist practice. A proliferation of nursing specialty competency documents are available; additionally, the ANF published competency standards for the advanced nurse in 1997, which have subsequently been revised and validated as the competency standards for the advanced RN (ANF, 2006). The terminology associated with specialist and advanced practice remains confusing despite being addressed comprehensively in a publication by the National Nursing and Nursing Education Taskforce (Heartfield, 2006).

The use of competency standards is contentious and, while their stated intent is to indicate a minimum standard of practice, provide evidence to the public that professionals are competent in meeting a standard of care and guide curriculum content, little is actually known about their dissemination, uptake or how they impact on specialist nurses and/or practice settings (Hendry et al., 2007).

EVIDENCE-BASED PRACTICE

Nursing **research** is essential to providing optimal patient care and ensuring that patient outcomes are based on contemporary knowledge. It is critical that nursing care be evidence-based and that nurses know how to access research, interpret it and then implement findings as appropriate. Excellence in the delivery of quality nursing care is achieved by translating research into **evidence-based practice** (EBP) and then evaluating its effectiveness in terms of patient outcomes.

Becoming a consumer of research

The Joanna Briggs Institute is an international research and development agency, made up of 26 interdisciplinary collaborating centres, incorporating nursing and midwifery research findings. Membership is required to access most of its materials. The Cochrane Collaboration is an easily accessible resource for nurses and contains a large number of research reviews. Although largely medically focused, the Cochrane Collaboration provides summaries of the latest research findings that may be useful to nurses. The Cochrane Collaboration uses systematic reviews of the effects of health care interventions to provide the latest information to improve health care delivery.

In order to use these resources effectively and incorporate research into clinical practice, nurses need to be able to appraise research. In the workplace, nurses need to be confident in their skill level in the critical analysis of research and evaluation. Experience in conducting literature reviews and searching databases assists in building confidence. Increasingly, this knowledge is gained via formal postgraduate education. Other reliable sources of information are specialty specific journals, such as the *Journal of Advanced Perioperative Care* (JAPC), *Journal of Perioperative Practice* (JPP) and *AORN Journal*; other sources include the *Journal of Clinical Nursing*, *Journal of Advanced Nursing*, *Australian Journal of Advanced Nursing* and *The Collegian*.

The benefits of evidence utilisation are well documented in the literature and most health care facilities now have an emphasis on the provision of cost-effective quality care. This means that perioperative nurses must make judgements about the appropriateness and possible effectiveness of different treatment regimens, while at the same time taking cost into account. Confidence in the effectiveness of the nursing intervention is also an important factor. This requires that nurses know how to quickly search and access the data, evaluate the latest findings and make considered judgements about treatment options for best outcomes. Areas of perioperative nursing practice that have proved of interest to researchers include examining hand antisepsis practices (Tanner et al., 2007) double gloving (Tanner & Parkinson, 2002), the surgical count (Hamlin, 2005) and communication in the operating room (Lingard et al., 2002).

While EBP is increasingly being used by nurses, the role of professional associations in undertaking or supporting the dissemination of results or otherwise using research findings is very limited (Holleman et al., 2006). In their study of international professional associations, including Australia, Holleman et al. (2006) discovered that most EBP activities were competence- and attitude-oriented, suggesting that an effective course of action would be for organisations to target members to establish a link between their association membership. A level of commitment on the part of members could be made and then a stronger professional profile promoted.

FUTURE PERIOPERATIVE ROLES

In an era of rapid technological advancement, the delivery of a safe and efficient health service requires a highly educated and flexible health workforce. Several reviews of the Australian health workforce have been undertaken in recent years. These include:

- *The perioperative workforce in Australia* (AHWAC, 2006)
- *Our duty of care: the national review of nursing and nursing education* (Australian DEST, 2002)
- *The patient profession: a time for action* (Senate Community Affairs References Committee, 2002)
- *Australia's health workforce: Productivity Commission research report* (Productivity Commission, 2006).

All reviews have made numerous recommendations, including some related to advanced practice. The most significant report was *Australia's health workforce* from the Productivity Commission (2006). It identified the need for workforce innovation, with a particular emphasis on the development of roles that cross professional boundaries. In the perioperative environment, roles that might cross professional boundaries of doctors include perioperative Nurse Practitioner roles, and ancillary workers' roles, which might cross the professional boundaries of nurses. The report warns that changes in one area can have flow-on effects in other areas; for example, 'enhancing the ability for nurses to substitute for doctors in some areas could exacerbate an existing nursing shortage' (Productivity Commission, 2006, p 58).

The RCNA (2007) acknowledges the need for these workforce innovations and supports a collaborative approach to the development of new roles, advising that this must be primarily in response to the changing health care needs of the community. The RCNA advocates for regulation of any new roles as a means of ensuring public safety and providing uniformity with new practice boundaries.

This is a complex issue for the perioperative environment, where ancillary workers, doctors and nurses work effectively in many combinations and teams. Ancillary workers have varying levels of education and skills sets, and work as assistants in nursing, and as orderlies and healthcare assistants. Unlike doctors and nurses, these roles are not regulated, and without regulation there may be a lack of clarity about professional boundaries, as well as limited accountability, in the delivery of patient care. However, national, competency-based education packages at certificate and diploma level have been developed and published recently (CS&HISC, 2007), which is an important step. Clear policies and practice guidelines, as well as collaboration and multidisciplinary educational support, are required to ensure that all members of the perioperative team continue to have the knowledge and skills required for safe patient care.

In Australian and New Zealand operating rooms, ancillary workers represent a small but important part of the workforce. ACORN's position on ancillary workers is that they must work under the supervision and management of appropriately educated and experienced RNs at all times (ACORN, 2006c), providing indirect patient care only. It remains to be seen if this position is sustainable in the future, especially as it is not the case in the United Kingdom, where the RN works in a team that includes diploma-prepared, non-nurse, operating department practitioners who undertake activities traditionally completed by nurses. Similarly, in the United States, the non-nursing role of the scrub technologist is one that is supervised by the RN circulating nurse. In many US states, legislation has been enacted to ensure that there is at least one RN present in the operating room, working as the circulating nurse (AORN, 2006a, 2006b, 2008a, 2008b), to oversee nursing care and supervise these workers.

Discussions about professional boundaries in the perioperative environment remain controversial, both here (NSW Operating Theatre Association, 2007) and overseas. Letters to the editor from nurses and operating department practitioners in Australian and British publications suggest that opinions are diverse and the debate seems likely to continue for some time (Anonymous, 2008; Fletcher, 2008; Goodley et al., 2008).

Advanced practice

Advanced practice can be defined as practice in which the nurse uses an extended knowledge and skills base to initiate the delivery of complex nursing care, either autonomously or in a model of collaboration with the health care team (RCNA, 2006). However, there is no absolute consensus; for example, the National Nursing and Nursing Education Taskforce (N3ET) draws the distinction between practice that is 'extended', such as the performance of tasks (medication administration), and practice that is 'advanced', such as the performance of a role at an advanced level (N3ET, 2005b).

The advanced RN demonstrates critical reflection, decision-making and problem-solving skills and functions within a nursing framework that includes assessment and diagnosis, planning, implementation and evaluation of care. Further, advanced practice is the foundation from which the Nurse Practitioner role develops (ACORN, 2006b; ANMC, 2006b; Nurse Practitioner Advisory Committee of New Zealand, 2006; RCNA, 2006). The Nurse Practitioner role has evolved over the last two decades or so in Australia and New Zealand, with Nurse Practitioners authorised to prescribe medications, order diagnostic tests and make referrals, which are activities traditionally performed by medical practitioners. Thus, Nurse Practitioners work at an advanced practice level in an extended role (N3ET, 2006). In Australia, the title and role of Nurse Practitioner is protected by legislation (ANMC, 2006b). ACORN recognises advanced practice perioperative nursing roles and supports those nurses who are in transition towards Nurse Practitioner roles. ACORN's position is underpinned by the views of both the RCNA and the ANMC, and acknowledges the legislative and regulatory framework in which Nurse Practitioner must work (see Ch 11). As mentioned previously, the National Nursing and Nursing Education Taskforce has also completed work more generally on advanced practice roles and the role of the Nurse Practitioner (N3ET, 2005a).

Even though Nurse Practitioner roles are slowly emerging within the Australian perioperative workforce (Michael, 2007; Ward & Hamlin, 2006), advanced practice roles already exist for both the RN and EN. The perioperative nurse surgeon's assistant (PNSA) is perhaps the most recognised advanced practice role for the RN, and the instrument nurse is an advanced practice role for ENs. Advanced practice roles also exist for anaesthetic and PARU RNs in areas such as pain management and intravenous access. Advanced practice roles may develop without the support and structure of formal education; however, completion of a recognised program may be a requirement of employers or professional bodies (ACORN, 2006a).

Advanced practice registered nurse

The PNSA is an advanced practice role for RNs and includes all stages of patient care delivery. Most notably during the intraoperative stage, the PNSA provides surgical and technical support, such as tissue retraction and dissection, haemostasis and wound closure as the surgeon's first assistant (ACORN, 2006a). While many consider this to be a new role, nurses have assisted with the technical aspects of surgery in the past. Today, the role of the PNSA may extend into the preoperative stage and include patient assessments, patient history taking and patient education (Brennan, 2001). The PNSA may also evaluate the patient's care during the postoperative stage and collaborate with the surgical team in preparation for the patient's discharge. However, there is no published evidence about the number of PNSAs or how their roles are enacted.

Educational preparation of the PNSA has been provided in Australia since 2000 as a result of an innovative collaboration between ACORN and the Southern Cross University in New South Wales (Brennan, 2000). This university remains the single provider for the PNSA course in Australia. The role has been picked up mostly by the private sector and in rural areas of Australia, complementing the dwindling supply of general practitioner surgical assistants (Brennan, 2001). Even though nurses develop the knowledge and skills required of the PNSA role as a result of informal, on-the-job education and instruction, the ACORN position description for the PNSA nurse stipulates that a PNSA course is a mandatory qualification for the role (ACORN, 2006a). It is important to note that, during surgery, while the PNSA may also be a perioperative nurse, he or she should not concurrently function as the instrument nurse. Equally, the perioperative nurse should not perform the activities of the surgical assistant without the appropriate education and credentials (Campbell, 2001). It is important to note that, while the PNSA is recognised as a perioperative advanced practice role, it is not a Nurse Practitioner role and does not have prescribing or referral privileges. ACORN acknowledges, however, that the PNSA role has the potential to develop into a perioperative Nurse Practitioner role (ACORN, 2006b).

Internationally, there are many other advanced practice roles for the perioperative nurse, many of which have been developed in response to the current and expected workforce shortages of medical staff (see Table 12-3). In the United Kingdom, the National Health Service Knowledge and Skills Framework (NHS KSF) was implemented in 2004, in response to the 'Agenda for Change'. This involved a single pay system for the health workforce, excluding doctors and dentists, and was expected to simplify the development of extended roles and to provide greater flexibility across all roles (UK Department of Health, 2007). Not all stakeholders, however, have viewed these new roles in a positive light, particularly when these roles are seen to cross the professional boundaries of doctors. In a recent development in the United Kingdom, nurses have been trained to perform surgical procedures in some National Health Service hospitals, a move which some surgeons and consumer groups have labelled as dangerous and unnecessary (Laurance, 2005).

Table 12-3 Advance practice roles	
Australia	Perioperative Nurse Surgeon's Assistant (PNSA)
United Kingdom	Surgical Care Practitioner (SCP) (or Healthcare Practitioner: Surgery) Advanced Scrub Practitioner (ASP) Perioperative Specialist Practitioner (PSP)

United States	Registered Nurse First Assistant (RNFA)
	 Perioperative Advanced Practice Nurse (including Nurse Practitioner,
	    Clinical Nurse Specialist [CNS], Certified Registered Nurse
	    Anesthetist [CRNA])

Nonetheless, in response to the European directive on junior doctors work hours, and political will, many initiatives have evolved, and will continue to (Kneebone et al., 2006). One example of an innovative approach has been taken in the United Kingdom at the Good Hope Hospital NHS Trust. This work was driven by the need to manage the flow of surgical emergencies more efficiently (Radford et al., 2003). The result is a clinical nurse specialist role that 'navigates' the complex path that emergency patients travel, from admission through to the operating room and beyond. Preoperatively, nurses in this role are authorised to order diagnostic tests, interpret results, make referrals to other specialist services and plan for surgical intervention and postoperative care.

The nursing professions in Australia and New Zealand are endeavouring to develop advanced practice and Nurse Practitioner roles within a nursing framework, with roles focused on improvements of health outcomes for patients and the greater population (NSW Health, 2007a) rather than simply acting as doctor substitutes.

Several state health departments and the NZ Ministry of Health provide advice to those nurses seeking to develop Nurse Practitioner roles. One example is the development and planning of a paediatric orthopaedic Nurse Practitioner role, with a focus on the perioperative environment (E. Harford, personal communication, 2007). Ward and Hamlin (2006) have also described an advanced practice role in New South Wales, which is currently a transitional perioperative Nurse Practitioner, similar to that described by Radford et al. in the United Kingdom (2003). With a scope of practice that extends beyond the operating room, this truly 'perioperative' role provides nurses in Australia and New Zealand with an appropriate model for the development of the perioperative Nurse Practitioner role.

Advanced practice enrolled nurse

As a result of the work being undertaken around nursing skill mix and the evolution of a more flexible nursing workforce, opportunities are emerging for suitably qualified ENs to work in advanced practice roles. These new roles have developed, in part, as a result of the development of advanced practice roles for RNs and, in Australia, partly because of the recent nationalisation of the EN qualification. This nationalisation itself has occurred as a result of the scope of practice of ENs recently being extended to incorporate medication administration.

The nursing profession and national organisations have recognised that extended and advanced practice roles need to be supported by the appropriate education, regulation and policy framework. Examples are listed below.

• The ANF acknowledges that ENs are being deployed in a broader range of practice environments and, as such, has developed competency standards for advanced practice ENs (ANF, 2007).

- The ANMC has developed a national framework to guide the decision-making process required when working within new scopes of practice and the subsequent need for the safe delegation of care by the RN (see Ch 11) (ANMC, 2007c).
- The Enrolled Nurse Professional Association (ENPA) of New South Wales has endorsed a position statement on the employment of ENs in specialised units (ENPA, 2006). ENPA supports the employment and retention of ENs in acute care and critical care areas, such as intensive care, special care nurseries and perioperative units. The Association views this employment as dependent upon the EN being endorsed for medication administration, as well as the provision of orientation, appropriate supervision and opportunities for ongoing education.

The last few years have seen the formalisation of an EN advanced perioperative practice role: the EN instrument nurse in New South Wales (Sutherland-Fraser, 2007). Even though the instrument nurse role has been performed by ENs in other parts of Australia and also internationally, it is a role that traditionally has been performed in New South Wales by RNs (NSW Health, 2007b). In 2003, a large area health service developed and piloted an in-house clinical program, known as the Perioperative Education Program for ENs (PEPEN). The successful pilot was followed by equally successful new PEPEN programs offered annually, with evidence that suitably selected and educated ENs in the instrument nurse role add to the flexibility of the nursing team and enhance patient care (Sutherland-Fraser, 2007).

In recognition of its success, a certificate course for this advanced practice role has been developed and offered by the College of Nursing since 2006 as part of its continuing education program (College of Nursing, 2007). In other states, such as Queensland, similar education programs are being developed to support this EN advanced practice role (Vargus, 2007).

Nationally, there are other providers of education programs for the perioperative EN, most notably TAFE institutions in New South Wales and South Australia. Currently, these programs do not prepare the EN for advanced practice roles; however, these certificates are valuable in terms of ongoing professional development for ENs and in preparation for employment in the perioperative environment.

CONCLUSION

This chapter has provided an outline of the perioperative nursing workforce and opportunities for entry to practice, as well as the importance of both formal and informal education. A brief overview of the development of nursing organisations and their role noted that specialist nursing organisations provide many valuable functions that contribute to the development of the nursing profession, as well as individual members. They have a key role in the development of standards for practice that, combined with evidence-based nursing, contribute to better patient outcomes. Finally, this chapter has considered the future for the perioperative nurse and explored the development and value of advanced practice roles.

CRITICAL THINKING EXERCISES

1. Professional associations

You have commenced employment in the operating suite and are keen to join a professional association.

- Conduct a search on the internet and list the organisations that appear to best suit your needs. Find out more about each of them, such as when and where they meet, and when their next conference or study day is to be held.

2. Further education

You are a nurse new to perioperative nursing and would like to participate in a formal education program in your area of perioperative nursing.

- List the agencies and the courses they offer and put this on the noticeboard where you work.

3. Evidence-based practice

Identify one aspect of perioperative nursing practice that you have participated in or observed and consider the available evidence that supports this practice.

- How much of the practice is evidence-based?
- How much is based on professional standards or health department/hospital policy?
- Is this practice 'the way we've always done it around here'?

4. Nurse Practitioner role

You think you would like to become a Nurse Practitioner in the operating suite. List your reasons for this, considering the following:

- How will a Nurse Practitioner improve patient care?
- How do you envisage the role being enacted in your operating suite and how could it be developed?
- What knowledge, skills, competencies and capabilities do you have now, and what further education and training will you need to meet the needs of your envisaged role?
- Where would you locate information about becoming a Nurse Practitioner, and what other resources do you need?

RESOURCES

American Association of Nurse Anesthetists
    www.aana.com
American Nurses Association
    http://www.nursingworld.org
American Society of PeriAnesthesia Nurses
    www.aspan.org
Australian Nursing and Midwifery Council
    http://www.anmc.org.au
British Anaesthetic & Recovery Nurses Association
    www.barna.co.uk
Cochrane Collaboration
    www.cochrane.org.au
International Council of Nurses
    www.icn.ch
International Federation of Perioperative Nurses
    www.ifpn.org.uk
Joanna Briggs Institute
    www.joannabriggs.edu.au
National Association of Assistants in Surgical Practice
    www.naasp.org.uk
New Zealand Nurses Organisation
    National enrolled nurses
    http://www.nzno.org.nz/Site/Sections/Sections/Enrolled_Nurses/default.aspx

Perioperative nurses
http://www.nzno.org.nz/Site/Sections/Colleges/Perioperative/default.aspx
Operating Room Nurses Association of Canada
www.ornac.ca

REFERENCES

Andrews, G. J., Brodie, D. A., Andrews, J. P., Wong, J., Thomas, B. G. (2002). Place(ment) matters: students' clinical experiences and their preferences for first employers. *International Nursing Review, 52,* 142–153.

Anonymous. (2008). Inequality between theatre nurses and ODPs. *Journal of Perioperative Practice, 18(2),* 40–41.

Association of periOperative Registered Nurses. (2006a). *Position statement on allied health care providers and support personnel in the perioperative practice setting.* Retrieved February 15, 2008, from http://www.aorn.org/PracticeResources/AORNPositionStatements/Position_HealthCareProvidersAndSupportPersonnel/.

Association of periOperative Registered Nurses. (2006b). *Position statement on one perioperative registered nurse circulator dedicated to every patient undergoing a surgical or other invasive procedure.* Retrieved February 15, 2008, from http://www.aorn.org/PracticeResources/AORNPositionStatements/Position_RegisteredNurseCirculator/.

Association of periOperative Registered Nurses. (2007). *Periop 101 information packet.* Retrieved December 1, 2007, from http://www.aorn.org/Education/Periop101.

Association of periOperative Registered Nurses. (2008a). *Position statements.* Retrieved February 15, 2008, from http://www.aorn.org/PracticeResources/AORNPositionStatements/.

Association of periOperative Registered Nurses. (2008b). *Registered nurses as circulator for ASC grid 2-4-08.* Retrieved February 15, 2008, from http://www.aorn.org/PublicPolicy/CurrentLaws/

Australian College of Operating Room Nurses. (1999). Competency standards for perioperative nurses

Australian College of Operating Room Nurses. (2006a). Nursing role 5: Perioperative nurse surgeon's assistant PNSA. *ACORN standards for perioperative nursing 2006.* Adelaide: ACORN.

Australian College of Operating Room Nurses. (2006b). Position statement 1: Advanced practice nursing and nurse practitioner roles. *ACORN standards for perioperative nursing 2006.* Adelaide: ACORN.

Australian College of Operating Room Nurses. (2006c). Position statement 2: Ancillary workers. *ACORN standards for perioperative nursing 2006.* Adelaide: ACORN.

Australian College of Operating Room Nurses. (2007). *Perioperative careers.* Retrieved December 1, 2007, from http://www.acorn.org.au/index.php/content/view/102/83.

Australian Department of Education, Science and Training. (2002). *National review of nursing education: our duty of care.* Retrieved December 1, 2007, from http://www.dest.gov.au/archive/highered/nursing/pubs/duty_of_care/Duty_of_care.PDF.

Australian Health Workforce Advisory Committee. (2006). *The perioperative workforce in Australia.* Sydney: AHWAC. Retrieved December 1, 2007, from http://www.health.nsw.gov.au/amwac/reports.html.

Australian Institute of Health and Welfare. (2005). *Nursing and midwifery labour force, 2003. National health labour force series: number 31.* Canberra: AIHW.

Australian Nursing Federation. (2006). *Competency standards for the advanced registered nurse.* Melbourne: ANF.

Australian Nursing Federation. (2007). *Competency standards for the advanced enrolled nurse.* Retrieved December 12, 2007, from http://www.anf.org.au/anf_pdf/Competency_Standards.pdf.

Australian Nursing & Midwifery Council. (2006a). *Country profiles for the Nursing and Midwifery Regulatory Authorities of the Western Pacific and South East Asian Regions.* Retrieved December 3, 2007, from http://www.anmc.org.au/wpsear/country_profiles.php.

Australian Nursing & Midwifery Council. (2006b). *National competency standards for the nurse practitioner.* Retrieved December 2, 2007, from http://www.anmc.org.au/professional_standards/index.php.

Australian Nursing & Midwifery Council. (2006c). *National competency standards for the registered nurse* (4th ed.). Retrieved April 23, 2008, from http://www.anmc.org.au/docs/Competency_standards_RN.pdf.

Australian Nursing & Midwifery Council. (2007a). *A national framework for the development of decision-making tools for nursing and midwifery practice.* Retrieved February 9, 2008, from http://www.anmc.org.au/professional_standards/index.php.

Australian Nursing & Midwifery Council. (2007b). *Continuing competence framework. Draft 1.* Retrieved November 9, 2007, from http://www.anmc.org.au/projects/current_projects.php#continuingcompetence.

Australian Nursing & Midwifery Council (2007c). *Project to produce a national framework for the development of decision making tools for nursing and midwifery practice.* Retrieved February 9, 2008, from http://www.anmc.org.au/professional_standards/index.php.

Bashford, A. (2000). Domestic scientists: modernity, gender, and the negotiation of science in Australian nursing, 1880–1910. *Journal of Women's History, 12(2),* 127–146.

Bessant, J., & Bessant, B. (1991). *The growth of a profession: nursing in Victoria, 1930s–1980s.* Melbourne: La Trobe University Press.

Board of Directors. (2007). Perioperative nurse guidelines. *Kai Tiaki: Nursing New Zealand, 13(5),* 35.

Brennan, B. (2000). PNSA Newsletter. Perioperative nurse surgeon's assistant, number 1. *ACORN Journal, 13(4),* 34–36.

Brennan, B. (2001). PNSA Newsletter. Perioperative nurse surgeon's assistant, volume 1, number 2. *ACORN Journal, 14(1),* 24–25, 27.

Brooks, I., & Berman Brown, R. (2002). The role of ritualistic ceremonial in removing barriers between subcultures in the National Health Service. *Journal of Advanced Nursing, 38(4),* 341–352.

Campbell, J. (2001). The evolving role of the PNSA role: social, professional and personal dimensions. PNSA Newsletter, 1 (3). *ACORN Journal, 14(2),* 22–24, 26–27.

College of Nursing. (2007). *Certificate courses for registered and enrolled nurses.* Retrieved December 8, 2007, from http://www.nursing.edu.au/Online_Course/ViewMainPage.aspx?CategoryID=12.

Community Services & Health Industry Skills Council. (2007). *Health training package HLT07.* Retrieved December 3, 2007, from http://www.cshisc.com.au/load_page.asp?ID=235.

Davies, M., & Hamlin, L. (2003). ACORN competency standards for the perioperative nurses: genesis, development and outcomes. *ACORN Journal, 16(2),* 27–30.

Dingwall, R., & Lewis, P. (1983). *The sociology of the professions: lawyers, doctors and others.* London: Macmillan.

Enrolled Nurse Professional Association of NSW. (2006). *Enrolled nurses working in specialised units.* Retrieved December 12, 2007, from http://www.enpansw.org.au/position3.pdf.

Fletcher, C. (2008). Periop skills review needed. *Nursing Review, February,* 30.

Frank, K. (2005). Benefits of professional nursing organization membership. *AORN Journal, 82(1),* 13–14.

Freidson, E. (1983). The theory of professions: state of the art. In R. Dingwall, & P. Lewis (Eds.). *The sociology of the professions* (pp. 19–37). London: Macmillan.

Freidson, E. (1994). *Professionalism reborn: theory, prophecy and policy.* Cambridge: Polity Press.

Frotjold, A., Hardy, J., Butler, M. (2007). New directions for transition: "Snapshot" hospital visits with clinician's support for final year undergraduate nursing students. *Nursing Monograph 2007.* Sydney: St Vincent's & Mater Health.

Gonczi, A., Hager, P., Oliver, L. (1990). *Establishing competency-based standards in the professions.* Canberra: Australian Government Publishing Service.

Goodley, A., Roberts, K., Toohill, S. (2008). Periop skills review needed. *Nursing Review, February,* 30.

Gutierrez, K., McCormack, C., Villaverde, M. (1989). Perioperative nursing in the college curriculum: a custom fit. *AORN Journal, 49(4),* 1052, 1054–1055, 1057–1058, 1060, 1062, 1064.

Guy, B. (2004). Perioperative nurses: stretch the boundaries. *Kai Tiaki Nursing New Zealand, 10(10),* 29.

Hamlin, L. (2005). Setting the standard: the role of the Australian College of Operating Room Nurses. Unpublished doctoral thesis. Sydney: University of Technology.

Happell, B. (2000). Student interest in perioperative nursing practice as a career. *AORN Journal,* 71(3), 600–605.

Heartfield, M. (2006). *Specialisation and advanced practice discussion paper.* Retrieved December 12, 2007, from http://www.nnnet.gov.au/publications.htm.

Hendry, C., Lauder, W., Roxburgh, M. (2007). The dissemination and uptake of competency frameworks. *Journal of Research in Nursing, 12(6),* 689–700.

Heywood, L., Gonczi, A., Hager, P. (1992). *A guide to development of competency standards for professions.* Canberra: Australian Government Publishing Service.

Hilbig, J. (1999). Validation of the ACORN Competencies research project report. *ACORN Journal, 12(3),* 18.

Holleman, G., Eliens, A., van Vliet, M., van Achterberg, T. (2006). Promotion of evidence-based practice by professional nursing associations: literature review. *Journal of Advanced Nursing, 53(6),* 702–709.

International Council of Nurses (ICN). (n.d.). *About ICN.* Retrieved April 28, 2008, from http://www.icn.ch/abouticn.htm.

Jones, J. M., & Sorrell, J. M. (1989). Undergraduate nursing students: are we meeting the need? *AORN Journal, 50(2),* 316, 318–320, 322, 324–325.

Kneebone, R., Chestel, D., Chrzanowska, J., Barnet, A., Darvi, A. (2006). Innovative training for new surgical roles: the place of evaluation. *Medical Education, 40,* 987–994.

Laurance, J. (2005). British nurses to train as surgeons. *Nursing Review, January,* 6.

Leicht, K., & Fennell, M. (2001). *Professional work: a sociological approach.* Boston, MA: Blackwell.

Lingard, L., Reznick, R., Espin, S., Regehr, G., DeVito, I. (2002). Team communications in the operating room: talk patterns, sites of tension and implications for novices. *Academic Medicine, 77(3),* 232–237.

Marenzi, B. (2006). What does the perioperative college offer surgical nurses? *Kai Tiaki Nursing New Zealand, 2(2),* 28.

McMullan, M., Endacott, R., Gray, M. A., et al. (2003). Portfolios and assessment of competence: a review of the literature. *Journal of Advanced Nursing, 41(3),* 283–294.

Michael, R. (2007). The perioperative nurse practitioner: reality or myth? A west and east state perspective. 2006 ACORN national conference abstracts: the editor's cut. *ACORN Journal,* 19(2), 15.

National Nursing & Nursing Education Taskforce. (2005a). *Nurse practitioners in Australia: mapping of state/territory nurse practitioner (NP) models, legislation and authorisation processes.* Retrieved December 12, 2007, from http://www.nnnet.gov.au/publications.htm.

National Nursing & Nursing Education Taskforce. (2005b). *Scopes of practice commentary paper.* Retrieved May 5, 2007, from http://www.nnnet.gov.au.

National Nursing and Nursing Education Taskforce. (2006). *Myth busters February 2006. What are the common myths about nurse practitioners?* Retrieved February 3, 2008, from http://www.nnnet.gov.au.

National Nursing Organisations. (2006). *Governance standards for specialist nursing and midwifery organisations. A report by NNO working group for the national nursing and nursing education taskforce.* Retrieved February 12, 2008, from http://www.nnnet.gov.au.

Nelson, D. (2006). To perform at your best, you must first know yourself well. *Kai Tiaki: Nursing New Zealand, 12(10),* 32.

NSW Health. (2007a). *Nurse practitioner.* Retrieved December 12, 2007, from http://www.health.nsw.gov.au/nursing/npract.html.

NSW Health. (2007b). *Perioperative enrolled nurse.* Retrieved December 12, 2007, from http://www.health.nsw.gov.au/nursing/periop_en.html.

NSW Operating Theatre Association. (2007). *New South Wales Operating Theatre Association 50th Annual Report 2007.* Sydney: NSW OTA.

Nurse Practitioner Advisory Committee of New Zealand. (2006). *Nurse practitioners in New Zealand: the facts.* Retrieved December 2, 2007, from http://www.nzno.org.nz/Site/Professional/Other/ANP/NPAC.aspx.

NZ Ministry of Health. (2006). *Clinical training agency nursing.* Retrieved 27 February, 2008, from http://www.moh.govt.nz/moh.nsf/pagesmh/4581/$File/1B46-nept-programme-mar07.pdf.

NZ Ministry of Health. (2007). *News: Nursing in New Zealand.* Retrieved 27 February, 2008, from http://www.moh.govt.nz/moh.nsf/indexmh/nursing-news.

Perioperative Nurses College. (2005). *Standards and guidelines for safe practice for perioperative nurses in NZ.* Retrieved February 13, 2008, from http://www.pnc.org.nz/Site/Sections/Colleges/Perioperative/Standguide.aspx.

Perioperative Nurses College. (n.d.). *About the College.* Retrieved February 13, 2008, from http://www.pnc.org.nz/Site/Sections/Colleges/Perioperative/About.aspx.

Productivity Commission. (2006). *Australia's health workforce: Productivity Commission research report.* Retrieved November 1, 2007, from http://www.pc.gov.au/study/healthworkforce/docs/finalreport.

Radford, M., Abbassi, A., Williamson, A., Johnston, P. (2003). Redefining perioperative advanced practice, scope of practice: measuring impact and sustainability. *British Journal of Perioperative Nursing, 13(12),* 504–511.

Richardson, M. (2004). *The history of ACORN: from little acorn's grow.* Melbourne: Latrobe University Press.

Rosenberg, C. (1987). *The care of strangers.* New York: Basic Books.

Royal College of Nursing, Australia. (2006). *Position statement: advanced practice nursing.* Retrieved December 2, 2007, from http://www.rcna.org.au/site/positionstatement.php.

Royal College of Nursing, Australia. (2007). Development of new roles—a question of safe, quality healthcare. *Nursing Review, October,* 9.

Schwirian, P. M. (1998). *Professionalization of nursing: Current issues and trends.* Philadelphia: Lippincott.

Senate Community Affairs References Committee. (2002). *The patient profession: a time for action.* Report on the Senate Inquiry into Nursing. Retrieved December 10, 2007, from http://www.aph.gov.au/senate/.

South Eastern Sydney Illawarra Area Health Service. (2006). *PIP: standardising education for the perioperative nurse.* Paper presented at the State Perioperative Managers' Forum, Perioperative Nurses Association of Queensland (PNAQ), Royal Pines Resort, Gold Coast, Qld, Australia.

South Eastern Sydney Illawarra Area Health Service. (2007). *Perioperative nursing in South East Health.* Retrieved December 2, 2007, from http://www.sesiahs.health.nsw.gov.au/publications/nursing/perioperativeBrochure.pdf.

Sutherland-Fraser, S. (2007). PEPEN: developing an educational pathway for the enrolled nurse instrument nurse in New South Wales. *ACORN Journal, 20(1),* 17–22.

Tanner, J., Blunsden, C., Fakis, A. (2007). National survey of hand antisepsis practices. *Journal of Perioperative Practice, 17(1),* 27–37.

Tanner, J., & Parkinson, H. (2002). Double gloving to reduce surgical cross-infection. *Cochrane Database of Systematic Reviews, 3,* CD003087.

UK Department of Health. (2007). *Agenda for change.* Retrieved December 12, 2007, from http://www.dh.gov.uk/en/Policyandguidance/Humanresourcesandtraining/Modernisingpay/Agendaforchange/index.htm.

Vargus, S. (2007). Enrolled nurses in the perioperative environment: working smarter—a private sector view. *ACORN Journal, 20(4),* 18–22.

Ward, K., & Hamlin, L. (2006). Lead or be led: are we ready to face the challenge? *ACORN Journal, 19(4),* 14–20.

Williamson, C., & Hill, V. (2007). Review of the competency standards for perioperative nursing. *ACORN Journal, 20(2),* 22–33.

FURTHER READING

Andre, K., & Heartfield, M. (2007). *Professional portfolios: evidence of competency for nurses and midwives.* Sydney: Elsevier.

Australian Nursing & Midwifery Council. (2007). *Development of a national framework for the demonstration of continuing competence for nurses and midwives: literature review.* Retrieved November 7, 2007, from http://www.anmc.org.au/projects/current_projects.php#continuingcompetence.

Barnard, A., & Locsin, R. (Eds.). (2007). *Technology and nursing practice concepts and issues.* Basingstoke, UK: Palgrave Macmillan.

National Nursing and Nursing Education Taskforce. (2006). *An atlas of the legislation and professional regulation of nursing & midwifery in Australia.* Retrieved December 1, 2007, from http://www.nnnet.gov.au.

Pratt, R., & Russell, R. L. (2002). *A voice to be heard: the first fifty years of the New South Wales College of Nursing.* Sydney: Allen & Unwin.

Reverby, S. (1987). *Ordered to care: the dilemma of American nursing, 1850–1945.* New York: Cambridge University Press.

Russell, R. L. (1990). *From Nightingale to now: Nurse education in Australia.* Sydney: Harcourt Brace Jovanovich.

Trembath, R., & Hellier, D. (1983). *All care and responsibility: a history of nursing in Victoria, 1850-1934.* Florence Nightingale Committee, Australia Victorian Branch. Melbourne: Globe Press.

GLOSSARY

Ablation: An amputation, an excision of any part of the body, or a removal of a growth or harmful substance.

Aboriginal: Refers here to both Aboriginal and Torres Straight Islander people.

Accountability: Nurses and midwives must be prepared to answer to others, such as health care consumers, their nursing and midwifery regulatory authority, employers and the public for their decisions, actions, behaviours and the responsibilities that are inherent in their roles. Accountability cannot be delegated. The registered nurse or midwife who delegates an activity to another person is accountable, not only for their delegation decision, but also for monitoring the standard of performance of the activity by the other person, and for evaluating the outcomes of the delegation.

Additional (transmission-based) precautions: Safeguards designed for patients who are known or suspected to be infected with highly transmissible or epidemiologically important pathogens for which additional precautions beyond standard precautions are needed to interrupt transmission in hospitals. There are three types of transmission-based precautions: airborne precautions, droplet precautions and contact precautions. They may be combined for diseases that have multiple routes of transmission, and, either singly or in a combination, are to be used in addition to standard precautions.

Advance directive: A document that expresses the patient's preferences for end-of-life issues.

Adverse event: An incident in which unintended harm resulted to a person receiving health care.

Asepsis: Absence of pathogenic microorganisms on living tissue.

Aseptic technique: Any health care procedure in which added precautions are taken to prevent contamination of a patient, object or area by microorganisms.

Allograft: Transplanted organ and tissue.

Arrhythmia: A broad term used to describe any rhythm other than sinus rhythm.

Atraumatic: Pertaining to therapies or therapeutic instruments and devices (e.g. needles) that are unlikely to cause tissue damage.

Australasian Donor Awareness Program Training (ADAPT): An Australasian program that provides a consistent and uniform approach to educating health professionals in the care and management of dying patients and their families, including patients who may become organ and tissue donors; in organ retrieval surgery; and in the organ and tissue donation process.

Australasian Transplant Coordinators Association (ATCA): An organisation that promotes communication and collaboration among organ and tissue donor and transplant coordinators, and promotes research, education and discussion of professional and ethical issues in the field in Australasia.

Australians Donate: The peak body for the organ and tissue donation sector in Australia. Members include state and territory organ donation agencies, independent tissue and eye banks, community groups, clinicians, policy makers, academics and ethicists.

Autonomy: The ethical principle of self-determination and independence.

Basic life support: The support of life by the initial establishment of and/or maintenance of airway, breathing and circulation and related emergency care.

Brain death: Death from confirmed irreversible cessation of all function of the person's brain and/or absent intracranial blood flow.

Bronchospasm: An excessive and prolonged contraction of the smooth muscle of the bronchi and bronchioles, resulting in acute narrowing and obstruction of the respiratory airway. The contractions may be localised or general and may be caused by irritation (e.g. secretions, airway equipment or pulmonary aspiration) or injury to the respiratory mucosa, infections, allergies, drug hypersensitivity or the rapid introduction of volatile anaesthetic agents. Bronchospasm is the chief characteristic of asthma and bronchitis. It is managed by increasing the level of inhalational anaesthesia, bronchodilators (e.g. salbutamol) and other drugs (e.g. steroids, ketamine or adrenaline) or repositioning the endotracheal tube in anaesthetised patients.

Cadaveric donor: Donor of tissue and solid organs after death.

Cardiac arrest: The cessation of cardiac mechanical activity with the absence of a detectable pulse, and unresponsiveness and apnoea (or agonal respirations).

Capnography: Graphical representation of expired carbon dioxide (CO_2), often termed end-tidal CO_2. Measurement assists in early detection of technical catastrophes (e.g. oesophageal intubation) or changes in patient's respiratory, circulatory or metabolic condition. An adaptor placed in the breathing circuit during general anaesthesia collects CO_2, which is then analysed and displayed as a wave form on a monitor.

Clinical decision making: The cognitive processes and strategies that nurses use when utilising data to make clinical decisions regarding patient assessment and care.

Clinical practice guidelines: Statements about appropriate health care for specific clinical circumstances that assist practitioners in their day-to-day practice.

Closed-wound suction: Any of several techniques for draining potentially harmful fluids (e.g. blood, pus, serosanguineous fluid or tissue secretions) from surgical wounds. Postoperative drainage aids the healing process by removing dead space and helping to draw healing tissues together. Closed-wound suction devices usually consist of disposable transparent containers attached to suction tubes and portable suction pumps.

Coagulopathy: Disorders of the clotting mechanism of the blood, which can be caused by pre-existing disease, medications (including herbal therapies), pathophysiological conditions (e.g. hypothermia and acidosis) or current treatments (e.g. massive blood transfusion).

Code of conduct: A collection of standards and rules of behaviour.

Cognitive impairment: Deficiency in the ability to think, perceive, reason or remember that may result in the loss of ability to attend to one's activities of daily living.

Cold ischaemic time: The time from cross-clamp to when blood supply is re-established to the organ during transplant surgery.

Compartment syndrome: A pathological condition caused by the progressive development of arterial compression and consequent reduction of blood supply. Clinical manifestations include swelling, restriction of movement, brown urine, myoglobinuria, vascular compromise and severe pain or lack of sensation. Treatment includes elevation, removal of restrictive dressings or casts and, potentially, surgical decompression (often in the form of a fasciotomy, to relieve the pressure).

Competence: Combination of skills, knowledge, attitudes, values and abilities that underpin effective and/or superior performance in a profession/occupational area.

Complementary therapies: Treatments that have not been considered part of standard Western medicine but are increasingly being used in combination with standard medical treatments. These may include therapies for pain (e.g. massage and relaxation techniques) and some nutritional therapies.

Confidentiality: The obligation of persons to whom private information has been given not to use that information for any purpose other than for the primary purpose for which it was given.

Cricoid pressure: see **Sellick's manoeuvre**.

Culture: A set of learned values, beliefs, customs and behaviour that is shared by a group of interacting individuals.

Cultural safety: the provision of effective health care to persons of dissimilar cultures, respecting difference and ensuring that care is not diminishing, demeaning or disempowering. Culture includes not only ethnicity or origin but also age, gender, disability, sexual identity, socioeconomic status, spiritual beliefs or migrant experience.

Debride: To remove dirt, foreign objects, damaged tissue and cellular debris from a wound or a burn to prevent infection and to promote healing. In treating a wound, debridement is the first step in cleansing; it allows thorough examination of the extent of the injury. In treating a burn, debridement of the eschar may be performed in a hydrotherapy bath.

Defibrillation: The application of a controlled electrical shock to the victim's chest in order to terminate a life-threatening cardiac rhythm.

Deontological: A philosophical view reflecting duty or a moral obligation to behave or act in a particular way.

Designated officer: According to Australian law, a person(s) appointed by the governing body of health institutions to authorise consent for non-coronial post-mortem examinations, and organ and tissue retrieval for transplant and research.

Donation after death: Also known as non-heart beating donation (NHBD): donor of selective solid organs and tissues after cardiac death rather than brain death.

Electronic health record (EHR) (or electronic medical record, EMR): an individual patient's medical record in digital format. EHR systems coordinate the storage and retrieval of individual records with the aid of computers. EHRs/EMRs are usually accessed on a computer, often over a network. It may be made up of electronic medical records from many locations and/or sources. A variety of types of health care-related information may be stored and accessed in this way. Integrated electronic health records are increasingly seen as the way to achieve quality and continuity in treatment, fill the gaps in public health research and contain costs; however, such systems have created many concerns about privacy.

Electrosurgical unit (ESU) (diathermy machine): The ESU generates a high-frequency electrical current, which creates heat in body tissue, resulting in coagulation or desiccation of tissue. This provides haemostasis and a bloodless field during a surgical procedure. There are two main types—monopolar and bipolar; use of the former requires the placement of an indifferent electrode (diathermy plate) on the patient's body, away from the operative site.

Endogenous: Microorganisms causing infection that originate from the body's own flora.

Endoscopy: Visualisation of the interior organs and cavities of the body with an endoscope, which may be rigid or flexible. The gastrointestinal tract, renal system, upper and lower airway and female reproductive system can all be examined, and cytological and histological samples collected, and some conditions treated via an endoscopic procedure.

Endotracheal tube (ETT): A large-bore, disposable catheter made of silicone or PVC tubing inserted through the mouth or nose and into the trachea to the point above the bifurcation of the trachea. It is used to deliver anaesthetic gases and oxygen directly into the trachea through the vocal cords. ETTs may have a single or double lumen (for lung surgery). Adult-sized ETTs have a cuff at their distal end, which, when inflated with air, seals off the trachea, permitting positive pressure ventilation and decreasing the risk of aspiration.

Epidural anaesthesia/analgesia: A type of central nerve anaesthesia block in which a local anaesthetic drug is injected via a fine catheter into the epidural space surrounding the dural membrane, which contains cerebrospinal fluid and spinal nerves. The catheter lies between the dura mater and ligamentum flavum at the L3–4 or L5–6 level. An epidural injection can be used to facilitate surgery of the lower half of the body and/or provide prolonged postoperative analgesia.

Error: A generic term to encompass all of those occasions in which a planned sequence of mental or physical activities failed to achieve its intended outcome, and when the failure cannot be attributed to the intervention of some chance agency.

Eschar: A scab or dry crust that results from trauma, such as thermal or chemical burn, infection or ulcerating skin disease.

Ethical/unethical: Right or morally acceptable/wrong or morally unacceptable.

Ethics: The study of morals and values.

Evidence-based nursing: The conscientious, explicit and judicious use of theory-derived, research-based information in making decisions about care delivery to individuals or groups of patients.

Exogenous: Microorganisms causing infection that originate from sources external to the body (e.g. other patients, staff or equipment).

General anaesthesia: Reversible, unconscious state characterised by amnesia, loss of sensation, analgesia and suppression of reflexes.

Haemodynamic monitoring: The measurement of pressure, flow and oxygenation within the cardiovascular system.

Haemostasis: The termination of bleeding by mechanical or chemical means or by the complex coagulation processes of the body, which consists of vasoconstriction, platelet aggregation, and thrombin and fibrin synthesis.

Health policy: A statement of a decision regarding a goal in health care and a plan to achieve that goal (e.g. a program for inoculating a population is developed and implemented to prevent an epidemic).

Heterotopic: Implantation of an organ into an abnormal anatomical position.

Incident: An event or circumstance that could have, or did, lead to unintended and/or unnecessary harm to a person, and/or a complaint, loss or damage.

Infection: Invasion of the body by pathogenic microorganisms that reproduce and multiply, causing disease by local cellular injury, secretion of a toxin or antigen–antibody reaction to the host.

Infection control: The policies and procedures of a hospital or other health facility to minimise the risk of spreading of nosocomial or community-acquired infections to patients or members of the staff.

Inflammation: The normal response of connective tissue and blood vessels to sublethal irritation or injury. Inflammation may be acute or chronic, the time scale relating to the nature of the injurious stimulus. The cardinal signs of inflammation are redness, heat, swelling and pain, often accompanied by the loss of function.

Informed consent: Authorisation obtained from a patient to perform a specific test or procedure. The concept of informed consent is a composite of: (a) consent to a procedure (or participation in a research study) and (b) the nature and extent of information that must be provided in order for the person's decision to be adequately informed. A broad indication of the nature and risks of the procedure is sufficient to defeat an action in trespass (assuming the other requirements of a valid consent are met, including voluntariness and competence of the patient).

Intraoperative: Pertaining to the period during a surgical procedure.

Justice: That which concerns fairness or equity, often divided into three parts: procedural justice, concerned with fair methods of making decisions and settling disputes; distributive justice, concerned with the fair distribution of the benefits and burdens of society; and corrective justice, concerned with correcting wrongs and harms through compensation or retribution.

Laparoscopy: The examination of the abdominal cavity and viscera with a laparoscope inserted through one or more small incisions in the abdominal wall, usually around the umbilicus. Laparoscopic surgery can be diagnostic or therapeutic (e.g. laparoscopic cholecystectomy, that is, removal of the gall bladder via the laparoscopic incisions). Also know as **keyhole surgery**.

Laryngeal mask airway (LMA): A device for maintaining a patent airway during general anaesthesia without tracheal intubation, consisting of a tube connected to an oval inflatable cuff that seals the larynx. Also called the Brain airway, after its inventor.

Laryngospasm: Spasmodic closure of the larynx. It may be caused by local irritation, such as the presence of secretions, airway equipment or pulmonary aspiration in the back of the pharynx, resulting in partial or complete spasm of the vocal cords and the inability of the patient to breathe effectively. Partial laryngospasm may be characterised by a 'crowing' sound made on inspiration. However, in total laryngospasm there is no sound made as no air moves into or out of the lungs; ineffective respiratory efforts will be noted in chest movement.

Laser: An acronym for 'light amplification by stimulated emission of radiation'. The energy generated by laser equipment can be used to destroy or refashion tissue. Laser beams can be harmful to the eyes of personnel activating and assisting with procedures, and protective goggles must be worn.

Latex allergy: Anaphylactic hypersensitivity to the soluble proteins in latex, most often seen in patients sensitised by repeated exposure to latex. Reactions range from irritant dermatitis and eczema to anaphylactic collapse.

Living donor: Donor of serum, tissue or solid organs while living.

Living will: An advance directive expressing individuals' wishes regarding health care if they become terminally ill and lose the ability to make decisions.

Malignant hyperthermia: Rare, life-threatening, autosomal dominant muscle disorder triggered by inhalational anaesthetic agents or muscle relaxant resulting in raised core body temperature, which can be fatal. Treatment involves the use of dantrolene sodium injection, removal of triggering agents and the application of temperature-reducing strategies (e.g. cooling blankets, cold intravenous fluids).

Māori: The indigenous people of New Zealand. They are Polynesian and comprise about 10% of the country's population. Māoritanga is the native language, which is related to Tahitian and Hawaiian.

Microorganism: Any tiny, usually microscopic entity capable of carrying on living processes. They may be pathogenic. Include bacteria, algae, protozoa, fungi (cellular), viruses and prions (acellular).

Minimally invasive surgery (MIS): Surgery done with only a small incision or no incision at all, as through a cannula with a laparoscope or endoscope. Also known as **minimal access surgery (MAS).**

Multi-organ donor: Donor of solid organs (e.g. kidneys, pancreas, heart, lungs, liver) and tissue.

Near miss: An incident that did not cause harm.

Negligence: A legal term defined as 'causing damage unintentionally but carelessly'. A court will determine negligence based on reasonable foreseeability that the damage might have been possible, the existence of a duty of care to the person damaged, a breach in that duty could be demonstrated and that damages were indeed experienced by the victim.

New Zealand National Transplant Donor Coordination: The central coordinating office for the retrieval of organs and tissues from deceased donors in New Zealand.

Nosocomial infection: Infection acquired at least 72 hours after hospitalisation. Also known as a hospital-acquired infection (HAI) or health care-related infection. Common causative agents include *Candida albicans*, *Escherichia coli* and hepatitis viruses.

Orthotopic: Implantation of an organ into a normal anatomical position.

Patient-controlled analgesia (PCA): A drug delivery system that dispenses a present intravascular dose of a narcotic analgesic when the patient pushes a switch on an electric cord. The device consists of a computerised pump with a chamber holding a syringe of drug. The patient administers a dose of narcotic when the need for pain relief arises in the postoperative period. A lockout interval automatically inactivates the system if a patient tries to increase the amount of narcotic within a preset period.

Personal information: Information by which individuals or collectives can be identified. This is defined in the *Privacy Act 1988* (Cth) as information or an opinion (including information or an opinion forming part of database), whether true or not, and whether recorded in a material form or not, about an individual whose identity is apparent, or can reasonably be ascertained, from the information or opinion.

Personal protective equipment (PPE): A range of equipment, such as gloves, eye protection, masks and plastic aprons, that is used to protect health care staff from infectious diseases.

Policy: A principle or guideline that governs an activity and that employees or members of an institution or organisation are expected to follow.

Postoperative: Pertaining to the period of time after surgery. It begins with the patient's emergence from anaesthesia and continues throughout the time required for the acute effects of the anaesthetic and the surgery or procedure to abate.

Practice development: A continuous process of improvement designed to promote increased effectiveness in patient-centred care. It enables health care teams to develop their knowledge and skills, transforming the culture and context of care.

Preoperative: Pertaining to the period before a surgical procedure. Commonly the preoperative period begins with the first preparation of the patient for surgery or other procedure and ends with the induction of anaesthesia in the operating suite.

Pressure (decubitus) ulcer: An injury caused by unrelieved pressure that damages the skin and underlying tissue, usually over a bony prominence.

Privacy: Control over the extent, timing and circumstances of sharing of oneself (physically, behaviourally or intellectually) with others. Implies a zone of exclusivity, where individuals and collectives are free from the scrutiny of others.

Professional practice standard: The standards of health professional care as determined by groups within the particular profession.

Protocol: A written plan specifying the procedures to be followed in giving a particular examination, in conducting research or in providing care for a particular condition.

Pulse oximeter: A device that measures the amount of saturated haemoglobin in the tissue capillaries. A beam of light is transmitted through the tissue to a receiver. This non-invasive method of measuring the saturated haemoglobin is a useful tool for determining basic respiratory function. A clip-like probe is usually placed on a finger, toe or ear lobe. As the amount of saturated haemoglobin alters the wavelengths of the transmitted light, analysis of the received light is translated into a percentage of oxygen saturation (So_2) of the blood, which is displayed on a monitoring device. A reading of 95% or above is considered a satisfactory value.

Quality improvement: The identification and adoption of continuous improvement strategies that are integrated into quality improvement activities as a normal part of the planning cycle.

Rapid sequence induction: A method of protecting the airway during induction of anaesthesia in patients at risk of aspiration of gastric contents, by minimising the time between loss of consciousness and intubation and applying cricoid pressure.

Regional anaesthesia: Anaesthesia provided by the injection of a local anaesthetic drug to block a group of sensory nerve fibres. Kinds of regional anaesthesia include axillary, brachial plexus, caudal, epidural, pudental, intercostal, paracervical and spinal anaesthesia.

Rejection: Destruction of the allograft due to the body's ability to identify self from non-self.

Research: Systematic, rigorous investigation to establish facts, principles and new knowledge.

Respect for persons: Has two fundamental aspects: respect for the autonomy of those individuals who are capable of making informed choices and respect for their capacity for self-determination; and the protection of persons with impaired or diminished autonomy (i.e. those individuals who are incompetent or whose voluntary capacity is compromised).

Risk: The function of the magnitude of a harm and the probability of its occurrence (i.e. the chance of something happening that will have an effect upon objectives). It is measured in terms of consequences and likelihood (AS/NZ4360:1999 Risk management standard).

Risk management: A function of administration of a hospital or other health facility directed towards identification, evaluation and correction of potential risks leading to injury of patients, staff members or visitors and resulting in property loss or damage.

Robotic surgery: Robots are remote, computer-assisted telemanipulators, developed for use in surgery to overcome some of the limitations associated with laparoscopic equipment. When merged with industrial robotic technology, three-dimensional (3D) visualisation systems and computer technology, robotic surgery is feasible. The advanced technology incorporates sophisticated mechanical equipment, which is used to hold and manoeuvre endoscopic instrumentation during minimally invasive surgery. The robotic devices can be remotely controlled by a surgeon, providing enhanced visualisation and precision in performing surgery.

Root cause analysis: A systematic approach whereby the factors that contributed to an incident are identified, and recommendations to prevent recurrence are generated. It is commonly applied to the health care setting, where a team of unbiased experts are called on to investigate how and why an error might have been caused by looking more at the system problems that emerged than at individual negligence.

Sellick's manoeuvre (cricoid pressure): A technique to reduce the risk of the aspiration of gastric contents during the induction of general anaesthesia. The cricoid cartilage is pushed against the body of the sixth cervical vertebra, occluding the upper end of the oesophagus and preventing passive regurgitation. The technique cannot stop active vomiting. Cricoid pressure is applied before tracheal intubation, immediately after the injection of anaesthetic drugs and as part of a rapid sequence intubation. Regurgitated gastric contents entering the lungs results in a condition known as Mendelson's syndrome.

Scope of practice: The full spectrum of roles, functions, responsibilities, activities and decision-making capacity that individuals within that profession are educated, competent and authorised to perform.

Sentinel event: Events that lead to serious patient harm or death.

Sepsis: A systemic inflammatory response to infection.

Sepsis-induced hypotension: A systolic blood pressure <90 mmHg or a reduction of ≥40 mmHg from baseline in the absence of other causes of hypotension.

Septic shock: A subset of severe sepsis, defined as sepsis-induced hypotension in the presence of perfusion abnormalities despite adequate fluid resuscitation.

Severe acute respiratory syndrome (SARS): The term given to a relatively new virulent respiratory infection.

Severe sepsis: Sepsis associated with organ dysfunction, hypoperfusion or hypotension.

Severity assessment code (SAC): A numerical score applied to an incident based on the type of incident, its likelihood of recurrence and its consequence. A matrix is used to stratify the actual and/or potential risk associated with an incident.

Skill mix: The relative mix of skilled and experienced staff in a team. For example, in the operating suite there may be experienced, qualified registered nurses (RNs) and enrolled nurses (ENs), less experienced RNs and ENs, new graduate/newly qualified RNs/ENs and various technical and other non-nursing personnel. Poor skill mix has a higher proportion of the lower order groups and/or less experienced staff; conversely, a good skill mix has a higher proportion of experienced and qualified staff.

Smoke plume: Smoke generated during cutting or coagulation of tissue while using electrosurgical equipment. This smoke has been shown to contain toxins, carcinogens and viruses. The use of high-filtration masks and smoke extraction units are recommended to protect the surgical team from inhaling the smoke plume.

Standard precautions: A range of strategies designed to reduce the transmission of microorganisms from both recognised and unrecognised sources. They involve safe work practices and the use of protective barriers (e.g. personal protective equipment). Standard precautions apply to blood, all body secretions (except sweat), non-intact skin and mucous membrane (including the eyes).

Sterile: Absence of all forms of microbial life.

Sterile field: The sterile field refers to the area around the surgical site that has been prepared by cleansing with an antimicrobial agent and surrounded with sterile drapes, which separate it from the rest of the patient's body. The sterile field also includes all furniture covered with sterile drapes, such as the instrument table, and the scrub team who are covered in sterile garb.

Sterilisation: The processes used to eliminate or destroy all forms of microbial life from equipment and surgical instruments, to prepare them for use during a surgical procedure. Methods to achieve sterilisation include the use of steam, ethylene oxide, dry heat, gamma radiation, peracetic acid and gas plasma.

Stress: A state of mental or emotional strain or suspense.

Sympathetic nervous system: A part of the autonomic nervous system or involuntary nervous system. It regulates tissues not under voluntary control (e.g. glands, heart, blood vessels and smooth muscle).

Surgical conscience: An individual's professional honesty and inner morality system, which allows no compromise in practice, particularly when breaches are noted in accepted behaviours or aseptic technique. These breaches must be corrected immediately, regardless of personal consequences or embarrassment.

Surgical site infection (SSI): An infection caused by the introduction of pathogenic microorganisms into a wound during or following a surgical procedure. Most commonly caused by bacteria (e.g. *Staphylococcus aureus*) or a strain of streptococci.

Thalamus: Mid-brain structure with a significant role in relaying information from the various sensory receptors to other brain areas.

Tidal volume: The volume of air that is moved into or out of the lungs with each breath.

Tissue-only donor: Donor of musculoskeletal tissue (e.g. femur, tibia, humerus pelvis, ligaments, tendons, fascia, meniscus) and/or cardiac tissue (e.g. bicuspid or tricuspid valves, aortic or pulmonary tissue) and/or eye tissue (e.g. cornea and sclera) and/or skin tissue.

Transplant Nurses Association (TNA): Formed to advance the education of nurses and other health professionals involved in the transplant process.

Transplant Society of Australia and New Zealand: A body with, as members, scientists, doctors, transplant coordinators and research students with an interest in all forms of transplantation.

Unconsciousness: A condition where a person fails to respond to verbal or tactile stimuli.

Utilitarian: Ethical theory that presupposes an action is right if it achieves the greatest good for the greatest number of people.

Voluntary: Free of coercion, duress or undue inducement.

Warm ischaemia: Time taken from withdrawal of ventilation and treatment, to the confirmation of death of a donation after cardiac death (DCD) donor, to the commencement of infusion of cold perfusion fluid and/or organ retrieval.

Work of breathing: The term applied to the physical effort a patient exerts to achieve spontaneous breathing. It is affected by lung compliance, chest wall resistance, muscle wasting (intercostals and diaphragm) and/or fatigue, and the use of secondary muscles to aid breathing.

INDEX

Page numbers followed by '*f*' denotes figures, '*t*' denotes tables and '*b*' denotes boxes.